Jeff Levin, PhD, MPH
Harold G. Koenig

Faith, Medicine, and Science
A Festschrift
in Honor of Dr. David B. Larson

Pre-publication
REVIEWS,
COMMENTARIES,
EVALUATIONS . . .

"**D**avid Larson energetically challenged a generation of psychiatrists to think differently about faith. Many wondered how he accomplished so much and where the science of religion and health would be without him. In this book are affectionate tributes to his humor, vision, generosity, and to the remarkable integration of his professional and family life. Drs. Levin and Koenig also include a collection of Dr. Larson's seminal papers and scholarly reflections of colleagues, providing valuable perspective on his legacy and on what remains to be done."

John Peteet, MD
Associate Professor of Psychiatry,
Harvard Medical School
Chair, APA Corresponding Committee
on Religion, Spirituality, and Psychiatry

"**T**his is a remarkable and moving tribute to the life and legacy of an extraordinary physician, scholar, and person. Colleagues, admirers, and family members reflect on Dr. Larson's life, faith, character, courage, and commitment to founding a field of study when most were dismissive of its significance. This book is a testament to that process, bringing together selections of Larson's writings that span two decades. It is a must-read for all who are interested in the history, development, and current thinking on the relationship between religious faith, healing, and personhood, and those who appreciate the occasional visionaries in our midst whose legacies continue to teach us in ways never imagined."

Allan Hugh Cole Jr., MS, PhD
Assistant Professor of Pastoral Care,
Austin Presbyterian Theological Seminary

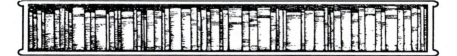

More pre-publication
REVIEWS, COMMENTARIES, EVALUATIONS . . .

"**D**r. David Larson and I attended residency together at Duke University in the 1970s. Ever since I knew him, he had a goal to help scientists better understand the spiritual dimension of man. Because I grew up in a very legalistic religious system, my goal was to help set people free from religious legalism yet maintain their spirituality and accept science, especially by feeling permitted to use psychiatric medication when needed.

Because we had different although related goals, we talked regularly from 1975 until his death on March 5, 2002. I have read his research from the beginning and I know how scrupulously careful and honest Dave was and how thorough he was in his research. Due to his work, Dave had a profound impact on my profession as a psychiatrist, and on me as a friend.

I am thrilled that *Faith, Medicine, and Science* is now available to satisfy each of our goals. Individuals can continue to grow in their understanding of the integration of faith, medicine, and science."

Paul Meier, MD
Founder of Meier Clinics,
Richardson, Texas

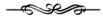

"**T**his is a most excellent reflection on the life of Dr. Larson, one of the world's foremost authorities on religion and medicine. This book allows the reader to travel with Dr. Larson through his passion for spirituality and its role in medicine and provides examples of his scholarly works."

Marvin L. Crawford, MD, MDiv
Assistant Professor of Clinical Medicine,
Morehouse School of Medicine,
Atlanta, Georgia

The Haworth Pastoral Press®
An Imprint of The Haworth Press
New York • London • Oxford

Faith, Medicine, and Science
A Festschrift
in Honor of Dr. David B. Larson

THE HAWORTH PASTORAL PRESS
Religion and Mental Health
Harold G. Koenig, MD
Senior Editor

Bioethics from a Faith Perspective: Ethics in Health Care for the Twenty-First Century by Jack Hanford

Family Abuse and the Bible: The Scriptural Perspective by Aimee K. Cassiday-Shaw

When the Caregiver Becomes the Patient: A Journey from a Mental Disorder to Recovery and Compassionate Insight by Daniel L. Langford and Emil J. Authelet

A Theology of God-Talk: The Language of the Heart by J. Timothy Allen

A Practical Guide to Hospital Ministry: Healing Ways by Junietta B. McCall

Pastoral Care for Post-Traumatic Stress Disorder: Healing the Shattered Soul by Daléne Fuller Rogers

Integrating Spirit and Psyche: Using Women's Narratives in Psychotherapy by Mary Pat Henehan

Chronic Pain: Biomedical and Spiritual Approaches by Harold G. Koenig

Spirituality in Pastoral Counseling and the Community Helping Professions by Charles Topper

Parish Nursing: A Handbook for the New Millennium edited by Sybil D. Smith

Mental Illness and Psychiatric Treatment: A Guide for Pastoral Counselors by Gregory B. Collins and Thomas Culbertson

The Power of Spirituality in Therapy: Integrating Spiritual and Religious Beliefs in Mental Health Practice by Peter A. Kahle and John M. Robbins

Bereavement Counseling: Pastoral Care for Complicated Grieving by Junietta Baker McCall

Biblical Stories for Psychotherapy and Counseling: A Sourcebook by Matthew B. Schwartz and Kalman J. Kaplan

A Christian Approach to Overcoming Disability: A Doctor's Story by Elaine Leong Eng

Faith, Medicine, and Science: A Festschrift in Honor of Dr. David B. Larson edited by Jeff Levin and Harold G. Koenig

Encyclopedia of Ageism by Erdman Palmore, Laurence Branch, and Diana Harris

Spirituality and Mental Health: Clinical Applications by Gary W. Hartz

Dying Declarations: Notes from a Hospice Volunteer by David B. Resnik

Maltreatment of Patients in Nursing Homes: There is No Safe Place by Diana K. Harris and Michael L. Benson

Faith, Medicine, and Science
A Festschrift in Honor of Dr. David B. Larson

Jeff Levin, PhD, MPH
Harold G. Koenig, MD
Editors

The Haworth Pastoral Press®
An Imprint of The Haworth Press
New York • London • Oxford

For more information on this book or to order, visit
http://www.haworthpress.com/store/product.asp?sku=5304

or call 1-800-HAWORTH (800-429-6784) in the United States and Canada or (607) 722-5857
outside the United States and Canada

or contact orders@HaworthPress.com

Published by

The Haworth Pastoral Press®, an imprint of The Haworth Press, Inc., 10 Alice Street, Binghamton,
NY 13904-1580.

Excerpt from THE COLLECTED POEMS OF WALLACE STEVENS by Wallace Stevens,
copyright 1954 by Wallace Stevens and renewed 1982 by Holly Stevens. Used by permission of
Alfred A. Knopf, a division of Random House, Inc.

Photo of David B. Larson by Sam Gray. All rights reserved ©2003 samgrayportraits.com.

Cover design by Kerry E. Mack.

Library of Congress Cataloging-in-Publication Data

Faith, medicine, and science : a festschrift in honor of Dr. David B. Larson / Jeff Levin, Harold G.
Koenig, editors.
     p. cm.
     Includes bibliographical references and index.
     ISBN 0-7890-1871-3 (hard : alk. paper)—ISBN 0-7890-1872-1 (soft : alk. paper)
     1. Larson, David B., 1947- 2. Mental illness—Religious aspects. 3. Spirituality—Health
aspects. 4. Health—Religious aspects. 5. Psychiatry and religion.
     [DNLM: 1. Larson, David B., 1947-2002. 2. Mental Disorders—psychology. 3. Religion and
Psychology. 4. Attitude to Health. 5. Mental Health. 6. Spirituality. WM 61 F174 2004] I. Larson,
David B., 1947-2002. II. Levin, Jeffrey S. III. Koenig, Harold George.
RC455.4.R4L3754 2004
616.89—dc22
                                                                          2004006930

To Susan, Chad, and Kristen Larson

CONTENTS

ABOUT THE EDITORS

Jeff Levin, PhD, MPH, an epidemiologist and former medical school professor, received his AB from Duke University, his MPH from the University of North Carolina, and his PhD from the University of Texas Medical Branch, and completed postdoctoral training in gerontology at the University of Michigan. His studies pioneered basic research in the epidemiology of religion and on the impact of religion on the health of older adults. He has been funded by grants from the NIH and private sources, including the AMA, totaling over $1 million in support. He has more than 135 scholarly publications and more than 130 conference presentations and invited lectures, mostly on religion in health and aging. He has published five books, including *God, Faith, and Health, Religion in Aging and Health,* and *Religion in the Lives of African Americans.* Dr. Levin lectures nationally and internationally, and has been featured in numerous stories in broadcast and print media, including multiple appearances on NPR and CBC and a cover story in *Time.* In 2001, a statement in praise of his work was read into the Congressional Record from the floor of the U.S. House of Representatives. In 2002, Dr. Levin was elected a Fellow of the Gerontological Society of America in recognition of outstanding career achievement and exemplary contributions to the field of gerontology.

Harold G. Koenig, MD, completed his undergraduate education at Stanford University, his medical training at the University of California at San Francisco, and his geriatric medicine, psychiatry, and biostatistics training at Duke University Medical Center. He is board-certified in geriatric psychiatry and geriatric medicine, and is a Professor of Psychiatry and Associate Professor of Medicine at Duke, where he is founding director of the Center for Spirituality, Theology, and Health. He has published extensively in the fields of mental health, geriatrics, and religion, with nearly 250 peer-reviewed articles and book chapters and 26 books. His research on religion, health, and bioethics has been featured nationally and internationally on approximately 50 TV news programs (including all major U.S. networks) and 80 radio programs (including multiple NPR, BBC, and CBC interviews), and in close to 200 newspapers or magazines (including three issues of *Readers Digest*). Dr. Koenig has testified before the U.S. Senate and the United Nations concerning the benefits of religion and spirituality for health, and has been twice nominated for the Templeton Prize for Progress in Religion.

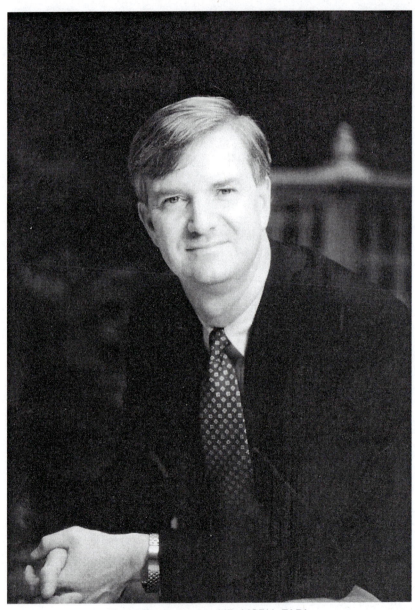

David Bruce Larson, MD, MSPH, FAPA
March 13, 1947, to March 5, 2002

About Dr. David B. Larson

David B. Larson, MD, MSPH, FAPA, an epidemiologist and psychiatrist, focused on understudied and potentially relevant factors which might help in prevention, coping, or recovery from illness. He had more than 270 professional publications and co-authored the *Handbook of Religion and Health,* published by Oxford University Press in 2001.

At the time of his death at age fifty-four, Dr. Larson served as an Adjunct Professor of Psychiatry and Behavioral Sciences at both Duke University Medical Center and Northwestern University Medical School, as well as an Adjunct Professor of Preventive Medicine and Biometrics at the Uniformed Services University of the Health Sciences, in Bethesda, Maryland. He was founder and president of the National Institute for Healthcare Research, which became the International Center for the Integration of Health and Spirituality.

Dr. Larson was formerly a captain in the U.S. Public Health Service Commissioned Corps. He served as a Senior Researcher in the Office of the Director of the National Institutes of Health, as a Senior Policy Analyst in the Office of the Secretary of the Department of Health and Human Services, and as a Section Chief, Primary Care Research Section, Mental Health Services Research Branch, at the National Institute of Mental Health during his ten years in the Corps.

In order to help eliminate selection bias when investigating research findings in controversial areas, Dr. Larson developed an objective, quantitative research methodology that he called the "systematic review." He received a Commissioned Corps Commendation Medal for developing this widely influential methodology—among the five Corps medals and awards that he received.

Dr. Larson helped pioneer the quantitative study of health and spirituality in the medical literature. His systematic reviews of research published in the middle 1980s brought recognition of the neglect of the potential relevance of religion and spirituality in research, medical education, and clinical health care. Dr. Larson stimulated critical new research examining the potential links of religion and spirituality with a variety of physical and mental health outcomes, including coping with chronic and serious illness, and prevention and recovery from depression. He directed seven national conferences which drew together leading researchers and medical educators, and he became a recognized expert on the relationship of religion and spirituality to physical, mental, and social health and well-being.

Dr. Larson graduated from Temple Medical School in Philadelphia. He completed his psychiatry residency, chief residency in psychiatry, and geriatric fellowship training at Duke University Medical Center. He received a three-year epidemiology fellowship from the National Institutes of Health during which he earned a Master of Science in Public Health in epidemiology from the University of North Carolina School of Public Health. He was Board Certified in psychiatry and was also certified as an administrative psychiatrist by the American Psychiatric Association. He was a fellow of both the American Psychiatric Association and the Southern Psychiatric Association, and a member of Sigma Xi Scientific Research Society.

In May 2002, Dr. Larson posthumously received the Oskar Pfister Award for outstanding career contributions to the interrelationships between religion and psychiatry from the American Psychiatric Association.

Foreword

"Dear Dr. Wilson, I hear you are a Christian psychiatrist. I want to be a Christian psychiatrist. Can I come and work with you? [Signed] David Larson."

This was my introduction to David B. Larson. Since I had promised the Lord that I would train students in how to integrate their faith, I wrote him back and offered him a student research fellowship for the summer. I would never have dreamed what the fellowship was going to do to his career. When he arrived in his Volkswagen "Bug" he came with piles of notes that he had collected during his first two years of medical school. It is not surprising as I look on his career now that he ended up being in demographic research. He loved detail.

We did some religious research that summer on the Christian family, and this got him excited about doing more in the future. During his senior year in medical school he came again to Duke and did a clinical elective with me. During the research fellowship and the elective he lived with us in our home. We made him part of our family and, since he was a "great big kid" at the time, he fit in nicely. Dave went everywhere I went during the workday and sometimes even went to church functions and to medical meetings with me. During our times together his inquiring mind made him ask questions about psychiatry and our faith. Together we were able to increase our knowledge of man as a spiritual being and how he, as a unity, can be spiritually diseased just as he can be physically and psychologically diseased.

Dave was a Presbyterian in his early life and never forgot the first article of the *Westminster Shorter Catechism*. He always remembered that man's chief aim is to glorify God and enjoy Him forever. He did this in his life and work, because it was his greatest desire. At the same time, he retained the humility he had when he drove up into our yard the first time. He said that he had come to learn and he kept that attitude throughout the rest of his life.

Dave was a very intense person. He was always jiggling his foot, which I interpreted as indicative of great energy. He used this great energy for the Lord. James Packer said that people who know God have great energy for God. Dave certainly showed evidence of having great energy for God, because he "shared Christ" with anyone who would listen. His enthusiasm resulted in many people coming to Christ. He energetically did research for the Lord and participated in his church and the Christian Medical Society at Duke.

In the same way, his energy translated into his research career. The enormity of his bibliography is evidence of that energy. Dave felt that the research he did would demonstrate the power of God in healing, and it has done just that. But mostly it has demonstrated the preventive medical aspects of a faith in the one true God.

When Dave lived with us he was physically active. I was amazed that each morning he did 100 sit-ups and 100 push-ups, and sometimes would jog, too. He continued this activity the rest of his life. He did not stop jiggling his foot in spite of this strenuous physical exercise.

When we decided to provide instruction for Christian medical students and residents, Dave took on responsibility for organizing seminars that we held outside of the medical center. We had a small committee who selected the subject matter and assigned the presentation to the residents who were available. We held thirty sessions a year, and he participated in them all.

When Dave finally finished his residency, he was asked to stay on the faculty and he did so. He was an excellent teacher and was well liked by the students and residents. He learned how to administrate during these years so that he became a well-rounded academician. I was dismayed when he left us to go to the NIH, but again he distinguished himself and was able to prepare himself for the part of his career that was to bring him the greatest fame.

Dave and I continued to maintain our relationship after he left Duke. He was like a son to me and I took great pride in his accomplishments.

It is only fitting that this book be published to honor him. I am glad that I had the opportunity to know him and to participate in his growth as a psychiatrist, researcher, and child of God. Kahlil Gibran said that the essence of a good teacher is that he will lead his student into a realization of his own mind. I believe that Dave truly came into realization of his. As you read this work, I pray that you realize what a remarkable man he was and how God used him for His glory.

William P. Wilson, MD
Professor Emeritus of Psychiatry
Duke University Medical Center
Durham, North Carolina

Preface

The late Dr. David B. Larson was a principal figure in the development of the religion and health field within academic medicine and public health. Along with the two of us, and several others, Dave was instrumental in the establishment of the field, its fertile growth and expansion, and what is coming to be its mainstream acceptance. But while we focused on our own scholarly careers, Dave devoted himself tirelessly to the work of field building. That the religion and health field is indeed a *field* is mostly Dave's doing. In fact, it would not be an exaggeration to state that the heightened awareness of the health effects of religious faith and participation among both clinicians and the lay public and the institutionalization of coursework on religion and spirituality within undergraduate and graduate medical education are owed in large part to Dave's vision and efforts.

When Dave died on March 5, 2002, at the age of fifty-four, the religion and health field lost its greatest proponent. As founding president of the International Center for the Integration of Health and Spirituality (ICIHS), formerly the National Institute for Healthcare Research, Dave sponsored conferences, symposia, research monographs, medical education funding programs, a speakers' bureau, and media outreach that served to raise faith-based issues to a prominent place in the consciousness of health professionals, biomedical researchers, social and behavioral scientists, journalists, and laypeople. The work of Dave and his beltway-based think tank extended considerably beyond promoting the role of faith in health and health care. He explored the impact of religious faith and identity on a wide swath of social issues, including criminal behavior, substance abuse, mental illness, juvenile delinquency, reproductive decisions, marital satisfaction and family functioning, and quality of life.

In putting together *Faith, Medicine, and Science,* we seek to honor the memory of our friend and colleague, and, more important, to document Dave's sweeping and encyclopedic contributions to science, medicine, and society. This book will serve both as a festschrift for Dave and as a permanent record attesting to the powerful role of religion, spirituality, and faith in God as potential resources for good in the lives of human beings.

Many people have generously devoted their time and energies to the production of this book. Festschrift books are not typically best-sellers, and so to keep expenses down this book was created without any budgeted funds. All of the nearly three dozen contributors offered their glowing words about Dave gratis, without any honoraria. Susan Larson's Oskar Pfister Award address and her essay about life with Dave are beautiful tributes to her late husband; words cannot express our gratitude for her generosity in allowing us to include these in this book. Likewise, our sincere thanks go to Dave's children, Chad and Kristen, whose beautiful eulogies to their father are also included. Tom Smith, Roz Brown, and Mary Milano, Dave's colleagues at ICIHS, were of invaluable assistance to us in so many ways, beginning when this book was just an idea and continuing through the writing, editing, and publishing stages.

The publisher of *Faith, Medicine, and Science,* The Haworth Press, graciously went ahead with this project despite a presumably limited audience. We would like to acknowledge the support and help of several people at Haworth. First, we owe a debt of gratitude to the publisher Bill Cohen, who agreed to publish the book and encouraged us throughout. We also thank Vice President of Publications Bill Palmer and his staff, Robert Owen, Amy Rentner, Rebecca Browne, Jillian Mason, Katy Kempf, and Peg Marr, for all of their help in preparing the manuscript and getting it into production. This book could not have been published without key contributions from each of these people. Their generosity, helpfulness, and patience are deeply appreciated.

Finally, we, the editors, have paid for our time and work on this project out of pocket, and are donating all royalties to an annual lecture fund named in Dave's honor at Duke University Medical Center. Every year forthcoming, the David B. Larson Memorial Lecture in Religion and Health will be given on March 5, the anniversary of Dave's passing, supported by the proceeds from *Faith, Medicine, and Science* and by the generosity of individual donors. The first Larson Memorial Lecture, "Religion, Health, and Healing: Controversies, Crossroads, and Cutting-Edges," was delivered in 2003 by Jeff Levin, one of the editors of this book. The other editor, Harold Koenig, is in charge of the lecture series, which is sponsored by the Duke University Center for Spirituality, Theology, and Health, for which he serves as director.

Both of us owe more to Dave Larson than we could ever fully detail. Less than twenty years ago the entire religion and health field was basically the three of us, and sometimes a few others, huddled together in a corner somewhere at various professional meetings. More soon followed, but we always felt a sort of unspoken kinship as the only three researchers reckless enough to actually devote our entire career to this field. Dave's passing is not only a devastating loss to medicine and science, to his colleagues, and to his family and loved ones, but to us personally, leaving us with a uniquely felt professional loneliness. That gap is unfilled. More than ever, our resolve is steeled to go forth and honor Dave's commitment by picking up where he left off and redoubling our efforts to spread the message that became the implicit byword of his life's work: faith matters.

I (Jeff Levin) would like to thank my beloved wife, Lea, for the blessing of her love and support as I took on the challenge of compiling this book. Also, I owe a great debt of gratitude to Harold Koenig for taking time from his incredibly full schedule to work with me on this project. It might come as a surprise to others in the field, but *Faith, Medicine, and Science* is the first collaboration of any type that Harold and I have ever published. That this belated venture should occur in a book honoring Dave Larson is only fitting. Finally, I offer thanks and praise to Almighty God for, to paraphrase the *shehecheyanu* prayer, giving me life, sustaining me, and enabling me to take part in this special project.

I (Harold G. Koenig) would like to thank Jeff Levin for his concept for this book with which he approached me shortly after Dave's death. It is such a privilege to be collaborating with Jeff, who has a gift for writing and power of expression that few possess, and is primarily responsible for crafting and editing *Faith, Medicine, and Science.* I immediately recognized that compiling this book was not only what we ought to do, but what we *must* do to honor this giant of a man. We both loved David and owe him more than mere words can ever express. He single-handedly opened doors that enabled us to pursue our dreams. Without Dave, those dreams could not have become a reality. Dave served God by serving others and sometimes sacrificed himself in the process: What greater legacy could anyone leave? I thank God for Dave and take comfort in knowing that now he is reaping his reward for that life of service.

PART I:
TRIBUTES TO DR. DAVID B. LARSON

If Dave Larson were merely a "father" of the religion and health field and a helpful facilitator of the research and writing of others, his legacy would be assured. To all who knew and appreciated him, however, he was so much more: an almost obsessively hardworking and committed scholar and researcher; a selfless, humble, and self-deprecating colleague and scientific pioneer who always made sure that others shared the credit for his efforts; an incredibly funny and quirky person who never took himself or his work seriously and could make even the dourest audience of skeptics smile; a deeply loving husband, father, and friend whose concern and compassion for those he cared about defy words; and a man of profound faith whose prayerfulness and devotion to Christ were foremost in his life and drove every action he undertook.

In Part I of *Faith, Medicine, and Science,* tributes are presented from friends, family, and colleagues. These include an original essay by the editors of this book offering reflections on Dave's life and career (Chapter 1); personal remembrances from people that Dave touched professionally and personally (Chapter 2); eulogies presented at his memorial service by his children, Chad and Kristen (Chapter 3); and, the Oskar Pfister Award Address, delivered by Susan Larson on the occasion of Dave's posthumous receipt of the award for career contributions in the field of religion and psychiatry given by the American Psychiatric Association (Chapter 4).

Together, these tributes paint a portrait of a man deeply committed both to his loved ones and to his life's work, which for Dave was a true calling—an extension of his commitment to God and to a life of service to others. Dave Larson left his mark on more people than he knew and on more institutions and fields than he was probably aware. His presence will be missed, but his work will continue.

Chapter 1

Faith Matters:
Reflections on the Life and Work
of Dr. David B. Larson

Jeff Levin
Harold G. Koenig

INTRODUCTION

Scholarly writing on the interface of religion and health is not a new development. While recent epidemiologic and clinical research studies have attracted the attention of scientists, physicians, and the popular media, discourse on the important connections between religious faith and religious institutions, on the one hand, and medicine, the healing arts, and the promotion of health, on the other, have been ongoing for more than a century. Published work in many fields, including psychology, pastoral care, psychiatry, and the history of medicine, has explored the valuable functions served by personal and collective expressions of religiousness for the advancement of mental and physical health and for the establishment of caregiving institutions and organizations.

Historians of medicine, science, and religion have documented in great detail the long-standing interconnections between religious and healing institutions. Discourse on matters related to human physiology, health, and medical treatment has always occupied a central place in both canonical and noncanonical writing within respective faith traditions,[1] and religions and religious organizations were the earliest sponsors of medical care institutions. Within the past two decades, several scholarly works have detailed these connections that have existed throughout recorded history between medicine and organized religions, East and West. Macmillan's two-volume *Caring and Curing*[2] and *Healing and Restoring*[3] comprehensively detail this rich heritage of attention to health, healing, and medicine within Judaism, nearly twenty denominations of Christianity, and a dozen of the world's other religious traditions.

Among Western religions, renewed attention has focused on religion-health and religion-medicine linkages. The Park Ridge Center for Health, Faith, and Ethics sponsored a series of monographs titled, "Health/Medicine and the Faith Traditions," which explored these connections within several major Christian denominations and Judaism.[4] In the Jewish tradition, especially, religious and medical authorities have written about the indivisibility of religion and medicine for centuries. Maimonides, for example, was a physician as well as a philosopher, and his writings on Jewish perspectives on the body, on health, and on medicine have been studied by scholars for more than 800 years.[5] In that time, a library of academic and popular writing on these topics has appeared, ranging from erudite commentaries on *halakhah* (or Jewish law) to *midrashic* commentaries to kabbalistic speculation. Most notable is Preuss' classic *Biblical and Talmudic Medicine,*[6] a 600-page compilation of biblical texts and commentaries organized like a medical textbook, which was translated into English by Rosner and republished in the United States and Europe.

Within Christianity, especially American Protestantism, the early to middle twentieth century witnessed the beginning of scholarly discussion of mental health, health care, and healing by prominent figures in the Christian pastoral counseling field. Important books include Hiltner's classic *Religion and Health,*[7] Oates' *Religious Factors in Mental Illness,*[8] Wise's *Religion in Illness and Health,*[9] Crowlesmith's *Religion and Medicine,*[10] and McCann's *The Churches and Mental Health,*[11] among many others. This work drew upon, and grew out of, earlier writing at the interface of medicine, psychology, and Christian theology that sought to identify etiologically and therapeutically significant factors in the religious life of Christians. This writing comprises the beginnings of what has come to be known in the clinical pastoral field as the "religion and health movement." Notable works in this genre date from Brigham's *Observations on the Influence of Religion upon the Health and Physical Welfare of Mankind,*[12] in the nineteenth century, to Worcester and colleagues' *Religion and Medicine: The Moral Control of Nervous Disorders,*[13]

Weatherhead's *Psychology, Religion and Healing,*[14] Walsh's *Religion and Health,*[15] and Holman's *The Religion of a Healthy Mind.*[16]

The latter work, and others in that vein, owe an obvious debt to philosopher William James, who contrasted the religion of "healthy-minded" and "sick-minded" souls in his *The Varieties of Religious Experience,*[17] a seminal work in psychology. James was by no means alone among early psychologists and psychiatrists in considering the value of religion and personal religiousness for human well-being. Freud, while antipathetic toward religious beliefs, nonetheless recognized their salience, for better or worse, for the psychological well-being of individuals.[18] Among psychiatrists, Jung[19] and Fromm[20] recognized the potentially salutary role of a religious outlook on life and of humanistic (as opposed to authoritarian) religion, respectively. Among psychologists, Allport[21] hypothesized that intrinsic religion serves an integrative function and thus benefits mental health, and Maslow[22] proposed that transcendent experiences (defined as peaks or plateaus of unitive consciousness) are more common among emotionally healthy individuals.

Despite the historically well-documented connections between religion and health and religion and medicine, and despite the traditions of writing on this topic within Judaism, Christianity, and psychology and psychiatry, as just noted, scholarly momentum waned by the late 1950s. This is not to say that nothing of importance was published during that period. Interesting symposia proceedings,[23-24] committee reports,[25-26] histories,[27] and edited books[28] and readers[29] and important scholarly works such as theologian Paul Tillich's classic essay on "the meaning of health"[30] continued to appear. But absence of a concerted collective effort to explore, empirically, the interconnections of religion, health, and medicine seemed to mirror the contemporaneous drought of academic writing in the psychology of religion.[31]

By contrast, another scientific field, gerontology, since its inception had paid considerable attention to religion and its ability to influence human lives for the good. Gerontology, the study of older adults and of the aging process throughout the life course, is a multidisciplinary field, and gerontological research typically has an applied or practical life focus. Accordingly, some of the earliest empirical studies in social gerontology, namely the stellar pioneering research of David O. Moberg[32] in the early 1950s, examined the impact of religion on the general well-being of older adults. Small-scale studies on this topic continued to appear over the next three decades,[33] but, as in psychology, systematic investigation was lacking.

Throughout this writing in gerontology, psychology, psychiatry, and other fields, once in awhile a published article or book would make reference to an actual empirical study of the putative effects of religion on physical or mental health. Such studies, it was presumed, were few and far between, and they were eagerly cited as evidence that a connection between religion and health might not only exist in theory but be empirically supported by data.

A few groups of epidemiologic studies garnered occasional attention through the years, according to a comprehensive review by Levin and Schiller.[34] These included investigations of rates of cancer and of colitis and enteritis in Jews, mortality patterns in the clergy, the morbidity of Parsis, Protestant-Catholic-Jewish differences in occupational-related morbidity, and the health of Latter Day Saints and Seventh-Day Adventists. Earlier epidemiologic reviews, as well, had included discussion of religious exposures as factors in morbidity or mortality, notably Kennaway's "The Racial and Social Incidence of Cancer of the Uterus,"[35] one of the finest review papers ever published in epidemiology.

Within psychiatry, likewise, a few studies of religious differences in certain disorders had become somewhat well known. An entire chapter of the book reporting on the famous Midtown Manhattan Study, published in 1962, documented differences in a variety of prevalence rates among Protestants, Catholics, and Jews by religious origin, parental religious-group identification, and parental religiosity.[36] An earlier study, published in the *American Journal of Psychiatry* in 1954, identified similar religious-affiliational differences in a variety of psychiatric diagnoses.[37] Enough of this kind of research and writing had accumulated by 1980 that the National Institute of Mental Health (NIMH) was able to publish *Religion and Mental Health: A Bibliography.*[38]

This type of research among epidemiologists and psychiatrists took its cue from some of the key pioneers of Western biomedicine. Benjamin Travers, an early British surgeon, first noted differences in rates of cancer between Jews and gentiles,[39] in 1837. John Shaw Billings, founder of *Index Medicus,* published one of the earliest epidemiologic studies of religious affiliation, in 1891.[40] William Osler, the father of U.S. medical education and instrumental in the establishment of the medical school at Johns Hopkins University, offered reflections on "the faith that heals,"[41] in 1910. The American Medical Association's official journal, *JAMA*, published an outstanding three-part series of articles on the topic of "religious healing,"[42] in 1926. But, again, as in other fields, systematic empirical exploration of a possible religion-health association appeared to have entered a state of limbo for the next several decades.

Throughout that time, a few thoughtful efforts were made to summarize existing findings and/or make sense of their meaning. Beginning in the middle 1970s, several prominent scholars and scientists, having encountered bits of this body of research and writing, sought to interpret and understand just what it was about religion that might be health promoting. Some of these reviews and theoretical papers made vital contributions and continue to be cited to this day. These include Vaux's[43] comprehensive effort to identify aspects of religious belief and practice that influence health-related behavior, Vanderpool's discussions of the possible "therapeutic significance" of religion[44] and of six major areas of interaction between religion and medicine,[45] Kaplan's[46] conceptual exploration of "the relevance of religious experience to heart disease," Bergin's[47] data-based "critical reevaluation" of the salutary role of religion for mental health, and Frank's[48] revisiting of Osler's "faith that heals."

DAVE LARSON, THE PIONEER

Aside from this handful of articles and books, there things sat for decades, until the middle 1980s when three scientists almost simultaneously—and completely independently—began to uncover, review, and write about existing studies of religion and health programmatically. One was an epidemiologist, one was a physician, and one was both. These three individuals were the two editors of this book and Dave Larson.

Contrary to popular presumptions, we discovered, much research had been done. An almost unbelievable amount of research, to be blunt. Despite commonly heard assertions that "nothing had ever been done" in this area, we found quite the opposite. The total included a couple of hundred epidemiologic studies of religion, as summarized in the Levin and Schiller review mentioned previously; another couple hundred studies of religion in psychiatry,[49] and nearly 300 scholarly publications about religion on topics related to aging, geriatrics, and clinical medicine.[50] According to another review of some of these studies that appeared about the same time,[51] the scope of published research on religion's impact on morbidity and mortality was broad, to say the least: studies had been conducted among Protestants, Catholics, Jews, Muslims, Seventh-Day Adventists, Latter Day Saints, Parsis, and Hutterites, among others, and in the general population. Oddly, epidemiologists and physician researchers, who had authored most of this work, seemed especially oblivious and dismissive.

Our responses to this treasure trove of information were quite different. One of us wrote detailed literature reviews, offered methodological critiques of existing studies, and developed a model of alternative theoretical explanations for findings, while conducting original empirical work among ethnic minority populations emphasizing the use of sophisticated social and epidemiologic research methods. Another of us emphasized the study of clinical populations and geriatric patients with medical and psychiatric illness, while producing two dozen books for clinicians, mental health providers, pastors, and laypeople, mostly written from a Christian perspective, and also establishing an academic center at Duke University. The third pioneer sought no less than to build a field from scratch—a network of clinicians, educators, and scholars from fields as diverse as medicine, nursing, public health, the social and behavioral sciences, religious and theological studies, ministry, bioethics, and the humanities—and to facilitate and promote the research and writing of all involved.

The first two people mentioned previously are the two of us, Jeff Levin and Harold Koenig; the third is Dave Larson. Although we would like to fall back on the scientist's conceit that the growth and institutionalization of the religion and health field are a direct result of our early research and of the outstanding studies by those others who have since taken up the call, the plain truth is that these efforts simply cannot account for all that has followed. As mentioned in the preface to this book, the fact that the religion and health field has indeed become a field is owed mostly to the vision, commitment, and single-minded dedication of Dave Larson. It is a sign of Dave's humility that, more than likely, he would vigorously protest this characterization and would attribute the emergence and growth of this field entirely to others and to God's grace.

Dave's curriculum vitae (see Chapter 16) details a remarkable, and strange, career trajectory. Twice in his professional life he radically changed course, undeterred, taking a huge leap of faith in order to pursue his dreams. First, in the early 1980s, he gave up a successful academic career for government service, leaving Duke University to enter the Public Health Service as a commissioned officer and to work in various policymaking and administrative capacities for the Department of Health and Human Services (DHHS), including stints at both the National Institutes of Health (NIH) and the NIMH. Nearly a decade later, in 1991, he founded the National Institute for Healthcare Research (NIHR), and in 1993 he left the government to serve full-time as NIHR's president, remaining there until his passing in 2002. Yet despite nearly two decades of only adjunct appointments in academic medicine, Dave's scholarly output exceeded almost everyone else in the religion and health field.

Dave and the two of us have several unusual shared connections. Each of us is part of the extended Duke University family. Dave came to Duke in 1974, completed his postgraduate work in psychiatry in 1977, followed by a postdoctoral research fellowship in 1979 and a clinical geropsychiatry fellowship in 1981, and then joined the faculty, rising to the rank of Adjunct Professor in 1985. Harold Koenig came to Duke in 1986, where he subsequently trained in geriatrics, biometry, psychiatry, and geropsychiatry, and has been a faculty member since 1992. Jeff Levin came to Duke in 1977 and is an alumnus of both the religion and sociology departments, class of 1981. Dave and Harold also have the additional connection of both being psychiatrists. Dave and Jeff have an additional connection as well: both are graduates of the University of North Carolina School of Public Health, Dave in 1982 and Jeff in 1983; both were trained in epidemiology; and both benefited from the mentorship of Berton H. Kaplan. Finally, all three of us, as so many others in the religion and health field, became gerontologists.

This is all worth mentioning because, despite these many connections, we stumbled into this area of research completely independently and without even knowing one another. Our work at Duke, for example, did not overlap and we only first met through professional circles. We have often speculated that perhaps something was in the air at the time, in the middle 1980s, as several other researchers besides us also began systematically to study religion and health. While the three of us each had been publishing scholarly papers on religion and/or health in peer-reviewed journals for several years, our first widely read articles on religion and health appeared almost simultaneously. Dave's famous literature review of religious research in psychiatry was published in 1986;[52] Jeff's much-cited literature reviews of epidemiologic studies of religion were published in 1987[53]; and Harold's well-regarded first three research papers on religion and aging were published in 1988.[54-56] Around the same time, Robert Joseph Taylor and Linda M. Chatters published the first of their collaborations in this field in 1986,[57] Ellen L. Idler published her first key paper on this topic in 1987,[58] Christopher G. Ellison[59] (also a Duke graduate, incidentally) made his first important contribution in this area in 1989, and David R. Williams[60] published one of the first longitudinal epidemiological analyses of religion, co-authored with Dave Larson, in 1991. These papers had overlapping themes and content, were gerontological in focus, and were written by investigators who had come to work in this field independently of one another.

For each of these scholars, the objective was that of the typical academic scientist: to further the field through advancing our own individual research efforts. Dave's objective, on the other hand, was to further the field by advancing the individual research efforts not of himself but of all of the rest of us, and of the countless others who followed. He became the tireless captain of a team of beleaguered sociologists, psychologists, epidemiologists, gerontologists, and physicians who shared not much else but a desire to do scholarly work, sometimes in collaboration and sometimes alone, in an area that most everyone else in academic medicine, public health, and the medical, social, and behavioral sciences, it seemed, derided or ignored. Dave in fact had a great sense of humor about this. In published writings, he more than once referred to this overt antipathy as a "taboo,"[61-62] one in which religion had become the unspoken "*R* word"[63] and, for academicians, something akin to an "anti-tenure factor."[64]

A short decade and a half later, a thriving field is in place. Empirical research on religion and health, if not yet fully accepted as mainstream in all disciplines, is fast becoming an accepted topic of investigation in several large fields of study. If peer-reviewed publications and funded research studies are good indications, these fields include gerontology and geriatrics, medical sociology, health psychology, public health, family medicine, and psychiatry. According to the *Handbook of Religion and Health,*[65] which Dave co-authored, by the year 2000 more than 1,600 scholarly publications had addressed the role of religion in health, mental health, general well-being, or quality of life, including at least 1,200 empirical studies.

Besides the names already mentioned, other prominent figures have devoted considerable time and effort to researching the connections between religion and health. These include Neal Krause, Diane R. Brown, Kenneth F. Ferraro, William J. Strawbridge, Kenneth I. Pargament, Linda K. George (a Duke graduate and professor), and Margaret M. Poloma. A second generation of scholars has emerged, as well, led by Michael E. McCullough, Marc A. Musick (a Duke graduate), and Amy L. Ai. Furthermore, especially within gerontology, dozens of other researchers with principal research foci elsewhere have nonetheless made important contributions to furthering the study of religion and health. This includes senior figures such as David O. Moberg, whose contributions to the field began in the 1950s; Dan G. Blazer and Erdman B. Palmore (both Duke professors), who started writing on the topic in the 1970s; Kyriakos S. Markides, who initiated a series of studies conducted both alone and in conjunction with Jeff Levin in the early 1980s; and George W. Comstock, dean of American epidemiologists, whose consideration of religious variables in his studies dates back decades. Also deserving of mention, in no particular order, are Stephen C. Ainlay, Andrew Futterman, Dana E. King, Keith G. Meador (a Duke graduate and professor), Byron R. Johnson, Herbert Benson, Harold Y. Vanderpool, George Fitchett, Dale A. Matthews (a Duke graduate), Stephen G. Post, Lawrence E. Gary, Preston L. Schiller, Andrew J. Weaver, Kimberly A. Sherrill (a Duke graduate), Gail Ironson, Peter H. Van Ness, Anthony Walsh, Christina M. Puchalski, Stanislav V. Kasl, Peter C. Hill, Elisabeth McSherry, and Harvey Jay Cohen (a Duke professor), each of whom has contributed significantly to the advancement of the field. Perhaps an underappreciated common element of so many important scholars in this field is a connection to Duke University!

Many of these named individuals now have endowed chairs or are department chairpersons, center directors, or deans. Most are tenured full professors. Thanks to Dave's tireless efforts to use NIHR to raise the profile of scientific research on religion and health and to foster its legitimization, taking time to conduct studies and publish in this area is no longer considered career suicide or a ticket to the academic fringes. Thanks also to his generally unrecognized efforts at DHHS beginning in the mid-1980s, the NIH and the private-foundation sector have come to acknowledge religion and health as a worthy topic for research funding and have supported the studies of many of the field's leading investigators. By virtue of Dave's work both behind the scenes and in the public eye, the once "anti-tenure factor" has been transformed more or less into a pro-tenure factor.

DAVE LARSON, THE PERSON

What kind of a man would put his own scholarly career off to the side in order to facilitate the work of others? This is a question that those of us who knew and loved Dave Larson have often reflected upon, with a mix of curiosity and gratitude. Perhaps the best explanation is that Dave was magnificently blessed with a sense of selflessness, lack of ego, and nonattachment to worldly gain more befitting a Buddhist monk or a Mother Teresa than the caricature of an academic medical scientist. He was *completely* committed to his life's work, his eye on the ultimate goal of transforming and respiritualizing the healing arts and sciences, and was able to maintain the long view in the face of ongoing highs and lows far better than anyone else in the field. As a result, he truly did care less about whether his name was attached to key advances than that such advances occurred. He was happy to deflect the credit to others, even where he himself deserved the lion's share.

How and why does a man choose to live his life this way? Perhaps the most important motivating factor for Dave was one that he was uncomfortable addressing in secular professional settings, although all of his colleagues were well aware of its salient presence in his life. Indeed, if Dave were still alive, he might wish we turned our attention elsewhere. He was always sensitive that he, and by extension every one of us working in the religion and health field, be seen as scientists first and foremost whose scholarly work could not be undermined or impugned by accusations of bias or speculations about our motives. Dave, we suspect, worried much more about this than any of the rest of us in the field. After nearly twenty years of dealing with naysayers, most of us by now have developed pretty thick skin.

Since Dave is no longer here among us in body, we will respectfully blow his cover. The secret to understanding Dave's profound dedication, commitment, and selflessness can be found in the words of his friend, Reverend Andrew J. Weaver, in his tribute to Dave included among the remembrances contained in Chapter 2 of this book: "Dave Larson was a Christian. He was not ashamed of the scandal of the Gospel. His piety was genuine and heartfelt. He had a desire for GOD."

In terms familiar to evangelicals, Dave was "sold out" to Christ. His faith in God was unwavering and all-encompassing. For his colleagues in the religion and health field, whose own faith commitments span myriad religious traditions and affiliations (including "none of the above"), Dave's love of God and devotion to being His faithful servant were never anything but an inspiration. For those of us committed to following Bible-based Judeo-Christian paths, Dave was a true role model of how to be both a scientist and a person of faith without ever sacrificing or compromising either identity. His success at this difficult balancing act is a lasting testament to his strength of character and great integrity as a person.

So, our apologies to Dave and to his wife, Susan, who has so carefully guarded his scholarly reputation. But without speaking of his Christian walk, the Dave Larson story would be terribly incomplete.

Elsewhere among the remembrances in Chapter 2 are other clues to what made Dave tick. The many words and phrases used to describe Dave paint a picture of a complex and exceedingly *good* person. Friends and colleagues spoke of his "modesty," "openness," "humility," "character and integrity," "incredible vivaciousness for life," "humor," "optimism," "innocence," "deep and abiding love for God and for all of mankind," "mentoring influence," "enormous energy," "vision," "enthusiasm," "inspiration," "full intensity," "characteristic vigor and zest," "profound gratitude," "support and encouragement," "fiery passion," "faith," "devotion and creativity," "kindness," "guidance and direction," "sincere interest in others," "heart for people," "rich wisdom," "deep insights," "idiosyncrasies," "strength of resolve," "courage," "great compassion and strong sense of purpose," "knowledge," "gift of discernment," and "characteristic generosity."

Dave was also described as "caring," "understanding," "at peace with himself," "dedicated," "a true believer," "intuitive," "confident," "a complete humanitarian," "godly," "interested and engaged," "a first-class networker," "unstintingly unselfish," "extraordinarily thoughtful and considerate," "influential," "earnest," "a totally genuine, engaging, humorous, dedicated, intelligent person," "eccentric, transparent, kind, insightful, and unique," "uncanny," "in so many ways at peace," "contemplative," "joyous," "successful," "easygoing," "not a pushover," "a total altruist," "gifted," "compelling," "humorous," "ingenious," "dedicated," "congruent," "a catalyst," and, most accurately of all, "inimitable, irreplaceable, unstoppable."

Dave Larson wanted little more than to be of service to his fellow scientists and clinicians in their quest to integrate faith and spirituality into their work. In so doing, he hoped, the culture of medicine and of medical science could begin to experience a transformation and renewal. Because of his constant efforts, and his selflessness, many of us have been able to experience professional success and even a little bit of celebrity while helping to fulfill Dave's dream. For those of us privileged to be carrying on in his place, his legacy of kindness and sacrifice are ever-present reminders of the moral standard that he set for scholars in the field that he helped to found.

DAVE LARSON, THE SCIENTIST

For someone who placed his own academic advancement beneath service to others, Dave actually was a very productive researcher. His most visible place in the scientific world was as a valued co-author to so many of us in the religion and health field. Dave gained a sterling reputation as a "manuscript doctor" without equal. Colleagues with an unpublishable scholarly manuscript on religion or any other controversial topic knew that they could send their paper to Dave, who would then work his magic and, in exchange for a co-authorship or an acknowledgment, produce a surefire gem. The two of us can personally attest to Dave's remarkable ability to see the good in an otherwise hopeless manuscript and bring it to the fore, resulting in a peer-reviewed journal article. We each benefited from Dave's magic.

This reputation actually disguises and undervalues Dave's own original work, which was impeccable, historically significant, and very influential. This, the reader will see, is a consistent theme of this book, underscored especially by the selection of many of his classic lead-authored papers included in Part II. Beginning with a series of papers written with William P. Wilson and published in the *Southern*

Medical Journal starting in 1980,[66-69] Dave embarked on a program of research and writing focused squarely on elucidating the role of religion, broadly defined, in preventing and treating psychiatric illness and in promoting mental health. Eventually, this body of work was extended to include physical as well as mental health, and also a variety of social and quality-of-life indicators impacted by religion. For more than twenty years, Dave was a nonstop source of theoretical essays, scholarly reviews, and empirical studies arguing for a complete overthrow of the long-held belief that religion was on the whole a malign influence on human life—a tacit belief so characteristic of both psychiatry and the sorts of "opinion leaders" valued by the popular culture and by official Washington. Dave's work and its lasting influence led to national recognition with his receiving the American Psychiatric Association's prestigious Oskar Pfister Award in 2002 (see Chapter 4).

The first of Dave's scholarly articles reprinted in *Faith, Medicine, and Science* is his "Religious Life of Alcoholics" (see Chapter 5), one of several studies conducted with his mentor William P. Wilson. Together, this series of papers examined the impact of religious teachings, beliefs, practices, and experiences on psychiatric patients diagnosed with alcoholism, narcotic addiction, schizophrenia, and affective disorders. The paper on alcoholism, published in the *Southern Medical Journal* in 1980, identified considerable religious differences between alcoholics and nonalcoholics, especially developmentally. Although the families of alcoholics mostly attended conservative Christian churches, Dave and Dr. Wilson suggested that a failure of alcoholics and their families to practice what they preached, so to speak, created a discordance or dissonance that contributed to their greater risk of alcoholism.

The next paper included in this book is the classic systematic review that established Dave as the world's leading authority on the scope of published research on religion and mental health. Titled, "Systematic Analysis of Research on Religious Variables in Four Major Psychiatric Journals, 1978-1982" (see Chapter 6), and published in the *American Journal of Psychiatry* in 1986, this review was based on earlier presentations at the annual meetings of the Southern Psychiatric Association and the American Psychiatric Association. Co-authored with colleagues at Duke, North Carolina, the Medical College of Georgia, and the NIMH, this article summarized the use and misuse of religious measures in the 2.5 percent of studies containing a religious measure out of 2,348 empirical studies published in four major psychiatry journals. The verdict: psychiatric research was not paying much attention to religion, and, when it did, it was doing a generally lousy job.

This article set the stage for a series of reviews published over the next several years. Each examined a different aspect of the research literature on religion and mental health, and each was published in a top-tier psychiatry journal. "Religious Affiliations in Mental Health Research Samples As Compared with National Samples"[70] (see Chapter 7) and "Associations Between Dimensions of Religious Commitment and Mental Health Reported in the *American Journal of Psychiatry* and *Archives of General Psychiatry*: 1978-1989"[71] (see Chapter 8) were two of the most influential of these reviews. The first article, published in the *Journal of Nervous and Mental Disease* in 1989, pointed out that study samples used in psychiatric research on religion were typically unrepresentative of the general population. The second article, published in the *American Journal of Psychiatry* in 1992 and an extension of his 1986 paper in the same journal, examined the results of three dozen studies that included measures of religious commitment. In all, 72 percent of the analyses presented in these studies pointed to a positive relationship between religion and mental health, contrary to the historic presumptions of many famous psychiatrists.

Dave's interest in connections between religion and mental health included involvement in effecting policy-level changes within the psychiatric profession. He was one of many figures instrumental in shepherding the process that resulted in changes to how the *Diagnostic and Statistical Manual of Mental Disorders* (DSM) dealt with religion, culminating in a "religious or spiritual problems" category in the DSM-IV. "Religious Content in the DSM-III-R Glossary of Technical Terms"[72] (see Chapter 9), published in the *American Journal of Psychiatry* in 1993, identified blatant examples of insensitivity in how the DSM-III characterized religion. More often than not, when religion was broached in case examples and clinical reminders, religious patients were characterized as psychotic, delusional, incoherent, illogical, and hallucinating, as well as in other ways that indicated psychopathology. This influential article was one of the final nails in the coffin that preceded changes to the DSM.

Dave was especially interested in fostering linkages between religious and mental health professionals. He saw this as a means to many ends, notably improving access to and delivery of mental health services. His classic study, "The Couch and the Cloth: The Need for Linkage"[73] (see Chapter 10), published in *Hospital and Community Psychiatry* in 1988, used data from all five sites of the first wave of the Epidemiologic Catchment Area Study to investigate differences in the lifetime prevalence of psychiatric disorders by whether respondents sought care from mental health specialists only, clergy only, both, or neither. Dave and his colleagues found important differences and similarities in patterns of care-seeking depending upon diagnostic category, using the Diagnostic Interview Schedule. For example, individuals with major life-altering affective or anxiety disorders were more likely to seek care from both mental health specialists and clergy; those with cognitive, abnormal bipolar, schizophreniform, or somatization disorders were more likely to seek care from neither. These and the other results from this study underscored the need for formal linkages between mental health professionals and clergy.

Dave's research as a graduate student in epidemiology at North Carolina was concerned with how religious practices and perceptions of religion affected blood pressure. The major empirical results of his study were presented in an article titled, "The Impact of Religion on Men's Blood Pressure"[74] (see Chapter 11), published in the *Journal of Religion and Health* in 1989. This study's findings remain just as fascinating today as when they first appeared. Dave and his colleagues found that respondents who considered religion somewhat or not at all important had an average diastolic blood pressure (DBP) of 87.2 mmHg; those who rated religion as very important to them had an average DBP of 84.0 mmHg. Furthermore, those who rated their religion as unimportant *and* infrequently attended church had the highest average DBP: 88.2 mmHg; those who considered religion to be important *and* were regular churchgoers had the lowest average DBP: 83.8 mmHg. This article has proved to be a classic in the epidemiology of religion, and has helped to inspire subsequent research on religion and chronic disease morbidity.

Throughout his career, Dave applied his systematic review methodology to a variety of substantive topics besides psychiatric morbidity. As lead- or co-author, these reviews constituted a large share of his published scholarly output throughout the final decade and a half of his life. He reviewed the role and consequences of religion, broadly defined, for scientific and policy-related topics in fields as diverse as pastoral counseling, gerontology, criminology, child development, psychology, health services research, medical education, and primary care. Specific reviews focused on outcomes ranging from juvenile delinquency to television content to the impact of abortion. Scanning Dave's curriculum vitae (see Chapter 16) shows how far afield his commitment to understanding the effects of religious faith took him from psychiatry, the medical specialty in which he was formally trained.

Two of the best of these reviews are characteristic of the detail and insight that can be found throughout this work, as well as of the breadth of topics that Dave chose to investigate. "A Systematic Review of Nursing Home Research in Three Psychiatric Journals: 1966-1985"[75] (see Chapter 12), published in the *International Journal of Geriatric Psychiatry* in 1989, is typical of Dave's best work: a thorough, sophisticated, and damning critique of sampling, design, and analytical shortcomings of published studies. This review was unique for Dave in that it did not focus on religion, but instead was a precise methodological critique coupled with some sharp policy-related recommendations. "Mortality and Religion/Spirituality: A Brief Review of the Research"[76] (see Chapter 13), published in the *Annals of Pharmacotherapy* in 2002, summarized the epidemiological literature suggestive of a protective effect of religion for longevity. Written with his wife, Susan, and with the co-editor of this book, Harold Koenig, the article was an "old-style" literature review, containing a narrative summary of key studies, existing systematic reviews, and meta-analysis results, along with careful consideration of what these findings imply for scientific medicine.

The final article of Dave's that is republished in *Faith, Medicine, and Science* exemplifies another of his many talents: writing for popular audiences. Throughout his career, especially since founding NIHR, Dave consistently published interesting, provocative, and entertaining summaries of religious research in both professional and lay periodicals. "Have Faith: Religion Can Heal Mental Ills"[77] (see Chapter 14), published in the newsstand magazine *Insight* in 1995, was part of a "point-counterpoint"-style debate with the notorious skeptic, Albert Ellis. In his article,[78] Ellis railed against the idea of a salutary effect of religion, yet demonstrated little familiarity with any research on the topic of religion and mental health more recent than a paper of his from 1948. Dave's response was cogent and to the point:

> What is perhaps most surprising about these negative opinions of religion's effect on mental health is the startling absence of empirical evidence to support these views. Indeed, the same scientists who were trained to accept or reject a hypothesis based on hard data seem to rely solely on their own opinions and biases when assessing the effect of religion on health. (p. 20)

Dave Larson was a pioneering figure in medicine. He was also a wonderful friend and colleague, and facilitator of the research and career progress of others. But Dave's contributions to science extended far beyond his contributions to the work of others. It is our hope that his valued gifts of service to others neither obscure what an excellent and important scientist he was nor focus attention away from the unmatched contribution of his own research, a body of work that was central to the establishment of the religion and health field.

DAVE LARSON'S LEGACY

Dave Larson was richly blessed. Strengthened and empowered by a loving family, by devoted friends and colleagues, and by his faith in God, he devoted his life to healing the wounds left behind by the centuries-old divorce of the medical arts and the human spirit. Multiply credentialed as a physician, epidemiologist, psychotherapist, uniformed officer in the U.S. Public Health Service, and federal policymaker, Dave used each of his talents in tandem to help fashion a new scientific field. Through his efforts, alone and in conjunction with the colleagues he gathered around himself, Dave truly left his mark on the world.

Dave's contributions to medical and health-related research have already been documented in this chapter. Part II of *Faith, Medicine, and Science* contains, in full, the text of all of the important articles and studies synopsized in the last section. These ten papers are just a drop in the bucket—about one-thirtieth of his total published output. They are, however, among his most important scholarly publications, and they accurately represent the contributions for which he is best known. Even in death, this scientific juggernaut continues: according to the most recent list of his publications that we consulted in preparing the version of his curriculum vitae that appears in this book (see Chapter 16), another sixteen scholarly manuscripts have been completed and several of these are currently under peer review at academic journals.

Dave was also instrumental in changing how medicine and psychiatry are practiced. He was avidly sought as a speaker at medical and psychiatry grand rounds, as well as at spirituality and medicine conferences throughout North America. He loved to speak and was a masterful teacher who mixed humor and research facts in a remarkable manner. For years he served as a key faculty member and speaker for Harvard Medical School's "Spirituality and Medicine" continuing medical education program. He also developed and directed for many years a speaker's bureau at NIHR, which provided other speakers for religion, spirituality, and medicine conferences. In 1997, he accepted Jeff Levin's invitatino to co-author the first invited essay on the topic of religion and spirituality in medicine to appear in *JAMA (Journal of the American Medical Association)* in over seventy years.[79]

Finally, Dave's efforts to effect change in the education of young medical students and residents in training may come to represent his most lasting contribution. In 1992, only three medical schools had coursework or instruction related to religion or spirituality. Then, in 1994, Dave obtained a grant from the John Templeton Foundation to start a curricular awards program that gave out $25,000 grants to medical schools in order to fund undergraduate medical courses devoted to the interface of religion, spirituality, and medicine. He put Dale A. Matthews in charge of running this program, which gave out its first awards in 1995.[80] Today, nearly two-thirds of the 125 medical schools in the United States have such coursework, and this is almost entirely due to the results of this innovative program and to the connections that Dave established within the Association of American Medical Colleges.[81] In addition, Dave developed training curricula for residents in psychiatry and primary care, which have been used as guidelines in many residency programs throughout the country, and started two additional curricular awards programs for the same constituencies.[82] All of the curricular awards programs that Dave initiated continue to the present day, now housed at the George Washington

Institute for Spirituality and Health under the direction of Christina M. Puchalski.

The last time that the principal editor of this book, Jeff Levin, spoke with Dave was during a radio panel interview conducted as part of the book tour for Jeff's *God, Faith, and Health*,[83] in the summer of 2001. The name of the radio program, was "Faith Matters." This very much could have been Dave's motto: faith matters. It matters for our health and well-being and it matters for life in general; it matters for all of us individually and for our families and it matters for society as a whole. Faith mattered to Dave Larson, and, because of this, he was driven to live a life of service, committed to sharing the importance of faith in God to all who would listen. Unlike evangelists, who count their harvest in souls reaped, Dave was a scientist. For him, victory was measured not in souls won or lives transformed, but in minds changed.

When Dave began researching and writing about the role of religious faith in mental and physical health, few people in academic medicine professed to believe that the two things were at all related. Now, two decades later, as a result of his life's work, the "religion-health connection"[84] is close to tacit knowledge among identifiable segments of the medical world. More minds have been changed, and curiosities awakened, than any of us who labored alongside Dave could have ever imagined would be possible. In the words of Christ's parable recorded in the Gospel of Matthew, "Well done, good and faithful servant."[85]

NOTES

1. Spector RE. (1996). Healing: Magicoreligious traditions. Chapter 7 in *Cultural Diversity in Health and Illness,* Fourth Edition (pp. 133-168). Stamford, CT: Appleton and Lange.

2. Numbers RL, Amundsen DW. (Editors) (1986). *Caring and Curing: Health and Medicine in the Western Religious Traditions.* New York: Macmillan.

3. Sullivan LE. (Editor) (1989). *Healing and Restoring: Health and Medicine in the World's Religious Traditions.* New York: Macmillan.

4. Feldman DM. (1986). *Health and Medicine in the Jewish Tradition: L'Hayyim—to Life.* New York: Crossroad.

5. Rosner F, Kottek SS. (Editors) (1993). *Moses Maimonides: Physician, Scientist, Philosopher.* Northvale, NJ: Jason Aronson.

6. Preuss J. (1993). *Biblical and Talmudic Medicine* [1911]. Translated and edited by F Rosner. Northvale, NJ: Jason Aronson.

7. Hiltner S. (1943). *Religion and Health.* New York: Macmillan.

8. Oates WE. (1955). *Religious Factors in Mental Illness.* New York: Association Press.

9. Wise CA. (1942). *Religion in Illness and Health.* New York: Harper and Brothers.

10. Crowlesmith J. (1962). *Religion and Medicine.* London, England: The Epworth Press.

11. McCann RV. (1962). *The Churches and Mental Health.* Joint Commission on Mental Illness and Health, Monograph Series, No. 8. New York: Basic Books.

12. Brigham A. (1973). *Observations on the Influence of Religion upon the Health and Physical Welfare of Mankind* [1835]. New York: Arno Press.

13. Worcester E, McComb S, Coriat IH. (1908). *Religion and Medicine: The Moral Control of Nervous Disorders.* New York: Moffat, Yard and Company.

14. Weatherhead LD. (1951). *Psychology, Religion and Healing.* London: Hodder and Stoughton.

15. Walsh JJ. (1920). *Religion and Health.* Boston: Little, Brown and Company.

16. Holman CT. (1939). *The Religion of a Healthy Mind.* New York: Round Table Press.

17. James W. (1917). *The Varieties of Religious Experience: A Study in Human Nature* [1902]. New York: Longmans, Green.

18. Freud S. (1930). *Civilization and Its Discontents.* New York: Cape and Smith.

19. Jung CG. (1934). *Modern Man in Search of a Soul.* New York: Harcourt, Brace.

20. Fromm E. (1950). *Psychoanalysis and Religion.* New Haven, CT: Yale University Press.

21. Allport GW. (1963). Behavioral science, religion, and mental health. *Journal of Religion and Health* 2:187-197.

22. Maslow AH. (1964). *Religion, Values, and Peak-Experiences.* Columbus: Ohio State University Press.

23. Academy of Religion and Mental Health. (1959). *Religion, Science, and Mental Health: Proceedings of the First Academy Symposium on Inter-Discipline Responsibility for Mental Health—a Religious and Scientific Concern, 1957.* New York: New York University Press.

24. White D. (Editor) (1968). *Dialogue in Medicine and Theology.* Nashville, TN: Abingdon Press.

25. Shriver DW, Jr. (Editor) (1980). *Medicine and Religion: Strategies of Care.* Report #13 of the Institute on Human Values in Medicine. Pittsburgh, PA: University of Pittsburgh Press.

26. Committee on Psychiatry and Religion. (1976). *Mysticism: Spiritual Quest or Psychic Disorder?* Group for the Advancement of Psychiatry Publication No. 97. New York: Group for the Advancement of Psychiatry.

27. Kelsey MT. (1973). *Healing and Christianity in Ancient Thought and Modern Times.* New York: Harper and Row.

28. Kiev A. (Editor) (1964). *Magic, Faith, and Healing.* New York: The Free Press.

29. Belgum D. (Editor) (1967). *Religion and Medicine: Essays on Meaning, Values, and Health.* Ames: Iowa State University Press.

30. Tillich P. (1961). The meaning of health. *Perspectives in Biology and Medicine* 5:92-100.

31. Beit-Hallahmi B. (1974). Psychology of religion 1880-1930: The rise and fall of a psychological movement. *Journal of History of the Behavioral Sciences* 10:84-90.

32. Moberg DO. (1977). Religion and aging. In Ferraro KF (Editor), *Gerontology: Perspectives and Issues* (pp. 179-205). New York: Springer.

33. Fecher VJ. (Compiler) (1982). *Religion and Aging: An Annotated Bibliography*. San Antonio, TX: Trinity University Press.

34. Levin JS, Schiller PL. (1987). Is there a religious factor in health? *Journal of Religion and Health* 26:9-36.

35. Kennaway EL. (1948). The racial and social incidence of cancer of the uterus. *British Journal of Cancer* 2:177-212.

36. Srole L, Langner T. (1962). Religious origin. In Srole L, Langner TS, Michael ST, Opler MK, Rennie TAC, *Mental Health in the Metropolis: The Midtown Manhattan Study* (pp. 300-324). New York: McGraw-Hill.

37. Roberts BH, Myers JK. (1954). Religion, national origin, immigration, and mental illness. *American Journal of Psychiatry* 110:759-764.

38. Summerlin FA. (Compiler) (1980). *Religion and Mental Health: A Bibliography*. DHHS Pub. No. (ADM) 80-964. Washington, DC: U.S. Government Printing Office.

39. Travers B. (1837). Observations on the local diseases termed malignant. *Medical Chirurgical Transactions* 17:337.

40. Billings JS. (1891). Vital statistics of the Jews. *North American Review* 153:70-84.

41. Osler W. (1910). The faith that heals. *British Medical Journal* 1:1470-1472.

42. Paulsen AE. (1926). Religious healing: Preliminary report. *JAMA* 86:1519-1522, 1617-1623, 1692-1697.

43. Vaux K. (1976). Religion and health. *Preventive Medicine* 5:522-536.

44. Vanderpool HY. (1977). Is religion therapeutically significant? *Journal of Religion and Health* 16:255-259.

45. Vanderpool HY. (1980). Religion and medicine: A theoretical overview. *Journal of Religion and Health* 19:7-17.

46. Kaplan BH. (1976). A note on religious beliefs and coronary heart disease. *Journal of the South Carolina Medical Association* 15(5 Suppl.):63.

47. Bergin AE. (1983). Religiosity and mental health: A critical reevaluation and meta-analysis. *Professional Psychology: Research and Practice* 14:170-184.

48. Frank JD. (1975). The faith that heals. *Johns Hopkins Medical Journal* 137:127-131.

49. Gartner J, Larson DB, Allen GD. (1991). Religious commitment and mental health: A review of the empirical literature. *Journal of Psychology and Theology* 19:6-25.

50. Koenig HG. (Compiler) (1995). *Research on Religion and Aging: An Annotated Bibliography*. Westport, CT: Greenwood Press.

51. Jarvis GK, Northcott HC. (1987). Religion and differences in morbidity and mortality. *Social Science and Medicine* 25:813-824.

52. Larson DB, Pattison EM, Blazer DG, Omran AR, Kaplan BH. (1986). Systematic analysis of research on religious variables in four major psychiatric journals, 1978-1982. *American Journal of Psychiatry* 149:329-334.

53. Levin JS, Vanderpool HY. (1987). Is frequent religious attendance *really* conducive to better health?: Toward an epidemiology of religion. *Social Science and Medicine* 24:589-600.

54. Koenig HG, Kvale JN, Ferrel C. (1988). Religion and well-being in later life. *The Gerontologist* 28:18-28.

55. Koenig HG, Moberg DO, Kvale JN. (1988). Religious activities and attitudes of older adults in a geriatric assessment clinic. *Journal of the American Geriatrics Society* 36:362-374.

56. Koenig HG, George LK, Siegler IC. (1988). The use of religion and other emotion-regulating coping strategies among older adults. *The Gerontologist* 28: 303-310.

57. Taylor RJ, Chatters LM. (1986). Church-based informal support among elderly Blacks. *The Gerontologist* 26:637-642.

58. Idler EL. (1987). Religious involvement and the health of the elderly: Some hypotheses and an initial test. *Social Forces* 66:226-238.

59. Ellison CG, Gay DA, Glass TA. (1989). Does religious commitment contribute to individual life satisfaction? *Social Forces* 68:100-123.

60. Williams DR, Larson DB, Buckler RE, Heckmann RC, Pyle CM. (1991). Religion and psychological distress in a community sample. *Social Science and Medicine* 32:1257-1262.

61. Sherrill KA, Larson DB, Greenwold MA. (1993). Is religion taboo in gerontology?: A systematic review of research on religion in three major gerontology journals, 1985-1991. *American Journal of Geriatric Psychiatry* 1:109-117.

62. Weaver AJ, Kline AE, Samford JA, Lucas LA, Larson DB, Gorsuch R. (1998). Is religion taboo in psychology?: A systematic analysis of research on religious variables in seven major American Psychological Association journals: 1991-1994. *Journal of Psychology and Christianity* 17:220-233.

63. Larson DB, Sherrill KA, Lyons JS. (1994). The neglect and misuse of the *R* word: Systematic reviews of religious measures in health, mental health, and aging. In Levin JS (Editor), *Religion in Aging and Health: Theoretical Foundations and Methodological Frontiers* (pp. 178-195). Thousand Oaks, CA: Sage Publications.

64. Sherrill KA, Larson DB. (1994). The anti-tenure factor in religious research in clinical epidemiology and aging. In Levin JS (Editor), *Religion in Aging and Health: Theoretical Foundations and Methodological Frontiers* (pp. 149-177). Thousand Oaks, CA: Sage Publications.

65. Koenig KG, McCullough ME, Larson DB. (2001). *Handbook of Religion and Health*. New York: Oxford University Press.

66. Larson DB, Wilson WP. (1980). Religious life of alcoholics. *Southern Medical Journal* 73:723-727.

67. Cancellaro LA, Larson DB, Wilson WP. (1982). Religious life of narcotic addicts. *Southern Medical Journal* 75:1166-1168.

68. Wilson WP, Larson DB, Meier PD. (1983). Religious life of schizophrenics. *Southern Medical Journal* 76:1096-1100.

69. Bishop LC, Larson DB, Wilson WP. (1987). Religious life of individuals with affective disorders. *Southern Medical Journal* 80:1083-1086.

70. Larson DB, Donahue MJ, Lyons JS, Benson PL, Pattison M, Worthington EL, Blazer DG. (1989). Religious affiliations in mental health research samples as compared with national samples. *Journal of Nervous and Mental Disease* 177:109-111.

71. Larson DB, Sherrill KA, Lyons JS, Craigie FC Jr, Thielman SB, Greenwold MA, Larson SS. (1992). Associations between dimensions of religious commitment and mental health reported in the *American Journal of Psychiatry* and *Archives of General Psychiatry*: 1978-1989. *American Journal of Psychiatry* 149:557-559.

72. Larson DB, Thielman SB, Greenwold MA, Lyons JS, Post SG, Sherrill KA, Wood GG, Larson SS. (1993). Religious content in the DSM-III-R Glossary of Technical Terms. *American Journal of Psychiatry* 150:1884-1885.

73. Larson DB, Hohmann AA, Kessler LG, Meador KG, Boyd JH, McSherry E. (1988). The couch and the cloth: The need for linkage. *Hospital and Community Psychiatry* 39:1064-1069.

74. Larson DB, Koenig HG, Kaplan BH, Greenberg RS, Logue E, Tyroler HA. (1989). The impact of religion on men's blood pressure. *Journal of Religion and Health* 28:265-278.

75. Larson DB, Lyons JS, Hohmann AA, Beardsley RS, Huckeba WM, Rabins PV, Lebowitz BD. (1989). A systematic review of nursing home research in three psychiatric journals: 1966-1985. *International Journal of Geriatric Psychiatry* 4:129-134.

76. Larson DB, Larson SS, Koenig HG. (2002). Mortality and religion/spirituality: A brief review of the research. *Annals of Pharmacotherapy* 36:1090-1098.

77. Larson DB. (1995). Have faith: Religion can heal mental ills. *Insight* (March 6):18-20.

78. Ellis A. (1995). Dogmatic devotion doesn't help, it hurts. *Insight* (March 6):20-22.

79. Levin JS, Larson DB, Puchalski CM. (1997). Religion and spirituality in medicine: Research and education. *JAMA* 278:792-793.

80. Matthews DA, McCullough ME, Larson DB, Koenig HG, Swyers JP, Milano MG. (1998). Religious commitment and health status: A review of the research and implications for family medicine. *Archives of Family Medicine* 7:118-124.

81. Puchalski CM, Larson DB. (1998). Developing curricula in spirituality and medicine. *Academic Medicine* 73:970-974.

82. Larson DB, Lu FG, Swyers JP. (1996). *Model Curriculum for Psychiatry Residency Training Programs: Religion and Spirituality in Clinical Practice— A Course Outline.* Rockville, MD: National Institute for Healthcare Research.

83. Levin J. (2001). *God, Faith, and Health: Exploring the Spirituality-Healing Connection.* New York: John Wiley and Sons.

84. Ellison CG, Levin JS. (1999). The religion-health connection: Evidence, theory, and future directions. *Health Education and Behavior* 25:700-720.

85. Matthew 25:21, 23 (RSV).

Chapter 2

Personal Remembrances

The thirty-one remembrances that follow serve as a collective tribute to Dave Larson. These heartfelt reflections from close friends and professional colleagues provide a glimpse at the widespread impact that Dave's life and work had on others. Some of these comments document Dave's enormous contributions to medicine and science. Others offer a personal take on what Dave, as a human being and as a committed Christian, meant to those who loved and appreciated him.

I have never had the type of friendship like the one I shared with David, one with such a profound connection but so minimal contact. Although we never met, we appreciated each other's work for years.

Back in 1998, I proposed him as a speaker for his leadership role in medicine and faith when I was on an Executive Planning Committee for a symposium at the University of Michigan Medical School. Although he was not invited, we began our e-mail exchanges. David became familiar with my research on the effects of faith on cardiac rehabilitation. He wanted to meet me in Washington, DC, and I promised to contact him if I visited there. From then on, I knew that he was closely watching my work and reading my articles. While I was struggling at the onset of my NIH-funded project, I sensed his support and learned that he had reviewed my grants favorably. In 1999, the Templeton Foundation called and asked me to be a candidate for its Director of Science and Religion position, but I could not leave my faculty position. I learned that Dave was on the search committee.

Finally, David called me in 2001 and we had our first very long conversation as old friends. David was very caring and encouraging. As he appraised my study as exactly the direction he wanted for the field to move toward, he surprised me by his understanding, modesty, and openness. He complimented my article on spirituality and education, and asked how it was that I could do both advanced empirical research and theoretical work. "My multidisciplinary background and collaboration with renowned colleagues," I said.

I shared the high costs I had paid and the tenure risks I had taken. David told me that I was not alone, and offered examples from his own life. At the close of the conversation, he enthusiastically expressed his desire to offer strong support for my future research grants and to develop collegial work. Unfortunately, this conversation was our last one.

Roz informed me of his sudden demise while I was launching my new proposal. She said, "He enjoyed so much working with you!" On March 8, the night before his funeral, David came to me in my dreams and had a discussion with me. On awakening, I was deeply saddened by the tremendous loss of this friend, yet felt privileged to be asked to carry on his unfinished dream with the same spirit of commitment.

Amy L. Ai, PhD
Assistant Professor
University of Washington
Seattle, Washington

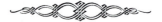

My sadness on the passing of David Larson is mixed with emotions of gratitude that I had the opportunity in a small way to interact with a man of such character and integrity. Despite his international success, he took time for me, a fledgling researcher from a small Canadian university and treated me as a colleague and peer. He helped direct my research, encourage me, and critique my research in his flamboyant manner—making sure to balance the criticism with eternal optimism. He gave me very wise, practical advice that will serve me well throughout my career. Although our relationship was primarily through phone calls and e-mail, he was truly a mentor to me for which I will be forever thankful.

Dave's keen insight into human nature, his awareness of his own shortcomings, his humility, humor, energy, and incredible vivaciousness for life are a legacy for those who had the privilege of knowing him. He was a man at peace with himself, who knew his priorities and ensured that he understood where I was coming from in order to help me with my priorities as well. He instilled a passion for research but made sure it was not at the expense of family.

A few months before his death he sensed I was particularly discouraged when we were discussing the progress of a research piece. I asked if he ever felt there were forces out there not wanting this research to go ahead. It was in the depth of his response that I had a sense of what he had faced to advance the research in this field. Though we still have our own battles to face, Dave has made the way much easier for us. The last e-mail to me the day before his death ended with, "Keep up the good work and continue well." I have lost a mentor but I hope that I, and all involved in this field, may keep up the good work and continue well.

Marilyn Baetz, MD, FRCP(C)
Assistant Professor of Psychiatry
University of Saskatchewan
Saskatoon, Saskatchewan, Canada

I was privileged to be a colleague of David Larson for more than ten years. He was a dedicated advocate of the health benefits of religious practice and beliefs. There is little question that he had an early, major influence on presenting the scientific data to support his theory. In fact, it is difficult to think of a more influential data-based advocate of the importance of religion on improving the prevention and treatment of medical problems.

David will be sorely missed as a spokesperson for this field and for a more inclusive, comprehensive medical practice. Personally I feel as though I have lost a close and valued friend.

Herbert Benson, MD
Harvard University
Boston, Massachusetts

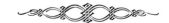

Faith matters! That describes Dave Larson perfectly. Much of this book is devoted to the scientific evidence that he either accumulated or facilitated, evidence that empirically demonstrates that faith matters. I will take a more personal view. I knew Dave for many years, dating back to the days when he was a medical student involved in a rotation with Bill Wilson at Duke. Dave was a true believer and such belief is axiomatic for someone who wishes to demonstrate that faith matters. Perhaps the reader doesn't agree with this proposition. Perhaps the study of the value of faith in facilitating health and mental health is best undertaken by someone truly neutral, truly objective. I beg to differ. Dave Larson is the reason I believe faith matters in the study of faith and health.

Dave came to the study of faith and health with the intuitive understanding of faith that only a true believer can possess. His personal faith shaped his questions. Questions of faith and health must in part be shaped by persons who believe as well as persons who are skeptical. Science always begins with theories based in belief and intuition, theories later translated into testable hypotheses. A science without belief is a sterile and boring science.

Yet Dave exhibited another quality that is essential to the scientific inquiry of the relationship between faith and health. His personal faith provided him with the confidence to incorporate the scientific method and accept the results regardless of the nature of the results. He was an honest yet persistent scientist, a true believer in the scientific method as well as his faith tradition. Dave never pushed aside findings that apparently contradicted his hypotheses, but rather pursued these findings. He was confident that the inevitable successive approximations necessary to approach truth would lead us toward a greater understanding of truth. Time properly devoted to the investigation, in time, would lead to the pathways and mechanisms by which faith supports health.

Dave was a true believer in yet another sense. His confidence, optimism, and genuine love of his colleagues and friends pushed those colleagues and friends to explore questions they otherwise would not have explored. Dave believed in the ideas of others even when those others at time did not believe in themselves. In this way he was perhaps the ideal ambassador for the maturing science of faith and health. We will miss him sorely, yet he worked so hard and so successfully during his short time on this earth that he has bequeathed us a mature, not an infant, field of study. If we fail to carry forth his work, we have only ourselves to blame.

Dan G. Blazer, MD, PhD
J. P. Gibbons Professor of Psychiatry and Behavioral Sciences
Duke University Medical Center
Durham, North Carolina

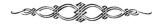

David Larson, MD, MSPH, had developed a very strong following at the University of North Florida at Jacksonville. He gave talks there on spirituality and health during the fall of 2000 and the spring of 2002, slightly before his untimely death. His candor and his humor contributed to his creditability. His interactive style of presenting and on occasion vigorously defending his research were hallmarks of his character.

Dr. Larson was truly a man of innocence, humility, and scientific accomplishment. He was a courageous pioneer investigator; he opened many eyes, hearts, and minds. He contributed to the maturation of a new science and his place in the annals of spirituality and health is assured.

His presence has made the world a better place.

J. Brooks Brown, MD, DHL
Chairman
Brooks Health System
Jacksonville, Florida

I had the pleasure of meeting and spending an afternoon with Dave Larson in early 2002. We were both quite familiar with each others' work, and it was an opportunity for us to get to know each other personally. I was extremely impressed with his dedication to improving health care for everyone and to looking at the complete person. Many scientists have a tendency to want to leave out the spiritual aspects of the human being, and I think this is done to their great detriment. Dave, on the other hand, felt that this is perhaps the most important aspect of the human being and thought that we should consider ourselves in the medical profession as healers of the entire person rather than only one small aspect of one's existence.

Dave Larson proves that a person can be both a scientist and a complete humanitarian with a deep and abiding love for God and for all of mankind. His life will be an example forever and I am sure will continue to touch people throughout the coming centuries. I feel very privileged to have made his acquaintance.

Benjamin S. Carson Sr., MD
Director of Pediatric Neurosurgery
Professor of Neurological Surgery,
Oncology, Plastic Surgery, and Pediatrics
Johns Hopkins University School of Medicine
Baltimore, Maryland

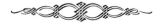

Today, throughout the medical research sciences and social sciences, critical masses of scholars and practitioners are taking religion and spirituality seriously. Very seriously.

It was not thus as little as two decades ago. Indeed, it was not thus as little as nine or ten years ago. But now hardly anybody denies that faith, variously measured, is an important variable in explaining and predicting wide range of vital physical health, mental health, and social welfare outcomes.

What changed?

Call it the "Larson factor."

David B. Larson, MD, MSPH, was *the* pioneering research scholar who put religion back on the intellectual map. Dave did it first in one of the toughest places—medicine. He did it later with Byron Johnson and others in other hard-nut-to-crack fields including criminology.

Dave conquered medical schools and the academy, the media and the foundations, and, finally, the policy and civic worlds. He did it all by the sheer force of the accumulated empirical evidence. He let the data do most of the talking in papers and in speeches and at conferences and in the mass media, but he had an uncanny, irreplaceable ability to communicate hard evidence with a warm smile and a funny joke. He always came across in ways that impressed his fellow researchers and entertained all his listeners and interlocutors.

The Lord took Dave back to Himself on March 5, 2002, but Dave is still with all who knew him—knew and loved, for to know this great and good man was to love him. He helped inspire all I have done of any worth in these fields.

And, let the record show, the Larson factor is still hard at work—*everywhere!*

The Larson factor is in scientific research agendas that put religion front and center.

The Larson factor is in public policy debates that no longer leave faith at the civic altar.

The Larson factor is evident in improved spirituality and religion foundation giving patterns.

The Larson factor is alive in increased media attention.

Everywhere.

Even after we had known each other for years and had become friends, even after I had tried to recruit him and his NIHR crew to join me at Penn, Dave would often end one of our long, rambling phone conversations by saying, "Oh, oh, John DiIulio, I just can't believe we are working to do these things together. We're so blessed! I, oh, oh, I just feel so blessed to know you."

Well, as I told Dave the last time we talked, it was I, not him, who was honored, and blessed, and humbled, and in awe to know and work with him.

What President Richard Nixon said of Lord Keynes can now be said of Dave Larson: "We are all Larsonians now." "Oh, oh," I say, "Dave Larson!" Sterling scientist. Mentor to so many. Godly family man. Dedicated friend.

Praise God for Dave. Long live the Larson factor.

John J. DiIulio Jr.
Frederic Fox Leadership Professor
of Politics, Religion, and Civil Society
University of Pennsylvania
Philadelphia, Pennsylvania

and Senior Fellow
The Brookings Institution
Washington, DC
and Former Director
White House Office of Faith-Based and Community Initiatives
Washington, DC

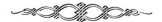

Faith matters. The lay public intuitively accepts the truth of this statement, but few scholars have dared to explore its implications. David Larson was one of the few who did, applying himself to examining the impact of spirituality on well-being, and welcoming the raised eyebrows his work elicited. And it did raise eyebrows. Scientists, particularly in the mental health arena, have long been uncomfortable with questions regarding faith.

Although I received excellent training in my early career, at no time did spirituality come up as a serious topic of discussion. The same exclusion was evident when I moved into the policy arena, in which faith was rarely part of the discussion on health care, mental health, or other vital issues. When it was mentioned, it was often in derogatory terms, as if spirituality were a deterrent to wellness. The consistent message seemed to be that this was a personal issue, not suitable for scientific evaluation or reasoned policy consideration. I tacitly accepted that view, although my years practicing in community mental health and my own experiences contradicted it.

Dave recognized the fallacy of the current orthodoxy. By modeling a scholarly approach to the issue he provided grounding for an intelligent discussion of the relevance of faith. However, although recognizing that his work had policy implications, he astutely avoided becoming a mouthpiece for a political cause. He cared about the issue because he cared about people, not because he had a religious or political agenda to promote. For that reason, his boldness in embracing the positive aspects of faith was tempered by an open discussion of the negative side of religiosity.

Since my own work has placed me at the intersection of practice, research, and policy, I found in Dave a kindred spirit. Because he exalted in being in the middle of the intersection, he never failed to spur me on as well, encouraging me to remain in the intersection when my instincts yearned to move me to the side of the road. His life and career served as examples of how to integrate personal values and professional activities. His voice will be sorely missed, but his place at the crossroads now has more, and better-informed, occupants because of him.

Daniel Dodgen, PhD
Public Policy Office
American Psychological Association
Washington, DC

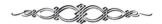

It was a crisp and cold but sunny winter day in Chicago. My hopes were high as I drove to O'Hare to pick up Dave Larson. He was in town for a few hours to give a lecture on religion and health research. Dave's reputation and important contributions to the field were well known to me. For the past few years, in collaboration with experienced investigators at the Medical Center, I had developed a small program of religion and health research. I was eager to meet Dave, to tell him about our research program, and make a good impression.

His plane was on time and we had no problems finding each other in the terminal, but the ride back to the Medical Center wasn't what I had expected. Dave seemed preoccupied. Rather than talking, his attention was focused on his notes for the lecture. It did not make sense. I was sure he had given this lecture dozens of times. I tried not to take his behavior personally.

At the Medical Center, Dave's lecture went well. There was a good turnout. Dave's presentation was animated and informative. He summarized a lot of important research and was appropriate in his claims for its significance. His humor helped people feel more relaxed and there were good exchanges during the discussion time.

After the lecture Dave joined me and my research colleagues for dinner. After introductions, we began to talk about our research—studies of the religious needs and resources of psychiatric inpatients, of spiritual well-being and quality of life in cancer patients, and of the role of religion in medical rehabilitation patients' recovery. Dave became very interested and engaged in the conversation, asking questions about our projects and sharing information about related work and the investigators conducting it. It was hard to interrupt the excitement and energy around the table to get him to O'Hare for his flight home. The drive back to the airport was very different from the earlier trip. Dave expressed encouragement for our research, offered suggestions for our program, and expressed his wish to stay in touch.

Several months later, a friend told me he had been to one of Dave's lectures. Did I know, the friend asked, that Larson referred to our study of psychiatric patients in several slides? I had not heard, but was delighted. In the following years, Dave continued to be interested in and enthusiastic about our research. I am very grateful for his friendship and encouragement and, like many others, will miss him.

George Fitchett, DMin
Associate Professor and Director of Research
Department of Religion, Health, and Human Values
Rush-Presbyterian-St. Luke's Medical Center
Chicago, Illinois

David Larson's last e-mail to me is still in my e-mail inbox. I scroll past his name every day. The brief message from him is some encouragement to me in an effort he was organizing to bring honor and recognition to a colleague. He had asked me to help him, and I was glad to do it. I frankly don't even know if the effort was ever successful— but the simple taking of the initiative speaks volumes about who Dave was.

In the first place, the effort was on behalf of someone else. Dave was a master at directing the spotlight away from himself and toward others. I was one of the (many) others. But without Dave there wouldn't have been a spotlight to shine. Dave was a first-class networker, but his networking was all about putting the members of his network in touch with one another. He loved seeing what happened when he did that. Dave was unstintingly unselfish with his time, extraordinarily thoughtful and considerate, and the best encourager I have ever met.

The second reason this little note tells a lot about Dave is that the effort had an uncertain outcome, but of course that didn't stop Dave. If anyone had told me in 1985, when I was working on my dissertation on religion and health, that there would one day be national conferences on the subject, I would have thought it preposterous. It *was* preposterous, but that apparently didn't occur to Dave or keep him from trying. Today, as I fly around the country lecturing on religion and health at medical schools, universities, and to the general public, I often think, "Dave did this." And he did.

Ellen Idler, PhD
Institute for Health, Health Care Policy, and Aging Research
Rutgers, The State University of New Jersey
New Brunswick, New Jersey

I was introduced to Dave Larson in 1993, by a mutual friend, Professor Walter Bradley, who happened to be conducting research in Washington, DC, while on sabbatical. Walter had known me for several years because we were affiliated with various Christian organizations that worked with academics. Having heard of Dave Larson's research linking religion and spirituality to health, he decided to look up Dave while in town. Unbeknownst to me, Walter had mentioned my name to Dave and, to my surprise, he was anxious to meet me. Walter then called me and told me that I had to meet this guy named David Larson. The meeting took place over dinner at the Larson's home in Rockville, Maryland. After dinner Dave wanted to show me his office and library in the basement of his house. I remember being astonished that someone would have in his home gargantuan commercial lateral file cabinets with revolving shelves. The cabinets were completely packed with thousands upon thousands of journal articles, systematically filed, and with multiple copies of each of the articles (not that Dave ever obsessed about things). I was fascinated with how much he had published, how passionate he was about research, and why he was interested in collaborating with a junior researcher like me. Little did I know that Dave Larson would become one of the most influential individuals in my life.

I was flattered by Dave's offer to collaborate with him on a research project. I soon discovered that part of Dave's vision was to mentor young academics in the art of getting research published. This is because Dave believed that published research was the most effective and appropriate way to influence public policy. It didn't take long for Dave to introduce me to Sir John Templeton, and then for Sir John to introduce me to my first major research grant. That was just the beginning. Dave began to teach me the skills that had helped him become such a prolific author in such a short time—he didn't really begin publishing until he was in his mid-thirties. Dave's tips on writing style, organizational layout, and detail were superb. He had a real knack for understanding what reviewers really wanted to see in a revised manuscript—and why. One of my fondest lessons learned from Dave was to understand the appropriate time to call a journal editor and the right argument to make when contesting an FLR (funny-looking review) or convincing an editor why he or she should overturn a negative publication decision.

Dave and I completed several grants together and published a number of papers over the past decade. We completed studies of at-risk youth and documented that religious commitment is a significant protective factor associated with reducing delinquency and improving pro-social or beneficial outcomes. We also examined the role of religion in rehabilitating adult offenders and subsequently found that religiosity helped reduce the recidivism rates of former prisoners. It is not an exaggeration to suggest that these published studies have had the effect of bringing religion and spirituality into the mainstream of American criminology and beyond. We can all be thankful that Dave's mentoring influence has been felt far and wide, as he has mentored young scholars in many disciplines, and we have hundreds of published studies to prove it.

I once heard someone say, "Don't spend your life—invest it." Dave's life was a living expression of this admonition. Thank you, Dave, for investing in me—and the many other young academics along the way. Thanks for helping us understand that producing scholarship is a calling well worth answering, and that it really is possible to change the world through research. I thank God for the legacy of David B. Larson, and the reward of seeing why it is so important not to spend my life, but to invest it.

Byron R. Johnson, PhD
Professor of Sociology and Director
Center for Religious Inquiry Across the Disciplines
Baylor University
Waco, Texas

and Fellow, The Witherspoon Institute
Princeton, New Jersey

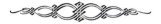

I had the privilege of advising David on his master's program and master's thesis in epidemiology. If I taught him as much as he taught me, we were even.

My first meeting with David revealed a great deal about David's future career. His bright energy and ebullient spirit were obvious. He expressed an earnest wish to link psychiatry to epidemiology. He expressed anxiety about the acceptability of his interest in religion and health. I assured him that his interests fit a very old and classic scholarly set of questions. At the end of our chat, I handed him my psychosocial codebook for the Evans County Heart Study. I ensured his access to my questions on religion. David developed his master's thesis from this discussion. He left my office relieved.

I left this conversation and other subsequent encounters thinking of David as an example of Wallace Stevens' idea of "the man with the blue guitar." I quote the verse that captures David's spirit:

> They said, "You have a blue guitar.
> You do not play things as they are."
> The man replied, "Things as they are
> Are changed upon the blue guitar."[1]

David played his own tune with a creative and affirmative affect on all he met. It is a joy to have had such a friend and colleague.

I will focus my brief comments on ideas from my last face-to-face conversations with David at a meeting he had organized on religion and health in Leesburg, Virginia, financed by the Templeton Foundation. My remarks were in the service of the larger challenges in studying religion and health. David was very open to these topics.

I will focus on one politically incorrect theme: the dark side of religion. In fact, I told David many times that his interests in religion and health were on target, a classic topic. I argued for equal attention to the study of the dark side of religion, an out-of-favor topic. Several examples will suffice:

William James put forth the concepts of the religious sentiments that encourage the religion of the healthy soul and, in contrast, the religion of the sick soul. The sick soul: "Such anguish may partake of various characters, having something more than the quality of loathing; sometimes that of irritation and exasperation; or again of self-mistrust and self-despair; or of suspicion, anxiety, trepidation, fear." Healthy-mindedness (or the healthy soul) is "the tendency which looks on all things and sees that they are good. . . ."[2]

More recently, Martin Marty puts forth a series of ten propositions for the most fruitful academic study of religion. His first two propositions fit James's thesis:

> "Religion motivates most killing in the world today."
> "Religion contributes to the most healing in the world today."[3]

Marty writes that less data were available on the second than the first proposition.

For a current historical account, Bernard Lewis's recent work, *What Went Wrong?*,[4] presents a careful examination of culture wars with religious origins. For a longer sense of history, Susan Jacoby's *Wild Justice*[5] argues that certain forms of Christian anti-Semitism formed the basis for the oldest revenge story in history. She documents the "curse" on the Jews as Christ-killers as revenge history. Finally, a more recent and more complete account of religiously sanctioned anti-Semitism and the Holocaust are James Carroll's *Constantine's Sword*[6] and Peter Gomes's chapter, "The Bible and Anti-Semitism: Christianity's Original Sin," in his *The Good Book*.[7]

Morris Cohen, one of the giants of twentieth-century philosophy, reminds us that the study of dark side of religion is a well-established theme in historical and philosophical literature. Cohen[8] details these dark sides or destructive aspects of religious history:

> (1) superstitions, demonic possession, and opposition to science; (2) historical crusades of war and hatred sanctioned by religion; (3) the "sacrifice" of heretics (e.g., during the Inquisition); (4) absolute claims that other faiths are heresy, in error, or "outside," as well as religious wars and justification of slavery; (5) the church normally siding with the powerful; and (6) inflicted spiritual agonies and terrors.

Cohen does not exclude the positive side of religion, but argues we cannot ignore the destructive in religion.

I never felt David rejected other questions about religion and health. His interests focused on the vital question of the contribution of religion to healing and health promotion. His contributions will endure in his written work and through those he stimulated.

I will end on one of the most generic questions about religion and adaptation. In Boris Pasternak's epic novel, *Doctor Zhivago,* the reader will find this much larger challenge to the understanding of religion and adaptation:

> Now what is history? It is the centuries of systematic explorations of the riddle of death, with a view of overcoming death. That is why people discover mathematical infinity and electromagnetic waves, that's why they write symphonies. Now you can't advance in this direction without a certain faith.[9]

Berton H. Kaplan, PhD
Professor Emeritus
Department of Epidemiology
School of Public Health
University of North Carolina
Chapel Hill, North Carolina

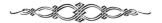

I first met David when I was asked to be a part of a conference that the Carrier Foundation sponsored in 1996. He was the keynote speaker for the conference. As we were driven back from Princeton to the Newark airport in a stretch limo, I had the good fortune of sitting next to him. When I shared with him that I had been diagnosed with ADD as an adult, we made an instant connection, for he resonated with the behaviors I described to him. I remember thinking after that trip that I had met a totally genuine, engaging, humorous, dedicated, intelligent person with enormous energy.

After that brief encounter, I was honored and surprised when he invited me to be a part of the conferences which produced *Scientific Research on Spirituality and Health: A Consensus Report,* a summary of the current state of research on health and spirituality based on a series of three conferences sponsored by the Templeton Foundation. For me, the conferences and the associations it led to were a turning point professionally.

I don't think that was untypical of him, for David had a way of meeting people, engaging with them, and then finding ways to foster their careers. And he did so in such a simple, selfless way.

Many others will no doubt comment on his intelligence, his vision, his courage, his dedication, his faith, but for me all of that is summed up in his ability to attend to each person with *presence*. And I must add that I cannot think of David without having Susan come to mind, for it seems whenever I saw him or think of him, I think of him in relation to her. It was a gift to know him.

Nancy Kehoe, RSCJ, PhD
Instructor in Psychology
Harvard Medical School
Cambridge, Massachusetts

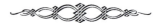

I remember the first time I spoke with David Larson. He called me on the telephone to congratulate *me* on the work I was doing. I had published two articles on the faith healing views of patients and physicians. David had published nearly 100 articles and reviews at that point. I couldn't get over the fact that he was calling me. His humility and enthusiasm were very evident from our first conversation. We spoke for a few minutes, then near the end of our conversation, he offered to pray for me. Our faiths were similar, and we had briefly discussed our religious backgrounds during our conversation. So I readily agreed to pray over the phone with David.

Later, as I reflected on our brief but memorable conversation, I realized that I had never prayed on the telephone with anyone before. I am a devout Christian, baptized at the age of seven, and have been involved in church life continuously since that time. Yet, it took a spirituality and health researcher to be the one to break down the barriers of societal expectations and pray over the telephone with me. I wonder whether it is the result of petitions and thanks that were offered to God that day that have been part of the reason for my continued interest and opportunities in the field of spirituality and health research since then. I am certainly grateful for the encouragement that David gave to me throughout my research career, and I will cherish the fond memories I have of him.

Dana E. King, MD
Associate Professor
Department of Family Medicine
Medical University of South Carolina
Charleston, South Carolina

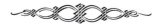

David B. Larson was a special person—eccentric, transparent, kind, insightful, and unique among all the people I have ever met. Of course, I was first drawn to David by his name, and that of his wife, Susan, which is also my sister's name. I had read a number of their writings in popular Christian magazines and appreciated his message of faith, prayer, healing, and the value of family. So when I heard that Dave would be speaking at an event sponsored by Christian Medical Association, I had to meet my namesake!

From that first exchange, it was obvious that we were on the same "wavelength"—like two old friends who hadn't seen each other for years. That was 1990 and the beginning of a long, close relationship that saw Dave leave his employment with the government and start NIHR. This was a very large step of faith for Dave and his family, but he felt that God was leading him down this path. I well remember the afternoon that Dave, Susan, and their daughter, Kristen, visited us in Wisconsin and he asked me to be the Chairman of the Board of this fledgling organization. At that point, I had no idea what paths our relationship would take, but one thing I would soon learn is that dealing with Dave is anything but predictable! His eating habits, exercise patterns, and our praying for each other while on the phone were all part of the David B. Larson persona that I came to love and appreciate.

As NIHR found its footing and began to make an impact on the secular world with which we are all so familiar, I found myself drawn to the message of faith, health, and family, but considered ways in which this could be applied in the world of the surgeon. Through encouragement (and a lot of coaching) by Dave, I was able to make numerous presentations to both national and regional surgical organi-

zations about the value of balance and faith in a surgeon's professional, personal, and family life. This message was, of course, one of
the major tenets of Dave's many contributions. I know that this "balance" concept was new and unique to many in the surgical world and
I believe that God equipped me through Dave to get this message to
my audience.

I loved David B. Larson as a brother and will always remember
him and his contribution to the specialty of plastic surgery.

David L. Larson, MD
Professor and Chairman
Department of Plastic Surgery
Medical College of Wisconsin
Milwaukee, Wisconsin

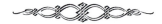

I first met Dave in January 1987, when I attended a NIMH workshop for young investigators in Rockville, Maryland. The night before the workshop it snowed tremendously, the roads were deserted,
yet Dave was there with his uncanny enthusiasm that amazed all who
attended. That same energy and enthusiasm was truly inspirational to
all who met Dave over the years, even if briefly.

We worked on several projects together through the National Institute for Healthcare Research that have transformed psychiatric education. One was a monograph titled, "A Model Curriculum for Psychiatry Residency Training Programs: Religion and Spirituality in
Clinical Practice," published in 1996. The accreditation standards
had just changed to include religion/spirituality among the didactic
topics to be taught. This monograph, with contributions from prominent psychiatric educators, was a landmark event. Subsequently, Dave
was able to start the Templeton Curriculum Awards for Psychiatry
Residency Programs to encourage the actual implementation of the
model. Twenty programs over the years have won an award. The programs have presented at the annual meetings of American Association of the Directors of Psychiatry Residency Training and the
American Psychiatric Association. Dave and I were part of those presentations. We also worked on organizing in 1997 the first conference
on teaching about these issues at Georgetown's Conference Center.

Both the Curricular Awards and the Teaching Conferences have continued under the able hands of Christina Puchalski, MD, at the George Washington Institute for Spirituality and Health (GWISH). She and Dave had worked together at NIHR before she started GWISH.

My last meeting with Dave was in late November 2001, when he accepted my invitation to come to UCSF to present Grand Rounds in the Department of Psychiatry. In one hour, he gave his usual *tour de force* presentation that masterfully summarized the key research in the field with that same gee-whiz enthusiasm and inspiration that I had seen in 1987. The next evening, he was at San Francisco General Hospital, my workplace for twenty-five years, giving a two-hour lecture with that same inspiration.

Finally, in May 2002, the American Psychiatric Association Committee on Religion and Psychiatry honored Dave posthumously with the Oskar Pfister Award for his contributions to the field. Susan, his wife, accepted the award at the APA Annual Meeting. Dave's spirit was there in all our memories of his love, devotion, enthusiasm, inspiration, and faith.

Francis G. Lu, MD
Professor of Clinical Psychiatry
Department of Psychiatry
University of California, San Francisco
San Francisco General Hospital
San Francisco, California

Thrown accidentally as I was into the world of health, faith, and ethics, when asked to co-found the Park Ridge Center, I not only had to catch up. I had to start from scratch. As a historian of religion I must have considered every topic under the sun as potentially approachable, so long as it had a past, the past being the only specialty historians have.

To my surprise, twenty years ago almost everyone who mattered also seemed to be starting from scratch. For all the discoveries in technical medicine, for all the refinements in philosophical ethics, for all the complexities in the delivery of care, something was being slighted. As I scanned the bibliographies and read desperately, it became clear to me that the patient was the partially overlooked figure in it all. This did not mean that researchers, physicians, nurses, and ethicists were inhumane; from the first, many of them impressed me with their generosity of vision and concern for most dimensions of patient life. But they, we, were not schooled to listen well to what was most deeply rooted in their experience, most anchored in their hearts, most ready to serve as a resource, a repository of options. Those three "mosts" signaled what we call spirituality, religion, faith.

After the first few years we wanted to see some certification that these things mattered in the world of science. Philosopher Michael Oakeshott reminds us that the differentia for the scientists is "measurement" just as for the historian it is "the past" (or for the poet, "the imagination"). Who was taking the measure of what could be measured in the places where faith, religion, and spirituality met in the patients' world? Three or four names rose to the top. We heard of the work of that then-"young" (and in my view, even after we have lost him, still young in spirit) David B. Larson. He was writing articles on how other articles overlooked religion and began asking why the neglect. I read everything I could find by him. He found plenty of barriers to his work, and would have been in a good situation to gripe.

One of the few absolutes at the Park Ridge Center can be summarized in a few commandments: No whining. No moaning. Don't just gripe; do something. David Larson was always doing something, mixing as he did scientific analysis related to measurement with humanistic, and in its own way, theological extrapolations, in language that people could pick up across the disciplines. David was the pioneer, was preeminent in that field, but he was also a collaborator, which is why his work will be carried on in his spirit. Most of the work has not yet been done. Newcomers in the Larson tradition can have the thrill of knowing how much is "out there" to discover.

Eventually, after much reading and correspondence, after times when I got to edit and publish him, we met. At sundry meetings the accident of alphabet set the man with the "L" next to this man with the "M." He always worked at full intensity. He had the gift (they tell me I have it too) of being able to listen to all the conference proceedings and still scribble outlines for future work. This he did in his famed microscopic script; his literary heirs will be deciphering for years.

We commiserated ("no whining") and joked about diagnosis of our malady or benison: ADHD? I don't know whether he ever had a formal diagnosis of his driveness; I know I didn't. I know that at prep school my nickname was "Kein Sitzfleisch," or at least that was the appellation in the yearbook: no "fat" to sit on, meaning no ability to sit still and endure. But whatever was there, David and I also knew how to "sit" at desk, and computer, or wherever else, as his astonishing publishing achievement bears out.

Every meeting with David Larson was a learning experience. He conversed and laughed and lectured and taught and inquired with intensity. So much energy got infused into his endeavors that I picture it still charging up his co-workers, his family, and others who mourn him, his associates and successors, and those who only can come to know him through his writings and the fellowship which will carry on the work.

In the world I come from and happily inhabit we say *Deo Gratias,* thanks be to God, and *Requiescat in Pace,* rest in peace, that is, if you can picture David, a man in so many ways at peace, ever stopping to rest.

Martin E. Marty, PhD
Fairfax M. Cone Distinguished Service Professor Emeritus
University of Chicago
Chicago, Illinois
and George B. Caldwell Senior Scholar in Residence
Park Ridge Center for the Study of Health, Faith and Ethics
Chicago, Illinois

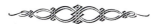

The National Institute for Healthcare Research, where I worked with Dave for four years, was located at 6110 Executive Boulevard in Rockville, Maryland. The 6110 building is an ordinary-looking, ten-story corporate office building—business parks all over the United States are teeming with them. Dave's ninth-floor office, in the northwest corner, had big, broad windows on its north and east walls.

Dave filled his days with activity. While the sun shone, he labored. So he and I typically found our time to talk in the evenings, when most everyone else had gone home. For those evening chats, Dave preferred to take a chair that allowed him to look through the northern window of his office. From his northern view, Dave could watch the sky grow darker as the sun fell below the horizon. As our conversations went on, and the sky grew mellow and beautiful, Dave would, from time to time, pause, sigh, and declare: "Isn't *that* a beautiful sight!" He would relax, become contemplative. Dave loved to watch the sunset, as does everyone, but I think this daily cosmic phenomenon was especially important to him. He seemed changed by it, or it marked a daily change in him. It not only was a cue for noting the passage of calendar time, but also an evening call to give thanks. Each day, at the end of the day, Dave's characteristic vigor and zest for what he wanted to accomplish took a backseat to his humility and profound gratitude for what he had been given.

With the passage of a few years since the last of our evening conversations, I have come to realize that they were actually the pretext for a short thanksgiving celebration. As our talk of work—were we not supposedly discussing work?—progressed, the conversation became increasingly punctuated by Dave's testimonials of thankfulness for all he had. He had two wonderful children and a wife who brought love, beauty, and meaning to his world. He had colleagues who energized and challenged him. He made a living doing what he enjoyed. Despite some persistent health problems, he was generally healthy. So with the sky nearly dark, the concerns of the day receded until all that was left was gratitude.

Even in the light of day, of course, Dave overflowed with thankfulness. He thanked everyone. He thanked his employees for merely showing up to work. He expressed gratitude to his collaborators for providing him with opportunities to make a difference. Indeed, many people can attest to the fact that it was difficult to end a conversation with Dave without being thanked for something. But with the setting sun, Dave's gratitude became more profound, more focused. At those times, I realized that Dave's gratitude was a serious and spiritual business.

Dave once told me that he felt as though he had been a beggar his entire career. This statement shocked me profoundly. Now, many sunsets later, I think I understand what he meant. Most of us take for granted the sun's own warmth until it leaves us at dusk, just as we take for granted the benevolence of friends, colleagues, employees, strangers, our families, and those who have come before us. Dave seemed determined not to take these things for granted. He could name a thousand people to whom he felt indebted. Unlike many of us, who waste our energy trying to liberate our self-images from the countless acts of love that have made us who we are—trying to signify to ourselves and the world that we are "self-made" men and women—Dave cherished his bonds of indebtedness because, collectively, they were a big part of his life story.

Neither did he view his life and work as an investment in the future, although it was. Rather, David Bruce Larson lived his life as a joyous, creative, lifelong exercise of acknowledging innumerable, inestimable debts that could not really be paid back anyway.

Michael E. McCullough, PhD
Associate Professor of Psychology and of Religious Studies
University of Miami
Coral Gables, Florida

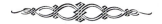

Dave liked to joke that his patron saint was Lt. Columbo of the Los Angeles Police Department because that typified his approach to research. He would always understate findings, and almost apologize for finding positive relationships between health and spirituality. He knew that he was often working in hostile waters, and went to great lengths to introduce his findings and move the field forward while arousing as little ire and resistance as possible.

Nowhere was this more apparent than in his speeches and presentations. Dave loved to pepper his talks with slides of his favorite cartoons. He would always say that if he could get people to laugh, he could "hook them" on the research. He was right. People loved to listen to him speak, and this funny, sometimes irreverent, researcher who just happened to find these crazy results linking spirituality to positive health outcomes, disarmed many resistant audience members.

But don't mistake his apologetic approach for a timid spirit. Dave was far from that. He was tenacious, determined, and relentless. He never gave up, never took no for an answer, and yet still managed to be a nice guy. He built up a large group of researchers and colleagues whom he mentored and counseled. More publications in this area ensued because Dave took the time personally to encourage and assist even fledgling researchers. He was determined to make a difference in the field of health and spirituality, and his legacy will continue because he took the time to invest in those around him.

Despite all of his successes and professional honors, Dave never lost his heart for people. Most people who had achieved the level of success he enjoyed had to do so at a great price—usually a personal one. Somehow, Dave managed to amass nearly 300 professional publications, crisscross the nation on speaking engagements, and mentor countless young researchers without suffering the loss of his personal life.

His wife, Susan, was a frequent collaborator with Dave, helping him in his writing projects and helping to "structure him," as he often put it. His children adored him, and he went to great lengths to make sure he got to spend time with them. We joked with his son, Chad, that Dave's travel and meeting schedule had to be worked around Chad's football schedule because Dave refused to miss a game. Dave put people first in his life and valued relationships. Perhaps he was so successful because he knew what really needed to come first.

Mary Greenwold Milano
Staff Writer
International Center for the Integration
of Health and Spirituality
Rockville, Maryland

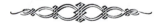

He was not just a colleague. He was a friend. Mentor. Example. Inspiration. This book is full of his professional accolades, but the greatest contribution he made to my life is so personal, it's a very difficult story to tell without confusing the issues. Yet it must be told, because from the telling comes the certainty that the gifts we give to others live on and on, long after we are gone.

I met Dr. David B. Larson in December 1998, when attending my first "Spirituality and Healing" conference at Harvard. In early 1998, I was an academic medical oncologist, deeply rooted in basic science and clinical research. By December, my existence had been irreversibly altered by having been a victim of complete violation, and the subsequent fight for survival. I knew that triumph over "victimhood" could only be accomplished by learning to lead others down the path of true healing I forged for myself. Though I can barely remember that year, changing career directions was my first step toward a future of hope and promise and true healing for others who face crisis.

Dave was the keynote speaker that year, animated and engaging the audience in a way that drove his points into our brains. (Later I would learn that his charismatic public speaking persona was one of the gifts he was most proud of.) Because verbal shyness has never been among my shortcomings, tracking him down during the break I introduced myself and essentially forced him to agree to help me make a break into the field of health and spirituality. But as easygoing as he seemed that day, Dave was not a pushover. I had to prove myself and pass his "critical eye" as any other person or scientific study had to do before gaining his approval and support.

During the following years, he helped Fusion Health Foundation become reality, first becoming a member of the Advisory Panel, then also teaming up to form an executive speaking team. As time went on, we both came to realize that we had to combine our different strengths and focuses in order to make inroads into traditional medical care. Medicine has changed. Those responsible for making the decisions about new programs have a different agenda than those doing the patient care. As all of us who are trying to address the issues of the importance of the spirit to health have learned, progress is slow and painstakingly difficult. To be an effective agent of change, we must understand how to get the attention of those who actually make the decisions. We were just beginning to get a handle on how to do this well when Dave died.

Selfishly, I must admit to feeling more than just grief. I wonder, how will all the progress we were beginning to make at Fusion Health continue on? Whereas there was once an aura of invulnerability to my gifts, courage, and vision, that illusion was shattered by proof of how vulnerable I truly was. That's when I learned the truth about my own human limits—as our bodies can die, so too can our spirits be mortally wounded. Dave's support helped strengthen my spirit again. Like everyone else, I, too, must learn to carry on without having him to turn to.

Physical healing is currently much easier than spiritual healing. Health care professionals know what can be done for the body, but have no clue how to attend the spirit—so they just don't do it. It's not because they don't want to, but because it's nearly impossible to learn or teach something that can't be defined and visualized. Leaning on Dave for support and feedback, we at Fusion Health developed a visual model to address this issue. In my estimation, lack of something visual/concrete which people can grasp and understand was the major roadblock to progress in this field. Eventually Dave agreed—though he constantly reminded me that any "model" had to be fluid enough to accommodate progress and change. I've never forgotten that.

Not turning back to the security of clinical oncology was difficult during the inevitable hard knocks one faces in trying to create a passage through uncharted territory. Dave kept me going during the darkest moments. As all healers know, belief in oneself is one of the hardest things to regain after being the victim of violation, but it is because of Dave's unshakable trust and belief in me that I was able to regain the confidence and courage to persevere. I'll never forget the intensely personal conversation we had one particularly difficult month. I asked him if he thought I was sane. He listened to my story, told his own, then said, "I believe in you, and I'm a great judge of character and ability." That was enough for me.

During that conversation, I asked him what drove him to choose this field professionally, and why he truly believed in God. He said, "By all rights, I shouldn't be here. The fact that I am alive and in this position is a true miracle not directly attributable to me." He went on to explain, but I already understood, for neither should I have survived what happened to me. His answer proved he was driven by deep inner truth, not the desire for notoriety that commands so many academic physicians. Dave knew he was in some way destined to use his gifts and talents to forge a new path for others to follow and take forward. He honored his inner truth above all, and for that reason could help others do the same. What greater difference can any of us hope to make?

It was after that conversation that we completed the model. Starting with a "whole" person, components of body, mind, and spirit were separated, with methods to address each fragment listed, ending with the pathway required to bring it all back together. Dave reviewed the model and liked it, but raised the issue that it would need to be tested to determine if it would be useful. Would it work? Who would foot the bill to try?

We spent the next several months trying to get a hospital or medical center to use the model in the clinical care setting. No one wanted to take the financial risk of being "the first." Once again, Dave kept giving encouragement, quoting *Field of Dreams* and insisting, "If you build it, they will come." Then on September 11, 2001, came the horror of the terrorist attacks that killed so many and wounded all of us. Watching President Bush on TV, I could actually feel his spirit hurting and in crisis. Yet, he was the man whose response to such violation would determine the future of this country, impacting the whole world. He was in desperate need of help. Luckily, we had already defined the path for crisis management for the model and presented it at a meeting in Detroit.

Without any other intention than to reach out to someone who was critically wounded and in need of help, I e-mailed President Bush a letter, forwarding a copy to Dave. In it I explained the importance of healing the spirit prior to making irreversible noncritical decisions. Using the model, I outlined a plan intended to guide President Bush through the process of healing first, then reacting to what had happened. The letter became the basis for President Bush's speech to Congress. Our model for healing became the model used to help heal this country. Certainly this doesn't qualify as passing any rigorous scientific testing, but it does mean we made a difference to so many we had only dreamed of.

In that moment, watching the speech, tears streaming down at the realization of what had come from my triumph over all I had been through in life, I thought of Dave and how the gift of his support and encouragement made it all possible. I thought about how making a difference that truly matters to humanity is all part of a cascade. It starts with one person making a difference to others, who in turn help others, and so on, until the truth is an unstoppable force. But in it, each of us is just a small part. I thought about the incomprehensible concepts of destiny and pre-destiny, whether such things really exist, and whether this was why Dave and I were meant to link our visions together. And then I felt great peace with my life. That link is now severed. At times the loss seems paralyzing.

His death leaves a void in the field of health and spirituality, as well as in the lives and hearts of all of us who were close to him. But all of us know death is a part of life. All of us know peace with such loss comes when we hold the spirit of those we lost inside ourselves as we go on. We must build upon the foundation Dave started laying for us. Time will go on, as it always does. Let us all continue to pass our strengths and gifts on to others, and hope they continue the cascade, and accept that in the end, each of us is but a small part of the whole. My son, Nathan David Palackdharry, was born October 30, 2002. May he also be part of the cascade.

Carol S. Palackdharry, MD, MS
President and CEO
Fusion Health Foundation
St. Charles, Illinois

He told them another parable: The Kingdom of heaven is like a mustard seed which a man took and planted in his field. Though it is the smallest of all your seeds, yet when it grows, it is the largest of garden plants and becomes a tree, so that the birds of the air come and perch in its branches. (Matthew 13:31, NIV)

As I reflected upon the life and legacy of David Larson in light of this festschrift, Jesus' parable of the mustard seed kept coming to mind. Dave had been given a mustard seed with a vision and a mission. Within a seeming short time, what had been seen only through the eyes of faith became a reality as the forgotten "faith factor" began to capture the interest of scores of scholars across the nation. Their collective research and writings are in part a legacy of Dave's vision of networking a community of scholars who share a passion for scientific research on religion and health.

I recall fondly my first encounter with Dave in the late 1980s when I met with him in his office at the National Institutes of Health. Jungians would note the synchronicity involved in a colleague telling me about Dave after hearing his paper presentation at a professional meeting. I had just begun my research on prayer and health in a field whose leading introductory text used prayer as an example of deviant activity. I felt like I was swimming upstream—alone. This colleague encouraged me to connect with Dave, which I did a few months later during an unexpected visit to Washington, DC. For me this encounter was not a serendipitous, random act. It was an act of divine providence.

For some reason, I half expected to meet a pompous self-centered scholar and psychiatrist who would have little time for or interest in my small research project. Instead I experienced a meeting of mind and heart with a down-to-earth man (eating an apple as we talked!) who had a passion for the forgotten "faith factor." He shared his dream with me that morning—a dream of some day bringing together scholars to share with each other as we were doing that morning. Then we prayed.

Dave's vision took institutional flesh in 1991 with the establishment of the National Institute for Healthcare Research (later the International Center for the Integration of Health and Spirituality). My recognition that the mustard seed was fast emerging into a tree of knowledge capable of bringing together scholars from diverse backgrounds came in April 1995, when I was privileged to participate in the Spiritual Dimensions of Clinical Research Seminar at the Lansdowne Conference Resort. I saw then how Dave's faith and vision were being "uprooted and planted" (Luke 17:6) in ways (as he later would share with me) beyond anything even he had expected.

Although most of our contacts over the years were by phone (save for the occasional opportunity to connect at professional meetings and conferences), Dave was a friend with whom I could share my professional endeavors and on whom I could count for encouragement and prayer. (Our conversations always ended with Dave suggesting that we pray.) David Larson didn't just study faith; he lived what he believed. His faith mattered! What has emerged from Dave's mustard seed of faith has played an important role in the paradigm shift that is underway in modern medicine.

Margaret M. Poloma, PhD
Professor Emerita of Sociology
University of Akron
Akron, Ohio

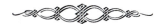

I was driving east on Route 80 toward Lewisburg, Pennsylvania, and stopped to check my telephone voice mail. There it was—a message about Dave's passing. Of course my thoughts went to his wonderful family, but also to how great a loss this was to me personally, for Dave was a wonderful friend, and to the field of religion and health, which he so ably created. Dave brought thousands of people together to develop a field that was enriched in every way imaginable by his devotion and creativity. He wrote many articles and gave talks from coast to coast, creating a legacy of excellence that few ever achieve. Just before he passed on he received an award from the American Psychiatric Association for his life's work.

But Dave understood people, and he nurtured hundreds upon hundreds of them with unlimited "agape" love. He was a total altruist, I think, and his most important accomplishment was in bringing people together. Others may come along who are as scientifically prolific as Dave, but no one will come along who can create the synergy-in-trust-and-love that was his special gift to the world. Dave was the father of his field, and his delight was always in the accomplishments of those many whom he so lovingly served as a loyal mentor.

In the early 1990s Dave and I co-authored a few articles, and eventually I had the honor of serving on the board of his National Institute for Healthcare Research. It was Dave who introduced me to the entire world of faith and medicine and in all respects gave me the confidence to speak and write in this area. He encouraged so many others like me to find a voice in the field, and to overcome adversity. It was Dave who introduced me to the universe of the Templeton Foundation, and this connection made much of my current work on the topic of love possible. Dave Larson saved me and a lot of other people in about as many ways as one human being can save another. He modeled creativity, courage, honesty, trust, and faith for us all.

Dave Larson mined the river of science, found gold nuggets of data, shouted Eureka!, and the whole wide world heard him. When he died, there were hundreds and thousands he had prepared to take up his cause.

Stephen G. Post, PhD
Professor of Bioethics, Religion, and Philosophy
Department of Bioethics
School of Medicine
Case Western Reserve University
Cleveland, Ohio
and President, Institute for Research on Unlimited Love
Cleveland, Ohio

I first made contact with Dave in 2001, when inviting him to come to give a guest lecture at the Royal College of Psychiatrists (UK) Annual Meeting. The previous year a Spirituality and Psychiatry Special Interest Group had been established within the College, and this would be a showcase event for us. As it turned out, we were never able to meet in person, since Dave rang the day before the talk to say his plane in the States had been grounded by storm conditions and how sorry he was about letting us down!

We had other speakers too, and in the event, we got off to a good start. But I soon was made aware of Dave's characteristic generosity when shortly after, he sent me two fully referenced papers he had written for publication on our new Web site where they can be seen to this day (http://www.rcpsych.ac.uk/college/sig/spirit/index.asp), and began a dialogue with me by e-mail which was consistently heartening to us in our endeavors on this side of the Atlantic.

In the United Kingdom, the field of spirituality and health is in its infancy, and Dave's great experience, his wisdom, and his unflagging encouragement were of enormous help to us. As our Group progressed, we began to submit detailed amendments to the Royal College in relation to the curriculum for training in the United Kingdom in psychiatry. Dave forwarded his Model Curriculum for Psychiatric Residency Training Programs to us, and together with the comprehensive research database that had been made available we felt able to bring heart and head together in our work for our submissions to the College.

We had high hopes of bringing Dave over to the United Kingdom in 2002 to explore ways and means of introducing spirituality into U.K. medical schools. Just the day before Dave passed on, he wrote, "Thank you for the good e-mail correspondence. Keep up the good energy and great work. I'm glad to hear you all are moving forward in the medical schools—very important step. As for the references, a recent cite you might find helpful is: 'The patient's spiritual/religious dimension: A forgotten factor in mental health.' We will mail you copy. Enjoy. Do take care." With the kind agreement of the co-authors, Susan Larson and Harold Koenig, and the publisher, Hatherleigh, we have just been able to publish this paper, one of Dave's last, on our Web site, where it will remain a testimony to his pioneering work.

When I heard with shock of Dave's sudden and untimely death, I felt I had lost a dear brother in spirit. The loss is small compared to those who knew and loved him most—his family and close friends and associates. Yet such was Dave's kindness, encouragement, and support that I had felt him to be with us every step of the way, a feeling that remains today as strong as ever. In gratitude, I can only say with heartfelt appreciation, "Thank you, Dave."

Andrew Powell, MRCP, FRCPsych
Founding Chair of the Spirituality
and Psychiatry Special Interest Group
Royal College of Psychiatrists
United Kingdom

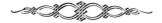

I first remember meeting Dave Larson in 1991. I was developing a new elective in spirituality and health at George Washington University School of Medicine (GW). The idea, while quite controversial at the time, generated a lot of interest from both colleagues at GW as well as professionals from the greater Washington, DC, area. One of my colleagues had heard of Dr. David Larson, who was doing research on religion and health at the National Institute of Mental Health (NIMH); he felt this person could bring an "interesting and important" perspective to the topic of spirituality and health.

It took me several weeks to track Dave down. He apparently had changed divisions at NIMH. It took careful navigating through the government maze to locate him. When we finally spoke, I felt an immediate kinship with Dave. Here was another physician who was committed to challenging theories about what might or might not be important in patient care.

Dave presented his talk to my class in spring 1992. He raised many challenging and provocative issues:

- Was religion harmful or helpful to patients?
- Was this even an area that could be researched?
- Was there a bias against religion in the medical establishment?

The session ran overtime as all of us engaged in a lively debate. From my perspective, Dave's lecture accomplished my goal: to get the students to question the accepted medical, disease-focused paradigm. Perhaps there were other factors in a person's life that could affect their health and illness—i.e., a more patient-centered focus of care.

Dave enjoyed the course. It was his first opportunity to share his research with medical students. It also inspired him to start an award program for medical schools in developing courses in "Faith and Medicine," as he called his program.

The course also was a beginning of a ten-year professional relationship for Dave and me. Several years later, I received one of the John Templeton Awards for the course at GW, which by then was being implemented not as an elective but as a required course. Dave recognized my passion for this field and quickly became my mentor. He empowered me to learn and grow in the field. His style of mentoring was to treat me as a colleague and give me the opportunity to be creative and develop a path for myself. He gave me the guidance and direction but did not hamper me by forcing me to follow his path as some mentors do.

One of my first tasks was to help Dave organize a national medical education conference on spirituality and health. He essentially gave me carte blanche to approach the project as I wished. His confidence in me inspired my confidence in myself.

Dave was truly a humble person. He freely acknowledged mistakes; he had an uncanny ability to laugh at himself. His humor was infectious and helped me to learn to take myself and the stumbling blocks I encountered with less seriousness.

Dave and I frequently discussed ideas and engaged in lively debates, sometimes disagreeing on issues. What I cherish most is Dave's ability to be challenged and grow from insights other people had. I suggested we broaden the award program title from "Faith and Medicine" to "Spirituality and Medicine." He listened to my argument, challenged my thinking even more, and then together, after some discussion, we changed the title. He taught me to be open to others' opinions whether from people more senior or junior than I. His model of mentoring is one I try to emulate to this day.

Dave loved to brainstorm, a trait we both have in common. I miss our evening chats, talking about ideas, developing plans, and delighting in creative joint ventures. Even now, as colleagues tease me about my brainstorming, I smile thinking that perhaps a little of Dave's influence lives on.

One of the most challenging times in our professional relationship was when I approached Dave about moving the education programs to a university. It became clear to both of us that in order to grow the programs they would need to be based in a medical school setting. It must have been hard for Dave to let go of something he helped initiate, but in his wisdom, he recognized that there is an appropriate time for change. So Dave, in his role as mentor par excellence, supported and helped me develop a proposal that the Templeton Foundation would later fund to move the education grant programs to GW in the form of an institute—the George Washington Institute for Spirituality and Health (GWISH). He never once shared any doubt or second thoughts. In fact, in my moments of insecurity, he only buoyed my spirits and encouraged me to move forward with the dream.

I am truly grateful to Dave for all he has done for me as well as for the many other students, researchers, and physicians who came to him for guidance. He will be forever remembered; his legacy will continue in all of our work.

Christina M. Puchalski, MD
Director
The George Washington Institute
for Spirituality and Health
Washington, DC
and Associate Professor of Medicine
The George Washington University
School of Medicine and Health Sciences
Washington, DC

My first encounter with Dave was during the summer of 1992 in Chicago at the Christian Medical and Dental Society National Student Convention when I was an incoming medical student and at which Dave was the highlighted speaker. I remember his impassioned appeal for students to take seriously a call into medical research as a means to bring glory to God and make manifest His Kingdom here in the "already and not yet." In his inimitable and gifted way, he gave his own story of failure and triumph, and as well swiftly and effortlessly summarized some of the research on health and religion. Dave presented a compelling reason to consider research as a career. As he is apt to do, in his fiery passion, I remember him reaching a rhetorical climactic moment and using a "four-star" curse word in the process! Though the buzz after his talk surrounded not only the content of his discussion but also the method of delivery (!), I swore an allegiance to that man on that day.

My second encounter with Dave was many years later as a rising second-year medical oncology fellow at Johns Hopkins where he asked me to write a chapter with him on "Cancer and Religion." Of course, I accepted. After much rigor and red ink, we produced a chapter we could be proud of. Dave stated that this third draft was encouraging and something we could publish. The second draft was not there and needed a lot of work. My first draft, however, he later confided in me, was nothing more than "an act of faith" that anything good could come out of it!

Dr. Larson . . . inimitable, irreplaceable, unstoppable. God has blessed us so.

Kent C. Shih, MD
Louisiana Hematology Oncology Associates
Mary Bird Perkins Cancer Center
Baton Rouge, Louisiana

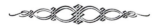

Most of us have individuals whose positive influence on our lives endures. If we are fortunate, such a person with an indelibly positive impression on us may have been a parent, a teacher, a coach, a clergyperson, or someone in our formative years worthy of our admiration and who cared enough about us to spend time and energy to leave a mark that would shape who we would become.

It is rare—perhaps once in a lifetime—that such an influential person crosses our paths as adults. Even months after Dave's untimely passing, I continue to attest to the wonderfully positive legacy he left for all of us on the staff of the International Center for the Integration of Health and Spirituality (ICIHS). Hardly a day passes without someone in the organization referring to one of Dave's idiosyncratic phrases, such as, "Thank you for coming to work today," or, "I'm so glad you're here." One can become dependent, if not addicted to such personal affirmation! As much as we continue to affirm each other, we still miss those strokes from Dave that were so consistent and effusive.

It wasn't just those of us who were privileged to interact on a daily basis with this man who could sometimes come across as a rather ordinary person, but who was often treated as a celebrity when he visited across the country to address important academic and professional meetings. His humility and sincere interest in others made dramatic impressions, even on individuals who met him only briefly.

Visitors to the office might spend an hour or so with him. A number of them would stop by my office on their way out and ask, "Is he for real?" They would have been so touched by an hour of conversation with Dave that their normal standards for evaluating such interactions were challenged. They needed a reality check because they sometimes concluded that if he were what they perceived him to be, he was too good to be true.

Dave was real, all right. He experienced life with a greater passion than most of us do. He let nothing interfere with his vision of what could be in the field of health care services if this notion of following the data rather than conventional wisdom could somehow catch on. But he honestly cared deeply for those in the trenches who were effecting change as well as those who would be beneficiaries of the change he was bringing to pass.

Upon his death, some of those people who had spent little more than an hour with Dave reported to me that their single hour with him had been one of the most important experiences in their lives. It wasn't necessarily his rich wisdom, deep insights, or sage advice that made those interactions so potent. It was his ability to focus on each person's gifts and unique strengths, accentuated by his obsessive optimism that allowed those he encountered to leave his presence renewed and revitalized.

In his humorous manner, Dave had the capacity to turn the greatest challenges to his views into an opportunity for dialogue. Instead of belittling those who complicated his life, he assumed the "one-down" position and sought more information in order to try to achieve common ground. Identifying Lieutenant Columbo of 1970s television fame as his "Patron Saint," he simply confessed, "I'm so sorry. All I am doing is reporting the data." What a powerful tactic that proved to be!

Chosen for the role of change agent, Dave gave it all he had. He didn't fit anyone's stereotype for leadership. His idiosyncrasies were all too apparent to anyone who knew him with any depth. And yet, he never allowed his idiosyncrasies to define him. In fact, he used them as bridges, allowing those with whom he would interact to gain a sense of importance in relating to him. It was an ingenious strategy. And it worked.

Most who found his peculiarities amusing simply took pleasure in the ways he would manage them. Others who found his habits annoying tolerated them because there was always more than enough to gain from the relationship that would more than compensate for them.

The fact is, however, that Dave's oddities were a function of his change-agent role. No one who "fits in" so as to be just like everyone else can cause major social change to occur. Being different was the price he paid in order to fulfill his destiny. Affirming and supporting others in loving ways, in addition to providing for numerous wonderful experiences for those who knew and worked with him, was his manner of maintaining contact with others.

Those chosen for such roles are rarely the ones our human wisdom would have selected. But in the providence of God, Dave was chosen for this vital role, and he not only performed his duty masterfully, he became the inspiration for any number of others as that "once in a lifetime" influence whose passion and strength of resolve will always endure as the model for creating change in the context of love.

How blessed all of us at ICIHS feel to have been allowed to be so closely associated with such greatness!

Thomas R. Smith, PhD
Senior Scholar
Interfaith Health Program
Emory University
Atlanta, Georgia

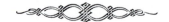

David Larson was my best early childhood friend. We lived in the small town of Hatboro, Pennsylvania, about a mile from each other. Most of the kids around us went to the public grammar school, but David and I were enrolled in the newly founded Willow Grove Christian Day school, a town away. We went to Willow Grove Christian School from first grade through fifth. There were no other Hatboro kids at our school, and so to all intents and purposes we were our own best—and practically only—friends in town.

We shared an avid interest in sports, but where I was going to be a professional baseball player, Dave was going into the NFL. I can still recall vividly how much I envied his Davy Crockett hat with the long coonskin tail and sporty cowboy boots. David's father had died when he was quite young, and I never knew him. By the sixth grade, David's mother decided to withdraw David from the Christian school and enroll him in Hatboro public school, where he excelled in the classroom and on the football field. Maybe he wasn't quite NFL material, but impressive enough to be elected to Hatboro High School's "Hall of Fame." Apart from seeing David's name in the local sports page, we saw virtually nothing of each other after fifth grade.

Until 1998. A former student of mine at Yale University began working for David and somehow my name came up. I got a letter from her asking if "Professor Stout was the same guy who used to be called 'Skippy.'" Indeed I was. From that happy coincidence David and I had several reunions at Yale, where I invited him to deliver endowed lectures and (the real reason) stay at my house and catch up on life. Those reunions are now precious memories.

Our last reunion came in the spring of 2000, when David and family arrived at our house on campus. We had a wonderful dinner at "Mory's," talked about our worst and best grammar school teachers (Miss Timmer was a terror, we both agreed), and talked with Chad about plans for law school. The next day the Larsons left and we were sure to get together again soon.

"Soon," I now realize is a relative term. Amidst all the sorrow and remembering, I hold on to the fact that soon in God's eyes is very different from soon in mine. Yes, we will reunite soon and pick up where we left off: best childhood friends.

Harry S. Stout, PhD
Jonathan Edwards Professor of American Christianity
Yale University
New Haven, Connecticut

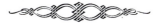

Worldwide, the health of people will benefit for generations to come by the dedicated work of Dr. David Larson and his wife Susan. As one of many examples, Dr. Larson proposed and managed a program subsidized by the John Templeton Foundation to encourage schools of medicine to offer courses on spirituality, medicine, and healing. In the first six years of the program, his work helped to increase the number of medical schools offering such courses from three to more than sixty. These courses train future doctors to help patients use their spiritual strength and resources to bring about healing in addition to medicine and surgery.

Sir John Templeton
Chairman
The John Templeton Foundation
Radnor, Pennsylvania

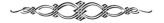

I knew Dave to do many things well. He was a careful researcher, a disciplined writer, and a persuasive public speaker. He invested his inquiries into the relationships between religion and health with deeper meanings born from his great compassion and strong sense of purpose. He had the rare gift of communicating these meanings to collaborators and younger scholars, thereby helping them to experience their research as an intellectual and moral vocation. As a professor in the field of religious studies I was well aware of the inspiring historical examples of medieval rabbis and monks who made their love of learning a way of serving their communities and glorifying

God. Yet I also experienced how the Weberian forces of bureaucratization and disenchantment too often make academic research less vital and productive than we would like it to be. Dave's example gave me courage. He left the accomplishments he had achieved at the NIH for the greater uncertainty but greater promise of founding his own research institution for documenting religion and health relationships. His encouragement and advice facilitated my transition from being a philosopher of religion at Columbia to being an epidemiologist of religion at Yale. For this I am deeply grateful.

As an epidemiologist, Dave respected empirical evidence. One of his most important achievements was to gather, summarize, and present evidence for the health benefits of various dimensions of religiousness in ways that persuaded medical colleagues to change their practices. That many medical schools now teach courses on spirituality and health, and that his psychiatric colleagues are less inclined to preemptively judge religious and spiritual concerns to be pathological, are due in large part to Dave's influence. He helped to make religious and spiritual ways of coping with illness more respected by health care professionals, and in doing so, he added to the self-respect of many ill people.

Yet Dave was not one to rest content with his successes. At the end of his life he was conversing with me about how religious communities addressing health needs might do so in a more reflective and informed way. He was advising me in my work for a faith-based program serving the needs of homeless addicts in recovery in New York City. I, like many others, shall miss his friendship and his wisdom, enthusiasm, and knowledge, but he will continue to shape the work we do and what we achieve will be our most respectful remembrance of him.

Peter H. Van Ness, PhD, MPH
Department of Epidemiology and Public Health
Yale University School of Medicine
New Haven, Connecticut

Dave Larson was a Christian. He was not ashamed of the "scandal" of the Gospel. His piety was genuine and heartfelt. He had a desire for GOD. He had the assurance of faith that comes from struggling to love and respond to GOD's call on your life. Although he was a devout Episcopalian, I joked with him about being "a closet Methodist." He sought to live by the advice that Mr. Wesley gave to his preachers in the eighteenth century: "Do all the good you can do, do as little ill as possible, and live by the commandments of GOD."

Dave knew that the Bible takes sides. He understood that we are required as people of the "Book" to speak up and work on behalf of those who are suffering and vulnerable. The passion in his work came from his "call" to say to his colleagues in medicine that a patient's faith should be acknowledged and affirmed—not ignored or belittled.

Dave encouraged others in their work and journeys of faith. He had the gift of discernment and was often wise in the ways of the world. He mentored many who will carry on his mission. He prayed for me from his heart on the phone at the end of our many conversations. I miss that very much. He enjoyed seeing others be successful in their work. Dave was an energizer. He was "long suffering" with prima donnas and could get us to work together in spite of ourselves.

As a Christian, you might not believe in the Resurrection of Christ every single day. However, a person of faith needs to believe in the power of divine love over death on days that people like Dave die. I must believe that the love of GOD has the last word, and that word connects us to the grace that we experienced in the life of Dave Larson.

Reverend Andrew J. Weaver
United Methodist Minister
Director of Research
Healthcare Chaplaincy
New York, New York

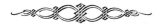

Faith mattered to Dave Larson. Dave was a man of vision, courage, and energy. Faith and values on health and religion were integrated seamlessly into his life. Dave knew that American people would turn toward God when they had health problems. His vision was to help medical practitioners in general, and psychiatrists in particular, be free to encourage people's religion and spirituality. He organized curricula, wrote scientific articles, and promoted meetings that helped build this vision. He wrote to the scientist, to the practitioner, and to the person in the street. He networked in a wide variety of communities.

Dave had courage. He was no stranger to controversy. When Dave began to write about religion, spirituality, and health, he was one of a few voices speaking in the wilderness. In the 1980s, most professionals and many lay people did not want to hear mental health professionals talk about religion and spirituality. Dave was undaunted. He wrote and spoke anyway despite this "anti-tenure factor." In the 1990s, he established the National Institute for Healthcare Research (NIHR) as a think tank. Even the name generated controversy. Many criticized the name as deceptively mimicking a federal agency. Dave's courage often came under fire.

Dave had boundless energy to pursue his vision. His phone was glued to his ear. He chased down grant makers and shared his vision. He was passionate about his vision because his faith mattered to him.

Dave was a catalyst. He worked with a wide network of collaborators. He inspired and encouraged them.

Dave was congruent. He valued religion and spirituality, and was active in his Episcopal Church congregation. Many times, he would end our phone conversations praying together. I have never had another colleague who so consistently, openly, and spontaneously prayed during the work day.

He valued mental and physical health. He was devoted to his wife Susan and his two children, and he took time to be with his family, carving out a safe place for his own mental health. He regularly (I almost said "religiously") lifted weights and ran on the treadmill. We spent three hours one evening at a conference talking. For the entire three hours that we were together, Dave did abdomen crunches. Just watching him made my stomach tired.

Dave integrated his faith and professional beliefs into his personal life, and was a model of integration for all who share those values. It was my honor to be a friend and a Christian brother with Dave. I'm sure that he has now heard the words from the Lord, "Well done, good and faithful servant; enter into my rest."

Everett L. Worthington Jr., PhD
Professor and Chair of Psychology
Virginia Commonwealth University
Richmond, Virginia

NOTES

1. Stevens W. (1972). The man with the blue guitar [1937]. In: Stevens H (Editor). *The Palm at the End of the Mind* (pp. 133-149). New York: Vintage Books.

2. James W. (1958). *The Varieties of Religious Experience* [1901-02]. New York: Mentor Books, pp. 126, 83.

3. Marty M. (1996). You get to teach and study religion. *Academe* (Nov.-Dec.):14, 15.

4. Lewis B. (2001). *What Went Wrong?* New York: Oxford University Press.

5. Jacoby S. (1983). *Wild Justice.* New York: Harper and Row.

6. Carroll J. (2001). *Constantine's Sword: The Church and the Jews.* New York: W.W. Norton and Company.

7. Gomes P. (1996). *The Good Book.* New York: Avon Press.

8. Cohen M. (1961). The dark side of religion. In Kauffman W (Editor). *Religion from Tolstoy to Camus* (pp. 279-297). New York: Harper and Row.

9. Pasternak, Boris. (1958). *Doctor Zhivago.* New York: Pantheon, p. 10.

Chapter 3

Eulogies

David Chad Larson
Kristen Joan Larson

This chapter contains two of the eulogies delivered on March 9, 2002, at Dave Larson's "Send-Off Service," held in the presence of loved ones, friends, and colleagues at St. James Episcopal Church in Potomac, Maryland. These eulogies were given by Dave's son, Chad, and his daughter, Kristen.

David Chad Larson, age twenty-three, was a senior at Princeton University when his dad graduated to heaven. He had played defensive line on the football team for three seasons. He majored in history, graduating with honors. Receiving a merit scholarship, he entered the University of Virginia School of Law the following fall.

This past Tuesday I learned that I will never again see the most important figure of the first twenty-three years of my life. David Bruce Larson was more than just a father to me. He was a mentor, a friend, and my Elijah.

If you asked my dad who he was, one of the first things he would tell you is that he failed his way into success. He would talk of countless ways that he messed up, but that God just kept blessing him.

But God did not bless my father despite his failures, but because of who my dad was. He was a man of faith who exuded thankfulness. If he believed God had called him somewhere, no matter the obstacle in his path, and there were many times that those obstacles seemed insurmountable, my dad would push, pull, strive, and strategize his way to go wherever God had led him. He would always tell me that you just need to trust God and that He would eventually reward you with more blessings than you could imagine.

My dad also knew how to accept God's gifts with a thankful heart. He would spend hours listening to psalms and praising God in our basement. With a sense of wonder, he would tell me that he had lived a better life than he could have possibly hoped for. He would specifically mention his dream job of research on spirituality as well as my mother, my sister, and me.

The three of us will never find a bigger fan than my dad. In our many talks together, my dad would reveal his love toward my mom and sister. About my mom he would say how thankful he was that she could think so rationally and clearly. By his own admittance, he was often illogical and a bit wacky, so he relied on my mom to complement his craziness. He would also say what a beautiful woman she is. But mostly he would talk about her wonderful servant's heart. He was always amazed at her seemingly boundless capacity to give of herself. He would usually finish by saying something like, "Chad, I've done nothing to deserve someone as wonderful as her."

About my sister, my dad would express his awe. He could not believe her spirited independence and her ability to discover the fun in any situation. In a family whose members have a propensity for people pleasing, my sister's independence made her stick out like a sore thumb. He was so proud of her, and was excited to behold the woman she is becoming. But he was proud of me, too.

My dad treasured the experience of being my father. No matter how far he needed to travel, or what engagements he missed, if I was playing in a football game, my dad was there. He or my mom would film the games, and, to be honest with you, I'm surprised those tapes still work. He spent countless hours watching them and couldn't wait to share his critiques. Oddly enough, these "critiques" always became a deluge of compliments for me. In fact, he would place every award I received in a position of prominence, and now my room looks like a shrine to me. All I did meant so much to him. Many times, when talking to others about my accomplishments, he would start to tear up, and I can't count the number of times he told me how proud he was of me.

Two of my favorite stories about my dad encapsulate his feelings for me. I had started to give my dad "the pound," which, for the uninitiated, involves the friendly tapping of fists between individuals. One day, when the time came for my mom and dad to hold hands for grace at dinner, my dad held out a fist. Understandably perplexed, my mom asked my dad what he was doing. He responded, "This is what Chad does." So my dad integrated "the pound" into his prayer life. Also, before undergoing surgery on his foot, his doctor asked him what he most looked forward to about being able to move about painlessly. He answered, "Going for walks with my son."

My dad and I spent hours together. Like when he used to read to me at night. I remember the pauses as he'd speed read through a paragraph and then give me a summary of what it was saying. He always had his own way of doing things. Junior High rolled around, bringing with it the classically adolescent issues of identity, and those nightly reading sessions turned into heartfelt conversations. I would share my fears, worries, and questions and he would respond with his own life experiences. These conversations continued until now. Last year when I lived at home, numerous days we would take hour-long walks just talking about life—sometimes twice a day. Of course, we would talk of less serious topics like history and sports, but I will remember our conversations on faith and life the most. We had more than a friendship, I knew his heart and he knew mine. It was my dad's dream to work together in some capacity in the professional world. I would have loved it, but the dream has been put on hold for the next life.

But in the next life, we won't just work, because if my dad taught me anything, it was how to laugh. My combination of intensity and sensitivity often lead me to have an overly serious outlook on life, believing that every little thing has eternal consequences. My dad's ability to joke helped teach me to loosen up and enjoy life. And he certainly loved jokes—both to make them and have them made about him (which was easy to do because he was so eccentric). My dad's love of laughter was infectious and thankfully he spread the wonderful contagion to me.

Although my dad has truly been my best friend and has taught me so much, it is his role as Elijah for which I am most thankful. The Gospel of Luke characterizes the spirit of Elijah as such: "And he will go before the Lord, in the spirit and power of Elijah, to turn the hearts of fathers to their children and the disobedient to the wisdom of the righteous—to make ready a people prepared for the Lord" (Luke 1:17).

My father embodied this spirit for me. My dad was a father who loved his child, turned me to righteousness, and prepared me to abide with my heavenly father. My dad certainly was not perfect and he would be the first to tell you his many faults, but he epitomized a man of faith who lived with a holy abandon and yet waited upon God—he had faith like a child, trusting that God would provide in all circumstances. In our relationship, he challenged me to take up his mantle of faith and obedience.

As I strove to take up this mantle, I found the greatest obstacle not to be sin but fear. And my dad never let me give in to fear. Christ doesn't say, "Stop sinning, have faith," but he continuously repeats, "Don't be afraid, have faith." Sinning is just what people do because they fear that God will not provide. Fears are funny things. If I ignore them, they don't really cause any problems. I might get a suspicion about them, but that suspicion will go away if I drown it out somehow. But when I face my fears, I find they are doubts that imprison me—false realities I believed were true and ran from my whole life. Faith is turning and facing those things I believe will destroy me. It is the declaration that they no longer have any power over me because I believe God will provide.

My dad encouragingly and lovingly pushed me to face my fears. The journey into the depths of one's soul to find the fears that control one's self is the hardest journey possible—not only because we have to face our fears, but because we have to find them. Years of compromising, giving into our fears, allows us, even if only subconsciously, to dress fears in a favorable light. But the man of faith stops at nothing, never compromising with falsehoods, to take up his cross, and nail his fearful self to it. He does so in order that his fears will no longer control him and that he can be reborn as one whose foundation is trust in God's love. Taking up that cross begins with trust, though, and I took it up because I trusted the loving, caring, and honest man who asked me to fight through my fears.

The past two years have been mentally, emotionally, and spiritually excruciating for me. I often have felt as if I was at the bludgeoning end of God's sledgehammer. I would cry out to Him in prayer, questioning why I felt so afflicted by Him, when I so sincerely sought to please Him. I now know that one of the reasons why I went through such a time of testing was that God was teaching me to totally put my faith in Him because my Elijah was going to be taken up to heaven.

My dad prepared the way for the Lord in my life. He taught me who God is by being a man of love, laughter, fellowship, faith, and truth. My adoring dad, my temporal representation of God, was going to be taken away from me, and it was time I matured to fully trusting in my perfect Heavenly Father. Due to my clutching onto God through my struggles and my father's preparing the way before God, I can quote with full assurance a slight paraphrase of Luke Skywalker: I am a man of faith as my father was before me.

If I had to guess what made my father such a man of faith, I would say it was the loss of his own father at the age of six. My dad often talked about what a loving individual and leader his own father had been, characteristics corroborated by numerous people who knew my Grandpa John. I think he missed his earthly father so much that he struggled with all his might to lay hold of his heavenly one.

David Bruce, I know you are with your Heavenly Father who you loved so much and with your earthly one with whom you are now making up for all those lost years. I also know that all the things I love about you have just been multiplied by infinity. I want to tell you I love you and I miss you. I can't imagine a greater honor in life than to be your son. Thank you for being my best friend and preparing me for my relationship with God. I know you are waiting in heaven for Mom, Kris, and I, but I want you to know that I'm waiting with breathless expectation for the days in which I can go on walks with my dad.

Kristen Joan Larson, age twenty-one, was a senior at Syracuse University at the time of her dad's graduation to heaven. She had a dual enrollment in the Newhouse School of Public Communications as a radio, TV, and film major, and in the School of Management with a major in entrepreneurship. She was scheduled to fly to Madison, Wisconsin, for an interview with Oscar Mayer the week that her dad passed away. Two weeks later, she was offered the year-long job of becoming a spokesperson for Oscar Mayer, doing media interviews and driving a Wienermobile around the United States.

I am filled with so much joy and I am so happy to have had a father like my dad. He was the most joyful person I have ever met. He was so positive about everything, and he was full of the Lord's grace. He had this uncanny ability to make everyone feel comfortable around him. So he got to know everyone, even our taxicab drivers.

Chad and I would always get asked, "What's it like to have Dave Larson as your father?" And we would always say, "Well, he's our dad. It's fun." There was never a dull moment.

One of the first things I thought about was when I was eight years old. We had just had a family over for dinner. Dad said, "Susan, Susan, the guests left their coats. Come into the living room." So my mom ran into the living room and let out this blood-curdling scream. Chad and I came running after to see what it was. My dad had taken this robotic, battery-operated hand with moving fingers and stuck it in his coat. He had it hanging over one of the chairs, and it had worked its way down the chair. It was hysterical. Making my mom scream seemed to be the brunt of many family jokes in the Larson household.

In elementary school, I would struggle so much with all the work. I didn't like school. Education was not my thing at that time. Dad would come to me and say, "Kristen, all you have to do is to learn how to make this work fun for yourself."

Living that statement out to the fullest, he would make friends with everybody he worked with. Everybody who called him loved him. They had genuine appreciation for him. He just loved them dearly. He cared so much for everybody.

When I was a high school freshman I decided to try out for softball, but I didn't really know how to play yet. It was dusk and Dad was throwing me tennis balls to hit since we didn't have any softballs. I'm trying to hit them, and of course I'm missing half of them. I finally hit one and it exploded. Dad made this typical "Dave Larson" face like he was stunned. It turned out he had pitched me an unripe tomato from our tomato vines. For one second, at least, I thought I was Wonder Woman.

But even though Dad had so much fun with us, he would push us. He knew that Chad needed to be pushed and I needed to be tamed.

A way of doing this was he would always threaten us that if we misbehaved, we would have to help him spray fertilizer on the azalea bushes. To a six-year-old, fertilizing is the worst thing ever. You turn all blue with the spray. My dad knew what we hated. There were various other things, of course, but that was the worst.

In high school, he totally let up on us. He was an amazing parent because he knew that we needed a strict setting as children. But as we grew up he understood he had to let us go and make our own mistakes. He would let me say whatever I wanted to say to him—which was good and bad. He would take it like a pro. He was probably the only person I could completely let my guard down around. I could say anything to this guy and he would take it from me. He just loved me for it. "That's Kristen. That's who she is." He didn't have this great ego you could step on.

When we were younger, he took Chad and me to the Sierra Nevadas to a rock-climbing course called Summit Adventures. Children go with their fathers to bond with each other and other families. This was funny because my dad has always hated heights. So, why did he do this? Because he wanted to be with us. So it was probably the most cherished experience I ever had with my father. I personally had the time of my life.

When we went rock climbing they had this competition between dads and their kids. You each rappel down a cliff and try to get to the bottom first. So here I am, his seven-year-old daughter in these pink corduroy pants. My dad is standing there, scared to death, holding his rope so tight. He was the only person beat by his kid down to the bottom. But you know what? He loved it, because everybody poked fun at him after that. Making people laugh was one of the aspects he enjoyed most in life, even if it was at his expense.

Dad was amazing. He just knew how to appreciate people. He always said how much my mom did for him. Dad's thoughts bounced everywhere, and it was hard to follow his train of thought. He'd say one thing, and then another, and you'd wonder, "How did that relate?" He'd say, "I'm just trying to get everything out, thinking out loud." My mom was his voice of reason. She was so good for him. She was his stability.

Dad talked about how much he loved the people he worked with at ICIHS and how much they meant to him. He'd say how he could never have gotten nearly so far without these people behind him.

And the cool thing about my dad is he never needed to tell you that he was proud of you or appreciated you. He was one of those people who would just look at you and you could see in his eyes what his heart was saying. I love that in a person. He never needed to say that he was proud because he just showed it so clearly.

He was so successful in everything he did, and the only reason for that was because of his faith in God. He said that every day was a blessing because he was surrounded by people he loved.

As Chad has mentioned, Dad's own dad died of melanoma at a young age. So after Dad was age thirty, he said every day was a blessing because he got to be here with his family and ones that he loved.

One verse that reminds me so much of my dad is Colossians 3:23: "Whatever you do, put your whole heart and soul into it, as work done for the Lord and not merely for men."

My dad is not dead. He just doesn't need his body anymore. I rejoice that he is so happy right now. He couldn't be in a better place. The joyful man that was here is now ten times more joyful.

Chapter 4

The Nearly Forgotten Factor in Psychiatry: What a Difference a Decade Makes: The Twentieth Annual Oskar Pfister Award Address

Susan S. Larson

These remarks were delivered by Susan S. Larson, MAT, on May 22, 2002, at the 155th Annual Scientific Meeting of the American Psychiatric Association (APA) in Philadelphia, Pennsylvania. The occasion was the celebration of her husband, Dr. David B. Larson, becoming the twentieth recipient of the Oskar Pfister Award, presented by the APA's Committee on Religion and Psychiatry in collaboration with the Association of Professional Chaplains, with funding by the Harding Foundation.

Oskar Pfister (1873-1956), a Swiss pastor, was a Lutheran theologian and pioneering psychoanalyst. He was known for encouraging his patients to express themselves creatively, and for discerning religious themes in works of art. Published correspondence between Pfister and his mentor, Sigmund Freud, has become an important starting point for discussions at the interface of psychoanalysis and religious faith for generations of psychotherapists.

The Oskar Pfister Award is presented by the APA for outstanding career contributions to the interrelationships between religion and psychiatry through research, publications, and clinical practice. Prior recipients, beginning in 1983, have been Drs. Jerome D. Frank, Wayne E. Oates, Viktor E. Frankl, Hans Küng, Robert Jay Lifton, Oliver W. Sacks, William W. Meissner, Peter Gay, Robert Coles, Paulos Mar Gregorios, Paul R. Fleischmann, James W. Fowler, Prakash Desai, Ann Belford Ulanov, Ana-Maria Rizzuto, Allen E. Bergin, Don S. Browning, Paul Ricoeur, and Irvin D. Yalom.

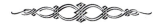

I feel extremely honored to accept the Oskar Pfister Award on behalf of my husband, Dr. David Larson. Dave knew he had been named to receive this award before he so suddenly passed away this past March. He was tremendously grateful for this honor. I would like to thank the committee, especially Dr. Irv Wiesner, chairman, for giving this award to him here in Philadelphia, which also happens to be Dave's hometown. Presenting with me today are Dave's colleagues, Dr. Michael McCullough, associate professor of psychology at Southern Methodist University, and Dr. Harold Koenig, associate professor of psychiatry and of medicine at Duke University Medical Center. Dr. Koenig, Dr. McCullough, and Dave collaborated as the three co-authors of the Oxford University Press book, the *Handbook of Religion and Health*, published last year, which reviews more than 1,200 studies.[1]

We will also be viewing two excerpts from a video of today's award winner.

I'd also like to refer you to an article published in *Directions in Psychiatry* written by Dave, myself, and Dr. Koenig, which reviews the topic of the patient's spiritual and religious dimension, and has the added benefit of providing continuing medical education credits.[2]

During his career, Dave desired to objectively investigate the potential relevance of spirituality and religious beliefs and practices for physical and mental health. An epidemiologist, Dave liked to quantify, to collaborate, and to help bring consensus through research. He had the honor of working with many of you on various professional publications. He so relished these collaborative relationships with you. I thank you for being here and for being such a crucial part of his life.

I also want to thank the APA for furthering this focus on understanding the relevance of patients' spirituality in treatment, training, and research. As Dave aptly stated, in past decades a patient's spirituality had often remained a "forgotten factor."[3]

APA guidelines during the past decade have underscored the importance of addressing what role a person's spiritual beliefs and practices may potentially play—for help or for harm—instead of letting these factors remain unrecognized. I hope the APA's efforts will continue to expand.

In this vein, I would like to quickly highlight why spirituality may be particularly relevant in the lives of the people whom mental health professionals serve here in the United States.

SPIRITUAL COPING AFTER 9/11: NEW ENGLAND JOURNAL OF MEDICINE *FINDINGS*

All of us in this country confronted a monumental crisis this past year. We as a nation felt the anguish of September 11's unexpected devastation, watching on national television as thousands lost their lives and thousands more lost treasured people they loved.

Where did many in our nation turn to cope?

A study published in the *New England Journal of Medicine* investigated levels of stress and coping mechanisms.[4] Using a national sample of 560 adults interviewed three to five days following the attacks, this study found that

- 90 percent reported symptoms of stress, and
- 44 percent had one or more substantial symptoms of stress.

The study also discovered that to deal with this stress religious coping was remarkably prevalent:

- 90 percent of respondents turned to prayer, religion, or spiritual feelings.

Further, the study found that a majority of these 90 percent relied on their spiritual resources to quite a sizeable extent:

- 57 percent said "a lot,"
- 37 percent said "a medium amount,"
- 15 percent said "a little," and
- only 10 percent said "not at all."

The substantial proportion—90 percent—of those who turned to prayer, religion, or spirituality at some level illustrates the frequency of spiritual coping when handling crises and stress.

IMPORTANCE OF RELIGION/SPIRITUALITY IN THE U.S. POPULATION

According to Gallup Poll data, religion and spirituality are important in the lives of most in the U.S. population, and thus stand out as significant factors to recognize when dealing with patients in the United States. Gallup data show that[5]

- 95 percent of those in the United States believe in God or a Universal Spirit;
- only 5 percent are atheist or agnostic;
- a substantial 85 percent of Americans consider religion "very important" or "fairly important" in their lives;
- 60 percent attend at least monthly at one of the half million places of worship in the United States, including churches, synagogues, and mosques; and
- about 40 percent attend religious services weekly or more.

Commenting on the prevalence of the importance of religion and spirituality in the United States, former Oskar Pfister Award winner, psychologist Dr. Allen Bergin observed that for more than 70 percent of the population for whom religious commitment is a central life factor

> Treatment approaches devoid of spiritual sensitivity may provide an alien values framework. . . . A majority of the population probably prefers an orientation to counseling and psychotherapy that is sympathetic, or at least sensitive, to a spiritual perspective. We need to better perceive and respond to this public need[6].

RELEVANCE OF RELIGION/SPIRITUALITY FOR MENTAL HEALTH PATIENTS

Gallup data reveal the relevance of spirituality in the life of the U.S. population in general, but what about those with mental health needs? Are spiritual and religious beliefs and coping relevant for those undergoing mental health treatment?

A study published in 2001 in *Psychiatric Services* explored the degree that persons with persistent mental illness might draw upon spiritual/religious beliefs in coping with their symptoms.[7] The study followed more than 400 patients served by mental health facilities in Los Angeles County and found the following:

- a large majority—80 percent—used some type of religious belief or activity to cope with their symptoms or daily difficulties,
- 30 percent stated that their religious beliefs or activities "were the most important things that kept them going,"
- 65 percent reported that religion helped them to either a large or moderate extent in coping with symptom severity, and
- almost half—48 percent—indicated that spirituality/religion became more important to them when their symptoms worsened.

Analyses further found that the number of years that patients had drawn on religious coping and the amount of their coping time which drew upon religious beliefs or practices were both correlated with less severe symptoms and better overall functioning.

In addition, a greater number of years and greater amount of religious coping were linked with lower symptom levels in six areas:

- obsessive-compulsiveness,
- interpersonal sensitivity,
- phobic anxiety,
- paranoid ideation,
- psychoticism, and
- total symptomatology.

Commenting on these findings, the researchers suggested that "religious methods of coping may be particularly salient for persons with mental illness, and they may be one of the more important strategies that enable these persons to persevere."[7]

A RESEARCH QUEST

Curiosity about the potential relevance of spirituality in patients' lives is what helped prompt Dave's quest to investigate spiritual and religious factors in quantitative research. Dave embarked on a career path of research—quantifying, collaborating, and consensus building. I would like to highlight a little of his journey as he developed a methodology to objectively approach an area which has often been fraught with controversy.

Here are a few words from Dave[8] about his mounting interest in the potential relevance of spirituality to physical and mental health:

> I got interested in this area first when I was a researcher at the National Institutes of Health. And really the area was "understudied variables" and their relevance to health and mental health. And there were social variables like religion, spirituality, and marriage and family that people weren't looking at much, but they seemed to have relevance to physical health and mental health and social health, as well.
>
> And so over time while I was at NIH I looked at more and more of these variables, and I found the one that really drew my attention was spirituality.

Early Theoretical Assumptions

To give a little further background, during Dave's psychiatric residency training in the mid-1970s, he noticed that a patient's spiritual/religious life appeared to be a "don't ask, don't tell" variable. He was advised as a therapist to avoid discussing patients' religious issues in treatment. Furthermore, the prevailing theory at the time was that religion and spirituality were primarily harmful to mental health. For instance, Freud[9] and psychologist Dr. Albert Ellis both theorized about religion and spirituality in terms of psychopathology. Ellis, best known for his groundbreaking work on rational-emotive therapy, wrote: "Religiosity is in many respects equivalent to irrational thinking and emotional disturbance. . . . The elegant solution to emotional problems is to be quite unreligious. . . . [T]he less religious they are, the more emotionally healthy they will be."[10]

This had been the premise of some theorists. However, research studies like that previously cited, and hundreds of others, have discovered benefits for mental health from spiritual coping.

Interestingly, after Freud published *The Future of an Illusion,* in which he described religious beliefs as illusions, he made the following comment in a letter to his long-time friend and correspondent, the Reverend Oskar Pfister, for whom this award is named:

> Let us be quite clear that the views expressed in my book form no part of analytic theory. They are my personal views, which coincide with many analysts and pre-analysts, but there are

many excellent analysts who do not share them. . . . In itself psycho-analysis is neither religious nor non-religious, but an impartial tool which both priest and layman can use in the service of the sufferer."[11]

Yet, despite Freud's disclaimer to Oskar Pfister, some of his other statements most likely helped contribute to the prevailing theory in the middle 1970s that religion was preponderantly detrimental to mental health.

Dave, however, while observing his patients, saw that a patient's religious beliefs at times seemed to help by giving them a sense of comfort and a feeling of hope which helped them both cope and persevere while experiencing the stress of their emotional illness.

When what he observed clinically did not totally align itself with the prevalent theory of detriment, Dave embarked on a data hunt. He decided to examine the research findings in psychiatry's leading journals to discover why religious beliefs and practices were primarily harmful.

Development of the Systematic Review
Research Methodology

To eliminate selection bias in what articles were surveyed, Dave developed an objective process called the "systematic review."[12] The Public Health Service Commissioned Corps at the National Institutes of Health later awarded him a Commendation Medal for developing this methodology. Unlike most research reviews that provide an overview based on articles a reviewer picks out to highlight, the systematic review avoids selection bias by looking at every single quantitative article published during a certain number of years in a particular journal to provide a comprehensive survey of findings. This makes the review process both objective and replicable.

The Forgotten Factor: Religion
and Spirituality Rarely Researched

In his systematic review of psychiatric research, which was published in the *American Journal of Psychiatry,*[13] Dave and his research team surveyed all articles published in the top four general psychiatry journals from 1978 to 1982. These included the *American Journal of*

Psychiatry, British Journal of Psychiatry, Canadian Journal of Psychiatry, and *Archives of General Psychiatry.* The review found that only three of 2,348 quantitative studies contained a religious variable as the central focus of the study, and only one used a state-of-the-art measure, a multidimensional religious commitment questionnaire previously tested for reliability. Only 2.5 percent of the quantitative studies included any religious variable, including denomination, with most using just a single item, inadequate for measuring the complexity of religious beliefs, attitudes, or frequency of practices. Dave discovered that this proportionately small number of studies of spiritual/religious commitment fell far short of the extensive research required to build theoretical constructs. This was indeed a "forgotten factor."

Next, Dave decided to explore those studies that did include a religious variable, to see how findings might confirm U.S. psychiatry's historical presumption of harm.

Patient Spirituality: Clinical Help or Harm?

A systematic review of all quantitative articles published in 1978-1989 in the *American Journal of Psychiatry* and *Archives of General Psychiatry* found that a large majority of articles—around 80 percent—indicated a positive clinical association between spirituality/religion and better mental health. A much smaller proportion of the research found negative associations.[14] This systematic review revealed that spiritual/religious commitment was more often linked with potential benefits to mental health rather than harm—the reverse of what previously was commonly assumed. Moreover, these were findings in psychiatry's own leading journals.

Dave was discovering that a patient's spirituality and religion were complex, potentially beneficial at times, and not necessarily harmful. In fact, associations with mental health benefits were far more frequent than associations with harm.

Let me pause here to say that Dave recognized both from a historical perspective and from research findings of harm that there is no doubt that religious activities, especially when taken to extremes, can adversely affect both physical and mental health, and at times encourage unquestioning devotion to single extremist religious leaders, as we saw in 9/11.

But as Dave and his colleagues further researched this area, they found that religious beliefs and activities that promote compassion, forgiveness, thankfulness, and hope are more likely to be associated with mental health benefits.[15] These beliefs may also promote the development of strong social support, encouraging reaching out to others in both giving and receiving emotional and instrumental help. They can also promote a sense of personal worth. Feeling loved and valued by God or a Higher Power can bring comfort and hope, especially when coping with the distress of emotional or physical illness.[16]

Psychiatric Residency Training in Spiritual/Religious Issues

Misunderstanding the role that religion plays in patients' lives could result in part from the lack of training concerning spiritual and religious issues during residency. The norm in psychiatric training had been to give scant attention, if any, to methods for addressing patient's religious/spiritual issues. A survey of psychiatric residency programs in 1988 showed that few included coursework on any aspect of religion, and that residency supervision infrequently addressed religious issues.[17]

More recently, in 2000, a random sample survey of members of the APA[18] found that

- 65 percent indicated that religious and spiritual issues were rarely or never addressed in their training, yet
- 92 percent of these graduate psychiatrists indicated that religious or spiritual issues came up in practice "at least sometimes," "often," or "a great deal," and
- 44 percent reported that "loss of purpose or meaning in life," which can have spiritual or religious relevance, was a focus of treatment either often or a great deal of the time.

To help close this gap in training, mandates of the Accreditation Council for Graduate Medical Education in 1994 required psychiatry residency programs to provide instruction about American culture and subcultures, and to include the issue of religion/spirituality as a relevant aspect of patient culture.

Model Curriculum

To meet the need for instruction in religious/spiritual issues, Dave helped work with a group of psychiatrists from various religious backgrounds—Buddhist, Hindu, Jewish, Christian, Moslem, and agnostic—to formulate a model curriculum,[19] released in May 1996, at the APA annual meeting.

Also, since 1997, the John Templeton Foundation has provided awards to outstanding academic programs in psychiatry and spirituality. Awardees include such prestigious institutions as Harvard, Baylor, Emory, and Georgetown.[20]

Risk of Misinterpretation

These training efforts are tremendously important. Without training to help understand a religious culture that may differ widely from a therapist's own culture, misunderstandings are much more likely to occur.

It can be quite difficult to properly interpret a language or an aspect of a patient's culture that is unfamiliar. Anyone who has tried to learn a foreign language realizes that idioms and expressions can certainly remain a puzzle, if not sound outright ludicrous, if taken literally. If someone from another culture heard the idiom "it's raining cats and dogs," they might think this response somewhat delusional.

Differing worldviews and the language used to express them can cause some of the same misunderstandings. For instance, when trying to illustrate the concept of delusion, the authors of the DSM-III-R "Glossary of Technical Terms" stated, "Delusion: Example, if someone claims he or she is the worst sinner in the world, this would generally be considered a delusional conviction."[21] Using the same logic, almost any hyperbole expressing depth of feeling could be regarded as a delusion if taken as a concrete statement, such as, "I am the happiest man alive." Language, particularly religious language, can express depth of feeling, rather than a concrete rating scale, but one unfamiliar with it might misinterpret it.

To point to this religious phrase as a delusion suggests a cultural misunderstanding. In fact, the Glossary showed a marked insensitivity by employing religion to demonstrate psychopathology in 22 percent of the case examples.[22] However, after these potential misunderstandings were pointed out by Dave and his colleagues in an article published in the *American Journal of Psychiatry*,[22] the next edition, the DSM-IV, removed the many examples using religious content to illustrate pathology.[23]

SUMMARY

To summarize, quantitative research has helped to identify salutary links with religious/spiritual vitality, as well as negative religious coping patterns and potential harmful effects. To identify current research findings and to map out future research directions, Dave helped spearhead a series of three conferences of more than seventy researchers, clinicians, and ethicists in the fields of physical and mental health, addictions, and the neurosciences. A consensus report culminated this collaboration.[24] It concluded that the data from many of the studies conducted to date were sufficiently "robust and tantalizing" to warrant continued and expanded clinical investigations.

Research findings were often significant despite use of a somewhat crude measure of assessing spiritual/religious commitment: the frequency of attendance at religious services. Dave often quoted Garrison Keillor to describe the inadequacy of this one measure to quantify depth of spiritual or religious commitment. Keillor remarked that, "If you think going to church makes you a Christian, sit in your garage and you will become a car."

Yet even when using this somewhat crude measure of frequency of attendance at religious services, a salutary link between spiritual/religious participation and mental health still often remains after controlling for numerous confounding variables.

Here's a concluding comment from Dave:

> When it comes to the research, this is still an emerging field. But there are some areas of great promise like mortality, like depression, suicide, delinquency, coping with illness, recovery from surgery, and I could go on more. But we see an emerging field where the research is showing some pretty solid findings, and we should take this and move it even on further.[25]

NOTES

1. Koenig HG, McCullough ME, Larson DB. (2001). *Handbook of Religion and Health*. Oxford, England: Oxford University Press.

2. Larson DB, Larson SS, Koenig HK. (2001). The patient's spiritual/religious dimension: A forgotten factor in mental health. *Directions in Psychiatry* 21:307-333.

3. Larson DB, Larson SS. (1994). *The Forgotten Factor in Physical and Mental Health: What Does the Research Show?: An Independent Study Seminar*. Rockville, MD: National Institute for Healthcare Research.

4. Schuster MA, Stein BD, Jaycox L, Collins RL, Marshall GN, Elliott MN, Zhou AJ, Kanouse DE, Morrison JL, Berry SH. (2001). A national survey of stress reactions after the September 11, 2001, terrorist attacks. *New England Journal of Medicine* 345:1507-1512.

5. Gallup GH. (1996). *Religion in America: 1996*. Princeton, NJ: The Gallup Organization.

6. Bergin AE, Jensen JP. (1990). Religiosity of psychotherapists: A national survey. *Psychotherapy* 27:6.

7. Tepper L, Rogers SA, Coleman EM, Maloney HN. (2001). The prevalence of religious coping among persons with persistent mental illness. *Psychiatric Services* 52:663.

8. Larson DB. (2001). Quoted in *The International Center for the Integration of Health and Spirituality* [Video]. Wilmore, KY: The Creative Group.

9. Freud S. (1962). *The Future of an Illusion* [1927]. London, England: Hogarth Press.

10. Ellis A. (1980). Psychotherapy and atheistic values. *Journal of Consulting and Clinical Psychology* 48:637.

11. Freud S, Pfister O. (1963). *Psychoanalysis and Faith: The Letters of Sigmund Freud and Oskar Pfister*. Edited by H Meng, EL Freud. Translated by E Mosbacher. New York: Basic Books, p. 117.

12. Larson DB, Sherrill KA, Lyons JS. (1994). Neglect and misuse of the *R* word: Systematic reviews of religious measures in health, mental health, and aging. In Levin JS (Editor), *Religion in Aging and Health: Theoretical Foundations and Methodological Frontiers* (pp. 178-195). Thousand Oaks, CA: Sage Publications.

13. Larson DB, Pattison EM, Blazer DG, Omran AR, Kaplan BH. (1986). Systematic analysis of research on religious variables in four major psychiatric journals, 1978-1982. *American Journal of Psychiatry* 149:329-334.

14. Larson DB, Sherrill KA, Lyons JS, Craigie FC, Thielman SB, Greenwold MA, Larson SS. (1992). Dimensions and valences of measures of religious commitment found in the *American Journal of Psychiatry* and the *Archives of General Psychiatry:* 1978 through 1989. *American Journal of Psychiatry* 149:557-559.

15. McCullough ME, Snyder CR. (Editors) (2000). Classical sources of human strength [Special Issue]. *Journal of Social and Clinical Psychology* 19:1-159.

16. Koenig HG, Larson DB, Larson SS. (2001). Religion and coping with serious medical illness. *Annals of Pharmacotherapy* 35:352-359.

17. Sansome RA, Khatain K, Rodenhauser P. (1990). The role of religion in psychiatric education: A national survey. *Academic Medicine* 14:34-38.

18. Shafranske EP. (2000). Religious involvement and professional practices of psychiatrists and other mental health professionals. *Psychiatric Annals* 30:525-532.

19. Larson DB, Lu FG, Swyers JP. (Editors) (1996). *Model Curriculum for Psychiatry Residency Training Programs: Religion and Spirituality in Clinical Practice.* Rockville, MD: National Institute for Healthcare Research.

20. Puchalski CM, Larson DB, Lu FG. Spirituality courses in psychiatry residency programs. *Psychiatric Annals* 30:543-548.

21. American Psychiatric Association. (1987). *Diagnostic and Statistical Manual of Mental Disorders,* Third Edition, Revised. Washington, DC: American Psychiatric Association, p. 395.

22. Larson DB, Thielman SB, Greenwold MA, Lyons JS, Post SG, Sherrill KA, Wood GG, Larson SS. (1993). Religious content in the DSM-III-R Glossary of Technical Terms. *American Journal of Psychiatry* 150:1884-1885.

23. American Psychiatric Association. (1994). *Diagnostic and Statistical Manual of Mental Disorders,* Fourth Edition. Washington, DC: American Psychiatric Association.

24. Larson DB, Swyers JP, McCullough ME. (Editors) (1998). *Scientific Research on Spirituality and Health: A Consensus Report.* Rockville, MD: National Institute for Healthcare Research.

25. Larson. Video quote.

PART II:
SELECTED WRITINGS
OF DR. DAVID B. LARSON

Dave Larson's reputation as a "manuscript doctor," discussed in Chapter 1 of this book, made him something akin to a legend among his colleagues in the religion and health field. His ability to rewrite and refocus a not-quite-ready-for-publication manuscript turned many chunks of coal into well-cited gems, and earned him scores of co-authorships and considerable gratitude.

This amazing skill, and the reputation that it brought him, however, may obscure in the eyes of Dave's admirers the priceless contribution of Dave's own original scholarly writing. Often overlooked within Dave's incredible curriculum vitae of almost 300 scholarly publications (see Chapter 16) is a body of vital and seminal theoretical and empirical writing that helped to establish religion as an accepted topic for clinical research and education.

In Part II of *Faith, Medicine, and Science,* ten of Dave Larson's classic first-authored papers are reprinted. These include one of a series of four early papers on religion and mental illness written with Dr. William P. Wilson while Dave was on the faculty at Duke University (Chapter 5); three extremely influential systematic reviews of religious research in psychiatry (Chapters 6, 7, and 8); an important critique of religious content in the DSM-III-R (Chapter 9); one of the most famous empirical studies published in the pastoral care field (Chapter 10); a much-cited study of religion and blood pressure based on Dave's graduate research in epidemiology at the University of North Carolina (Chapter 11); an example of the numerous systematic reviews that Dave conducted in nonmedical fields (Chapter 12); an example of Dave's many traditional-style literature review articles on religion and health (Chapter 13); and, a celebrated essay on the healing power of faith published in a national newsmagazine (Chapter 14).

This collection of articles demonstrates, finally and conclusively, that, quite aside from his prowess at field-building, Dave Larson was an absolutely first-rate scholar and scientist. He was, moreover, one of the most important writers on the interface of the human spirit and the healing arts to come along in the past several decades. Nobody researching or writing on religion and health, or on the broader topic of religion and science, can legitimately claim to have covered these issues in full without first discussing and citing his work.

Chapter 5

Religious Life of Alcoholics

David B. Larson
William P. Wilson

It has been documented that alcoholics often become abstinent after a religious experience. We have inquired into the religious teachings, beliefs, practices, and experiences of a group of chronic alcoholics. It was observed that alcoholics were less involved in religious practices, had less exposure to religious teachings, had fewer religious experiences, and withdrew from religion more frequently during adolescence than did a group of normal subjects. It is concluded that early-life religious experiences of an alcoholic are most conflictual and lead to religious confusion rather than commitment.

Before the founding of Alcoholics Anonymous, the fate of the alcoholic was dismal. Some 28 percent died as a direct result of their alcoholism, and another 51 percent drank for the rest of their lives, but a few did stop drinking. Eleven percent did so spontaneously and 7 percent had a religious experience which resulted in sobriety.[1] Alcoholics Anonymous brought hope for some alcoholics. Large numbers of alcoholics stopped drinking when they joined this group. Its success has been attributed to the spiritual dimension that is at the heart of its twelve steps to sobriety.[2] Despite its success, medicine has not always known how to use the power of AA. Usually it is invited into the medical and psychiatric care, but its participation is often appended to rather than integrated into the treatment. Medicine has been uncomfortable with syncretizing the spiritual (or moral) with the more tech-

Reprinted, with permission, from *Southern Medical Journal* 1980; 73: 723-727. Read before the Section on Neurology, Neurosurgery, and Psychiatry, Southern Medical Association, Seventy-Third Annual Scientific Assembly, Las Vegas, Nevada 4-7, 1979.

nical.[3,4] We believe there is a need to learn to use such a dimension within the full treatment, as past literature has substantiated.[4-6]

Students of human behavior generally agree that the nurturing environment is a powerful determinant of both healthy and unhealthy behavior. Two major factors that we see as important in this environment are teaching and experience. Teaching will determine the values held, and experience will determine the emotional significance of these values. Consistency of values taught with those experienced within a family setting will have a powerful impact on a person's spiritual health. We therefore have conducted a preliminary investigation designed to look at a few important aspects of how teaching and experience related to the spiritual lives of a group of alcoholics and a group of normal control subjects.

METHOD

The alcoholic patients included in this investigation were eighty-one men who were admitted to the psychiatric units of the John Umstead State Hospital in Butner, North Carolina, and the Veterans Administration Hospital in Durham, North Carolina. After detoxification and management of their physical complications, each patient was examined using a structured interview. We obtained topical data concerning the subject's age, sex, marital history, and socioeconomic status. Socioeconomic status was determined using the Hollingshead-Redlich two-factor index.[7]

In our investigation of the patient's early religious life we recognized that his knowledge of religion would be obtained from two sources: his parents and the church. We thus obtained a history of how the subject experienced both. The following religious data were obtained: the denominational preferences of the subjects and their parents, the beliefs of the subjects and their parents, and the church attendance of the subjects and their parents. Recognizing that children may passively accept religious teaching, only to later redefine or reject their faith in adolescence, we inquired as to whether there had been a change in religious interests during adolescence. As this change in interest might be influenced by the occurrence of a salvation experience, we inquired also as to whether the subjects had ever had such an experience and at what age it had occurred. It was of interest to determine under what circumstances this event had occurred, for such might reflect the influence of the home on the individual. We did therefore inquire whether the experience occurred outside the church, at ordinary church services, or at evangelistic church services. Even though we knew that our alcoholic patients were not healed by whatever faith they might have had, it seemed important to determine the basic Christian beliefs they held. Thus we inquired whether they believed in a God, that He had a son named Jesus, and if they felt there was a Holy Spirit who could dwell in people spiritually. To conclude our investigation we asked whether our subjects actually practice their faith. We operationalized the term "practice" by defining it as reading the Bible, praying at meal time, praying at other times, and telling others about their faith commitment.

Similar data were obtained from 107 normal subjects who were recruited from the same geographic area as the alcoholics. Volunteers were accepted into the study after it was determined that they had not been treated for psychiatric disease, had not had significant symptoms of psychiatric disease, and at no time had their work capacity been compromised by psychiatric symptoms. All data were recorded on IBM cards and subjected to computer analysis using a telestorage and retrieval system (TSAR).[8] Chi-square analysis was used to determine significance.

RESULTS

The demographic data are summarized in Table 5.1. The age range in the two groups differed in that 93 percent of the alcoholics were thirty to fifty-nine years old, while 48 percent of the normal subjects were in the same range. There was a large numerical difference in comparing the socioeconomic backgrounds of the alcoholic and control populations. In the control population, 87 percent had come from social classes 1 to 3. In contrast, 79 percent of the alcoholics came from classes 4 and 5. As shown in Table 5.2, the social class range of the children was similar to that of the parents, with 89 percent of the alcoholics coming from classes 4 and 5 and 69 percent of the normal subjects coming from classes 1 to 3.

The alcoholics were more frequently separated and divorced (42 percent of the alcoholics versus 11 percent of the nonalcoholics) at the time of the interview. Also, a larger number of alcoholics had

TABLE 5.1. Demographic Data

| | Age Distribution (%) | | | | | |
	10-19	20-29	30-39	40-49	50-59	60+
Alcoholics	0	7	28	23	36	5
Normals	4	24	9	22	17	25

| | Race Distribution (%) | | |
	White	Black	Asian
Alcoholics	74	25	1
Normals	83	16	1

| | Subjects' Social Class (%) | | | | |
	1	2	3	4	5
Alcoholics	2	5	14	24	55
Normals	23	31	33	8	5

TABLE 5.2. Demographic Data

| | Parents' Social Class (%) | | | | |
	1	2	3	4	5
Alcoholics	2	1	5	26	63
Normals	19	17	33	10	17

| | Marital Status (%) | | | | |
	Single	Married	Widowed	Separated	Divorced
Alcoholics	20	31	7	22	20
Normals	27	49	13	4	7

| | Came From Families of Broken Homes (%) | | | | |
	Father Missing	Mother Missing	Both Missing	Reared by Others	Not Broken
Alcoholics	48	6	6	10	30
Normals	9	3	3	5	80

N = 81 for alcoholics.
N = 108 for normals.

been married two or more times (24 percent of the alcoholics versus 11 percent of the nonalcoholics). The majority of the alcoholics (70 percent) came from broken homes, whereas 20 percent of the normals had. This last difference was significant ($P < .01$). In both groups it was usually the father who was missing (84 percent of the alcoholics and 92 percent of the normals).

The two groups differed significantly in their denominational loyalties. Three-fourths of the alcoholic patients were Baptist (Table 5.3). The control group had a greater mix, with one-third Baptist and one-third Methodist. The religious preference of the families of origin were quite similar. In both groups the fathers had "no religious preference" more often than did the mothers (20 percent of the fathers versus 4 percent of the mothers of the alcoholics, and 9 percent of the fathers versus 2 percent of the mothers of the normal subjects). Denominational loyalties can profoundly influence how one lives one's

TABLE 5.3. Religious Data

	Denominational Preferences (%)			
	Baptist	Presbyterian	Methodist	Other
Alcoholics				
Subject	70	11	7	11
Subject's father	57	7	10	20
Subject's mother	64	9	9	18
Average frequency per family	62	9	9	18

	Baptist	Methodist	Presbyterian	Catholic	Episco-palian	Other
Normals						
Subject	31	32	10	11	3	13
Subject's father	35	26	8	7	4	21
Subject's mother	35	31	9	7	7	13
Average frequency per family	34	30	9	8	5	16

religious life. We thus looked at what basic philosophic approach to living was lived out religiously by the subject's parents. More than 50 percent of the alcoholics' parents emphasized to their children to be good and do good (Table 5.4). On the other hand, more than 50 percent of the parents of the nonalcoholics believed that one had to be "born again," go to church, pray, and read the Bible to live out a successful life. This we called a conservative religious belief system.

There were more differences in the parents' frequency of church attendance (Table 5.5). In both groups the mothers attended church more often than did the fathers. The mothers of the alcoholics attended more regularly than the mothers of the normals (66 percent versus 54 percent), whereas the fathers of the normals attended more often than did the fathers of the alcoholics (43 percent versus 33 percent). As children, both the alcoholics and the nonalcoholics attended church. It is noteworthy that 89 percent of the alcoholics lost interest in religion during their teen years, in contrast to the normal subjects who either had an increased (48 percent) or unchanged (32 percent) interest in religion during their adolescence. The difference between the normal and the alcoholic group was significant at the .01 level of confidence.

There was a significant difference in the occurrence of salvation experience in the alcoholic and the normal populations (Table 5.6). In the normal population, 75 percent were found to have had a salvation experience, whereas only 46 percent of the alcoholics had. Again this difference is significant at the .01 level. In both groups this tended to occur before the age of thirty (80 percent of the control group versus 69 percent of the alcoholics), though a large number of alcoholics (28 percent) had such an experience after fifty. Only 11 percent of the control group had such an experience after fifty.

Most of the alcoholics reported that their salvation experience was not a lasting experience and they soon had "fallen away." It was infrequent that the salvation experience of alcoholics permanently influenced their drinking problem. Although 38 percent of the alcoholics reported a period of sobriety of six months or longer after a salvation experience, all of them returned to their alcoholism. Some 63 percent of the alcoholics had been able to stop drinking using their own willpower for a similar period of six months or longer.

The circumstances of the salvation experience in the two groups were different in that most of the salvation experiences of the

TABLE 5.4. Parents' Beliefs (%)

	Good Character, Good Works	Conservative	None Expressed	Atheist	Agnostic	Deist	Other
Alcoholics							
Father	52	23	6	3	3	6	7
Mother	56	36	3	0	0	6	0
Normals							
Father	26	48	7	0	2	12	5
Mother	19	66	7	3	1	4	2

TABLE 5.5. Parents' Church Attendance (%)

	Regular	More Than Occasional	Occasional	None	Not Expressed	Indeterminate	Not Applicable
Alcoholics							
Father	33	23	21	11	7	0	4
Mother	67	20	10	1	1	1	0
Normals							
Father	43	25	11	13	0	2	7
Mother	56	23	9	3	3	3	3

TABLE 5.6. Occurrence of Salvation (%)

	Salvation Experiences	
	Yes	**No**
Alcoholics	46	54
Normals	75	27
	Twenty-One Years Old at Occurrence of Salvation	
Alcoholics	47	53
Normals	55	45

	Circumstances of Salvation			
	Spontaneous	**Church**	**Revival**	**Other**
Alcoholics	6	46	34	14
Normals	23	23	24	30

alcoholics occurred in church. These were divided between regular church and church evangelistic services and amounted to 80 percent of the conversions. In contrast, only 57 percent of the salvation experiences of the normal subjects occurred in church.

The findings related to the personal aspect of the subjects' faith are shown in Table 5.7. Even though few of the alcoholics were practicing Christians, 80 percent of them held theologically Christian beliefs. On the other hand, 86 percent of the nonalcoholics held these beliefs.

Finally, the alcoholics practiced their beliefs with less frequency than did the normal subjects. The alcoholics did occasionally read the Bible, pray, and bless their food, but the normals were far more active in each of these practices. A very interesting finding was that only 3 percent of the alcoholics had ever publicly shared their faith with others, while more than 50 percent of the normals had done so.

DISCUSSION

The problem of alcoholism is believed to start before adulthood. Maddox[9] determined that individuals in the United States learn to drink during adolescence, and most adolescents are influenced in their

TABLE 5.7. Subjects' Religious Practices (%)

		Bible Reading			
	Daily	**Once per Week**	**Occasionally**	**Never**	**Not Applicable**
Alcoholics	1	14	68	14	1
Normals	40	19	31	10	0

		Prayer			
	Several Times per Day	**Once a Day**	**Occasionally**	**Only in Need**	**Never**
Alcoholics	20	33	15	27	5
Normals	57	15	10	12	7

	Prayer Before Meals		
	Yes	**No**	**NIA***
Alcoholics	57	40	4
Normals	80	19	1

	Public Confession of Faith		
	Yes	**No**	**NIA**
Alcoholics	3	97	0
Normals	56	40	4

	Subjects' Beliefs in Trinity and Eternal Life		
	All	**None**	**Combination**
Alcoholics	80	3	17
Normals	86	3	11

*No information available.

drinking by their family and friends. Kimes et al.[10] confirmed these findings, also demonstrating that one-third of youth are regular imbibers by the age of sixteen. McCord[11] further observed that the relationships of the alcoholic parents with the alcoholic are distorted during his childhood. The mother is often less affectionate than in normal families and the parents often interact differently with their alcoholic child as compared to normal families. McCord's findings were consistent with what we were considering in terms of the religious life of alcoholics.

Indeed, our data document the instability in the alcoholic's early life. Almost nine-tenths of the alcoholics came from socioeconomic classes 4 and 5, whereas in normal families far more of the children came from socioeconomic classes 1 through 3. Fewer than 20 percent of the nonalcoholics came from broken homes, whereas 70 percent of the alcoholics did. Such data can be interpreted to demonstrate that there was far greater discord in parental relationships within the family settings of the alcoholics.

It was in this environment that the mother most frequently attempted to present the religious teaching. Interestingly, she presented to her alcoholic son the necessity of "being good" in a predominantly Southern Baptist or religiously conservative milieu. Theoretically the church was conservative, yet in practice the mother encouraged a much less conservative religious lifestyle. Approximately 50 percent of the alcoholics tried salvation but few found any benefit. Why?

From our data we hypothesize that several factors might be causally related. The first factor is that the church seemed to be an area of unresolved conflict between parents. Sixty-six percent of the alcoholics' mothers participated regularly as opposed to 33 percent of the fathers. In the normal group the difference was much less, with 54 percent of the mothers participating regularly and 43 percent of the fathers. The differences between the mothers' and fathers' participation is noteworthy, for religion should have a goal of healing broken relationships. In the arena of the alcoholic's family, though, the church seemed to support the differences between the alcoholic's mother and father, with a 66 percent versus 33 percent difference. Then also, with 70 percent of the alcoholics coming from broken homes, the alcoholic had not seen the church dealing practically with such important issues as holding the marriage together.

A third point that needs to be made is that although the children were taken to conservative churches, the parents emphasized the more liberal approach to religion. Summing up this section, the church had not practically resolved broken relationships; indeed, it had maintained differences between the alcoholic's mother and father, and lastly it taught a message that was different from the message given to the alcoholic by his parents.

Returning to the salvation experience, almost half of the alcoholics experienced salvation. In addition, a great percentage of those who did so had it in a structured setting. The alcoholic seemed to be seeking more than salvation could really offer. Salvation is a first step, not the only step in terms of religious involvement.

The alcoholics did pray, bless their food, and read the Bible regularly, but they very infrequently shared their faith with others. Yet the alcoholics had a theologic belief that was quite similar to that of the normals. In essence, the alcoholics did not "practice what they preached." Such was not inconsistent with the family setting which they had grown up. In other words, in both the religious life of the alcoholics' parents and the religious life of the alcoholics themselves, there was a lack of syncretizing the theoretical and the practical belief systems.

In contrast to the alcoholics, the control subjects came from homes where there was less separation and divorce. The parents agreed more frequently with each other concerning staying married, religious beliefs, and religious practices. Because of the general atmosphere of the home concerning the church, the normals had an increased or unchanged interest in church at adolescence. There was a much higher incidence of salvation experience than among the alcoholics. We believe the presence of such a high and significant incidence of salvation linked with the very low frequency of psychiatric disorders further substantiates some past observations—that there are mental health benefits attached to the salvation experience.[12-14]

Material derived from the results mentioned could be used to assist the work of AA. If the alcoholic can link up emotionally with a model (an ex-alcoholic) who has abused alcohol and successfully "kicked the habit," this person would be consistent in his beliefs and practices of successfully terminating his relationship with alcohol. Thus the model might be in effect taking on a parental role and consistently supporting the alcoholic in giving up alcohol and discouraging further involvement with it.

CONCLUSION

It appears from the foregoing that the faith to stick to one's beliefs is very important if those beliefs are to be of benefit. This type of faith needs to be one in which the theory is consistent with the practice, with both parents supporting the same belief and practice style. This needs to be reinforced in the early home life and not just in the church. It is also important for the parents to choose a church whose teachings are quite similar to what they themselves are teaching their children.

In this study the alcoholic home lacked (1) parents who had the same religious practices, (2) a synthesis of practical daily living from the religious beliefs and the theoretical constructs of the religious beliefs, (3) a religion that had beneficial effects in the home (e.g., preventing marital separation or divorce), and (4) an agreement between what the parents taught the children religiously and what the church that they attended taught the children religiously.

Thus we found that the alcoholic, coming out of this environment, more frequently than the normal subject rejected his Christian faith in his adolescence, experienced a salvation that had few lasting effects concerning his major problem of alcoholism, and practiced his faith far less regularly than the nonalcoholic, though his theologic beliefs were quite similar.

NOTES

1. Lamere F: What happens to alcoholics. *Am J Psychiatr* 109:673, 1953.

2. Wilson B: The fellowship of Alcoholics Anonymous. *Alcoholism* (pp. 116-124). In Cantanzero E (editor), Springfield, IL, Charles C Thomas, 1968.

3. Coles R: Medical ethics and living a life. *N Engl J Med* 301:444-446, 1979.

4. Beck MN: Christ and psychiatry. *Can Psychiatr Assoc J* 18:335-362, 1973.

5. Vincent MO: Christianity and psychiatry: Rivals or allies? *Can Psychiatr Assoc J* 20:527-532, 1975.

6. Pattison EM: Psychosocial interpretations of exorcism. *J Operational Psychiatry* 8:5-21, 1977.

7. Hollingshead AB, Redlich FC: *Social Class and Mental Illness: A Community Study.* New York, John Wiley and Sons, Inc., 1958, pp. 393-394.

8. *TSAR Users Manual.* Computation Center, Duke University, October 1974.

9. Maddox GL: Drinking prior to college. *The Domesticated Drug: Drinking Among Collegians.* Maddox GL (editor). New Haven, CT, College and University Press, 1970, pp. 107-120.

10. Kimes WT, Smith SC, Mather RE: *Alcohol and Drug Abuse in South Carolina High Schools.* Columbia, South Carolina Department of Education, 1969.

11. McCord J: Etiological factors in alcoholism. *Alcohol* 33:1020-1027, 1972.

12. Wilson WP, Larson DB: The maltreated child grown up. (Unpublished data).

13. Wilson WP: Mental health benefits of religious salvation. *Dis Nerv Syst* 33:382-386, 1972.

14. Nicholi A: A new dimension of the youth culture. *Am J Psychiatry* 131:396-401, 1974.

Chapter 6

Systematic Analysis of Research on Religious Variables in Four Major Psychiatric Journals, 1978-1982

David B. Larson
E. Mansell Pattison
Dan G. Blazer
Abdul R. Omran
Berton H. Kaplan

The authors conducted a systematic analysis of quantitative research on religious variables found in four psychiatric journals between 1978 and 1982. Of the 2,348 psychiatric articles reviewed, fifty-nine included a quantified religious variable. In this research, the religious variable chosen was most often a single static measure of religion rather than multiple dynamic measures. In addition, other available religious research was seldom cited. Comparison with systematic analyses of religious research in psychology and sociology suggests that psychiatric research lacks conceptual and methodological sophistication. The data suggest that the academic knowledge and skills needed to evaluate religion have not been absorbed into the psychiatric domain.

Reprinted, with permission, from *American Journal of Psychiatry* 1986; 143:329-334. Presented in part at a meeting of the Southern Psychiatric Association, Hot Springs, Virginia, October 6-9, 1984, and the 138th annual meeting of the American Psychiatric Association, Dallas, May 18-24, 1985. The authors thank Dr. Barbara Burns, Dana Fennell, and Dr. David Moberg for their help. The views expressed in this paper are those of the authors and do not necessarily reflect those of NIMH.

Religious thought and behavior have moved dramatically into the forefront of American cultural concerns in the past decade. Because such religious concerns are likely to be important to the clinical practice of psychiatry, we have evaluated the theoretical and empirical measures of religion found in the psychiatric literature.

Our approach to this evaluation is based on the sociology of knowledge, which is concerned, in part, with the analysis of the types of information and the diffusion of information between different population sets. First, we were concerned about the disparity between the religious beliefs of psychiatrists and psychologists and the religious beliefs held by the general public. Second, we examined and compared the theoretical and empirical information base for the scientific study of religion in psychiatry and in two other behavioral sciences. For the latter evaluation, we systematically analyzed and compared our findings with those of similar analyses of behavioral science research.[1] Could the disparity between a theistic population and atheistic mental health providers be having an impact on rates of service delivery?

Over the last ten years, national surveys[2-5] have documented the substantial religious orientation of the population of the United States. More than 90 percent of those polled believe in God, more than 40 percent attend religious services weekly or more often, and more than 20 percent perceive religion to be very important in their lives. Therefore, psychiatric understanding of religion in normality and psychopathology seems to be clinically necessary.

A belief in God is less frequently found among psychiatrists or psychologists than in the general public. In a survey of the APA membership[6], 43 percent believed in God. This contrasted sharply with the more than 90 percent of the general public who professed belief. Yet, psychiatrists were far more theistic than psychologists; Ragan et al. (unpublished 1976 paper) found that only 5 percent of the American Psychological Association membership believed in God.

Although mental health professionals infrequently believe in God, their belief, or lack of it, should not influence who consults with them or comes to them for treatment. The few studies done demonstrate otherwise. In further analyzing Kadushin's referral data[7], we found that clergy members referred significantly more often to the religious-psychiatric clinic, while the psychologists and psychiatrists referred more to the psychoanalytic and hospital outpatient clinic

($p < 001$). In addition, if the clergy member was the first contact, the patient more often ended up at the religious-psychiatric clinic, whereas if the psychiatrist or psychologist was the first contact, the patient more often ended up at the psychoanalytic and hospital outpatient clinic ($p < .0001$). Concerning community consultations, psychiatrists providing services to the religious sector more frequently attended church ($p < .001$) and observed religious rituals or ceremonies ($p < .001$) than did those not providing services to the religious sector.[6]

As to who seeks care from mental health professionals, research has shown that those who have no religious beliefs are overutilizers,[8, 9] whereas those with more conservative Protestant beliefs attempt to find a therapist with parallel beliefs.[10]

The presence or absence of theistic beliefs not only influences patient choice about obtaining therapy, it influences therapist choice about obtaining their own personal therapy. Henry et al.[11] and Marx and Spray[12] sampled more than 3,000 mental health professionals, including psychiatrists (psychoanalytic and nonpsychoanalytic), psychologists, and psychiatric social workers. We reanalyzed their data and found that those with theistic beliefs had received therapy much less often than did those with atheistic, agnostic, or no religious beliefs ($p < .0001$). The same result ($p < .0001$) was found when the psychologists and social workers were excluded and only the more than 1,000 psychiatrists were analyzed.

These findings concern us. Previous research[13,14] has demonstrated that many in the U.S. population who need treatment do not obtain it. Since few studies assess how the respondents use both religious practices and mental health professionals to cope with their emotional problems, it becomes difficult to assess how many individuals substitute religious practices for mental health treatment. A recent national survey[2] permits a comparison of those using prayer versus mental health professionals for their emotional problems. Far more prayed than received treatment for their "unhappiness" or "worries." Between 1 percent and 2 percent had used mental health professionals for periods of either unhappiness or worries. On the other hand, prayer had been used by 20 percent to cope with their worries, while 30 percent prayed to cope with unhappiness.

It is also evident that there is a discrepancy between the public and psychiatric populations in the interpretation of religion. First, some of the most visible psychiatric opinions on religion have come from the psychoanalytic genre, perpetuating Freud's complex, contradictory, and confusing interpretations.[15,16] Such interpretation of religion frequently has been criticized as inaccurate because it is conceptually reductionistic.[16,17]

Second, the bulk of clinical psychiatric literature has focused on psychopathological and neurotic uses of religion among psychiatric patients—a skewed sample without a comparison group. The function of religion in normal lives presents different interpretations.[18-20] When the religion of the psychiatrically impaired was contrasted with community controls, the controls more frequently were associated with a church ($p < .01$) and attended church ($p < .01$).[21,22]

Third, compared to the general population, a substantial number of psychotherapists exhibit a model of "religious apostasy," a term coined by Henry et al.[11] Religious apostates grew up in homes holding to theistic beliefs but now profess to be atheistic or agnostic or have no beliefs. Of the more than 3,000 mental health professionals in the Henry et al. study, some 900 (29 percent) had become apostate. The highest rate of apostasy (40 percent) was among psychoanalysts, compared with 26 percent for the nonpsychoanalytic psychiatrists, clinical psychologists, and psychiatric social workers, a significant difference ($p < .0001$).

From 1944 to 1981, the Gallup Poll interviewed Americans a dozen times about their belief in God.[5] In 1944, 96 percent believed in God; in 1981 95 percent believed in God. The mean for the twelve surveys was 96.25 percent with a small standard error of 0.49 percent. Thus, for this thirty-five-year period, there was little change in the proportion of the population with theistic beliefs. Although the secularization thesis has come under much scrutiny in recent research,[23,24] it seems well substantiated among mental health professionals of this generation.

Two further points clarify the trend in the rate of apostasy among mental health professionals. First, if the proportion of those who became apostate was equal to the number of those who converted to theistic beliefs, the rates of theism would be constant, as they are in the general population. But in the Henry et al. study, of the 474 mental health professionals who came from nontheistic homes, only sixty-six (14 percent) had become theistic. This contrasted with the 907 apostates (29 percent) who had come from 3,147 homes ($p < .0001$).

Second, mental health training does not affect the religious beliefs of mental health professionals only. At least two studies[25,26] have shown that clergy who received mental health training became more committed to delivering therapeutic services and less committed to their religious responsibilities.

A number of mental health professionals have been attracted to alternative religious perspectives as represented in Eastern traditions, transcendental psychologies, meditation, and mysticism. This parallels the recent American trend to nontraditional religion termed the "consciousness reformation in America."[27] For both public and psychiatric adherents, this is an arcane religious knowledge, with less than 1 percent of the population adhering to these beliefs.[28]

In contrast, a sizable number of conventionally religious psychiatrists actively promote new approaches to psychiatry based on conventional religion. This approach is proffered as "religious psychiatry," an alternative to "conventional nonreligious psychiatry." In its present state, this is an attempt to reduce discrepant knowledge within a constrained informational base.

This cursory review suggests several important generalizations. First, there is a general disparity of knowledge in the types of perceptions of religion between the two populations. The general public appears to view and value religion as a major factor in their lives, whereas, in general, mental health professionals do not. Second, the public views mental health professionals as unknowing or unappreciative of the role of religion in their own lives (a perception supported by factions of "religious" psychiatrists), whereas many psychiatrists view the religious public as naive, neurotic, or unsophisticated. Third, as a problem in the sociology of knowledge, it appears that the two populations hold different interpretive knowledge bases on religion, and the two populations appear to possess inadequate or distorted information on religious knowledge in the other population.

RELIGIOUS RESEARCH IN PSYCHIATRY AND IN BEHAVIORAL SCIENCE

We turn now to our major concern, for we suggest that, at least for psychiatry, knowledge of religion should be grounded on an adequate conceptual and empirical base.

We examined five issues in our systematic analysis of the psychiatric literature: (1) the frequency of inclusion of religious variables in quantitative psychiatric research; (2) the robustness of statistical analysis; (3) the type of measure of religion used; (4) the conceptual basis for measurement of religion; and (5) awareness of the scientific database on religious research.

We selected four major psychiatric journals: the *American Journal of Psychiatry*, the *British Journal of Psychiatry*, the *Canadian Journal of Psychiatry*, and the *Archives of General Psychiatry* as representatives of current quantitative psychiatric research. We assumed that psychotherapy journals would yield few quantitative studies and that biological journals would yield few religious studies. All issues for the five-year period 1978-1982 were analyzed. A total of 3,777 articles were scanned. All articles without quantitative data were excluded along with seventeen quantitative studies on sects and cults. These seventeen studies were viewed as diverging from the more general considerations of religion in a Western context. After the exclusions, there were 2,348 articles. Of the 2,348 quantitative articles, only fifty-nine papers contained a quantitative religious variable. Of the fifty-nine, three included religion as a major emphasis of the study.[29-31] Thus in the five years reviewed, these four journals included seventeen articles on cults or sects and only three on traditional religious phenomena. We confine our analysis to these fifty-nine articles.

Robustness of data analysis was assessed by comparing the use of descriptive statistics (mean, percentage, standard deviation) versus inferential statistics (z, t, and F tests). Inferential statistics were considered a more robust method of data analysis.

An early measure of religion was a simple denominational denotation such as Protestant, Catholic, or Jewish. This measure is considered "static," since it ignores the diverse range of religious styles and practices within such broad categories. Denomination is currently considered a weak and ineffective measure of religious domain.[32]

Methodologists now prefer the use of more dynamic, "religiosity" measures.[33,34] These assess religious commitment by asking questions about religious beliefs, practices, or attitudes. Consequently, in the studies reviewed, we noted whether one static, denomination question was asked or if the more dynamic, religiosity measure was used. In the case of religiosity, we evaluated whether it was unidimensional, thus a single question, or if it was multidimensional, using more than one question.

We not only assessed if religious measures were denomination or religiosity questions, but we also evaluated if religiosity had been assessed using the state of the art—previously developed multidimensional religiosity scales. In a review that is now more than three years out of date Silverman[35] found 292 religiosity scales, combining at least two questions to arrive at a numerical result. We thus evaluated whether or not research was based on an appreciation of religion as a multifaceted conceptual domain. Religion is not a single measure of practices, beliefs, or attitudes, but a construct of multiple and interactive variables. The most well-known and widely used research categorization of religion is that of Glock and Stark,[36] who defined five dimensions of the religious domain: ideological, intellectual, emotional, sacramental, and consequential. Other categorizations have been recommended since then.[37-40] Therefore, we analyzed each article in terms of whether only one, or two (or more), "religiosity" variables were used to measure religion. This simple dichotomy is the lowest common denominator to infer whether the psychiatric researcher was minimally aware of the conceptual requirement to measure more than one dimension of the religious domain.

We were also interested in the extent to which scientific knowledge of research on religion had diffused into the psychiatric domain. We reviewed each of the fifty-nine articles to determine how many citations were made to religious research. We did not evaluate the relevance of such citations; we again applied the lowest common denominator—at least one reference would indicate greater awareness of the scientific base of religious research; no reference would indicate no awareness of the available religious literature.

RESULTS

First we consider frequency of publication. Of the 3,777 articles published by the four journals over the five-year period, 2,348 included quantitative data: the *American Journal of Psychiatry,* 914 (52.2 percent of all articles published during the period); the *British Journal of Psychiatry,* 637 (77.8 percent); the *Canadian Journal of Psychiatry,* 167 (37.3 percent); and the *Archives of General Psychia-*

try, 630 (83.1 percent). Of the quantitative studies, the American journal published eighteen articles (2.0 percent) including a religious variable, the British journal published nine (2.4 percent), the Canadian journal published eleven (6.6 percent), and *Archives* published twenty-one (3.3 percent). The major finding here is the uniformly low rate of quantitative studies that included at least one religious variable found in journals representative of general psychiatric research. The means ranged from 1.4 percent to 6.6 percent with an overall mean of 2.5 percent (59/2,348). Thus about one in forty quantified articles included at least a single religious measure.

Robustness of statistical analysis in the fifty-nine articles was determined by comparing the use of descriptive versus inferential statistics. For the quantitative articles overall, the ratio of descriptive to inferential statistical was 241/673 for the American journal, 86/551 for the British journal, 60/107 for the Canadian journal, and 65/565 for *Archives,* with less robust, descriptive statistics being used 19 percent of the time. For studies with a religious variable, the ratio was 21/38, with less robust descriptive statistics being used 55 percent of the time. Comparing the use of inferential versus descriptive statistics in the 2,289 articles without religious measures and the fifty-nine articles with religious measures, we found that the less robust descriptive statistics were more often used in the fifty-nine articles ($\chi^2 = 10.40$, df = 1, p < .001).

As to whether religion was assessed with denomination or religiosity questions, thirty-seven studies used denomination, seventeen used religiosity, and five used both types of questions. Regarding the number of religious questions, including both denomination and religiosity questions, forty-nine studies (83 percent) used only one religious question, eight (14 percent) included two questions, and two (3 percent) included three or more religious questions. Of the ten studies having two or more questions about religion, five included a question about denomination and religiosity, while the other five included two or more religiosity questions. Only one study[30] used a previously scaled multidimensional religiosity questionnaire.

In sum, the majority of articles used a single, weak denotative measurement (denomination), while a small proportion used appropriate multiple measures of religiosity.

The conceptual base of psychiatric research on religion might be inferred as inadequate when inappropriate measures are used. Another inferential evaluation is provided by analysis of the number of reference citations to religious research. Of the fifty-nine studies, fifty-one (86 percent) had no such references, two (3 percent) had one reference, and six (10 percent) had two or more. Next, we considered that the failure to use appropriate multiple religiosity measures might reflect ignorance of current research on religion. To test this, we compared the number of religiosity questions items with the number of literature citations. As predicted, the higher the citation rate, the higher the use of multiple religiosity questions ($\chi^2 = 13.96$, df = 2, p < .01). In brief, the low citation rates suggest that current state-of-the-art concepts and methods for research on religion have not diffused into psychiatric research.

Finally, we compared these findings with those of similar systematic analyses of related behavioral sciences journals. Beuhler et al.[41] analyzed research on religion in four major American sociological journals for the eighty-year period 1890-1969, while Capps et al.[42] analyzed fifty journals from the fields of social psychology and psychology for the twenty-five-year period 1950-1974. Although each study used somewhat different methods of systematic analysis, a comparison gives estimates of trends.

As shown in Table 6.1, the rate of publication of research with religiosity variables is markedly lower for psychiatry journals than for other behavioral science journals. In terms of methodology, we compared the use of denomination versus the use of the religiosity measures. Given the years of the three reviews, we expected psychiatry to include more religiosity measures, and psychology and sociology to include more denomination measures. Thus, we were surprised to find that other behavioral science research more often used religiosity measures of religion: sociology versus psychiatry ($\chi^2 = 35.2$, df = 1, p <.0001) and psychology versus psychiatry ($\chi^2 = 290.4$, df = 1, p < .0001). As expected, the psychology review more frequently included denomination measures ($\chi^2 = 11.97$, df = 1, p < .001). Surprisingly, psychiatry more often included denomination measures than did the sociology review ($\chi^2 = 7.95$, df = 1, p < .01). The religiosity-to-denomination ratios for sociology and psychology were much larger than psychiatry's: sociology's ratio was more than four times larger, while psychology's was more than seven times larger. Again, these results suggest that the most recent psychiatric research on religion is

TABLE 6.1. Comparative Analyses of Religious Research in Sociology, Psychology, and Psychiatry

			Number of Religious Studies		
Field	Years of Review	Total	Using Religiosity As Measure of Religion	Using Denomination As Measure of Religion	Religiosity-to-Denomination Ratio
Sociology (41)	1890-1969	9,485	219	100	2.2
Psychology (42)	1950-1974	1,869	242	66	3.7
Psychiatry[a]	1978-1982	2,348	22	42	0.5

[a]Five studies included both denomination and religiosity questions and, thus, were counted twice under the religiosity and denomination columns.

118

not consonant with less recent comparable research in other behavioral sciences.

To conclude, the overall results of our systematic analysis indicate that quantitative psychiatric research including religiosity has an absolute and relative low frequency rate when compared to other behavioral science research, uses methodologically inadequate measures of religion, and lacks appropriate use of current conceptual approaches to religious research.

DISCUSSION

We raise two issues for consideration. First, why does psychiatric research so infrequently consider religious variables, and when it does, why is the methodology so inadequate? Second, what implications, if any, do these results have for the field of psychiatry?

Several alternative explanations for our results are possible. First, these results could reflect an unusual distribution of quantitative research on religion in psychiatric journals for the years of our sample. However, other major literature reviews on religious research[43-46] do not support this. Second, the journals chosen may be unrepresentative in their rank of publication of quantitative religious research in psychiatric research journals. However, our combined knowledge of psychiatric journals does not suggest this to be the case.

As a third alternative, we suggest simply that psychiatric researchers are for the most part ill-informed about research on religious variables. This stands in juxtaposition to the current spate of very sophisticated psychosocial research studies on religion found in other behavioral science journals. The reasons for this discrepancy may be explained by information derived from Pattison's recent literature review.[47,48]

First, we note that religion is a highly salient variable in the theoretical structure of most behavioral science. Therefore, the other behavioral sciences have developed sophisticated conceptual and methodological approaches to the scientific study of religion. On the other hand, religion has a minimal place in psychiatric theory of human behavior. As a gross generalization, religion is viewed as a secondary derivative of structural psychic process. Therefore, we might expect psychiatric research to ignore state of the art research on religion if it is viewed as theoretically unimportant.

Second, although in general, behavioral scientists are much less religious than is the general population, their own personal valuation of religion does not preclude recognition of the importance of religion in human behavior. But to understand this will require knowledge, both theoretical and empirical, to explicate the functions of religion. On the other hand, the personal valuation of religion by psychiatrists may substantially affect their knowledge base. The data presented support this position. If psychiatrists do not personally value religion, they may conclude that knowledge of religion in general and knowledge of religion in their patients is irrelevant. Or, in the case of personally religious psychiatrists, they may approach knowledge of religion solely from their own idiosyncratic religious values.

We suggest that the clinical practice of psychiatry is ill-served by the current inadequacies in the psychiatric literature. Psychiatrists, without religious beliefs or ambivalent about their beliefs, in perusing the psychiatric literature may be reinforced in their belief that knowledge of religion is irrelevant and may thereby misinterpret the religious dynamics, whether healthy or harmful, of their patients' lives. For the religious psychiatrists, the same literature provides little demand to broaden *their* religious knowledge base beyond their sectarian personal knowledge; thus, they are just as liable to misinterpret their patients' religious dynamics.

Finally, in constructing a scientific base for understanding human behavior, research on religion cannot ignore the applicable research literatures that are available and far better developed in neighboring disciplines. In the case at hand, there appears to be little diffusion of theory and method articulated in behavioral science research on religion into psychiatric research. At a theoretical level, other behavioral sciences approach religion as both independent and dependent variables associated with both emotional illness and health. Psychiatry usually approaches religion as an independent variable, associated with a psychiatric disease outcome; it seldom assesses religion as a dependent variable. In addition, psychiatry knows little of the benefits of religion, since it seldom assesses it either as an independent variable in association with emotional health or as a dependent variable of a psychotherapeutic or psychosocial intervention. This has resulted in substantially different conclusions. For example, in its crassest form, psychiatry views religion as neurotic, immature, or a solace for the mentally disturbed. This is at variance with empirical generalizations from other psychosocial research which demonstrate that the mentally ill are less religious and engage in less religious activity, whereas the psychologically healthy are more religious and engage in more religious activities.[21, 22, 49-51]

We consider this state of affairs unfortunate. It is likely to continue the misinterpretations of religious knowledge between the public and psychiatry. It is likely to breed the proliferation of "religious brands" of psychiatric practice devoid of a sophisticated appreciation of the conceptual and empirical knowledge linking both psychiatry and religion. And it will likely perpetuate the disparity of the knowledge base between psychiatry and the other behavioral sciences.

The central issue raised here is trenchantly stated in a recent editorial in the *Chronicle of Higher Education:*

> The academic study of religion is not the practice of religion. . . . Religion has always been there, informing our self-understanding, our values, and our public life. It will always be there. The question is whether we will remain vulnerable to its abuse or will acquire the fundamental knowledge and skills to evaluate it.[52]

In summary, this analysis of psychiatric research reveals a considerable lag in the diffusion of academic knowledge and skills to evaluate religion in psychiatric theory, concept, and methodology.

NOTES

1. Light RU, Pillemer DB: *Summing Up: The Science of Reviewing Research.* Cambridge, MA, Harvard University Press, 1984.

2. Veroff J, Douvan E, Kulka R: *The Inner American.* New York, Basic Books, 1981.

3. Hadaway CL: Life satisfaction and religion: A re-analysis. *Social Forces* 57:636-643, 1978.

4. *The Connecticut Mutual Life Report on American Values in the Eighties.* Hartford, CT, Connecticut Mutual Life Insurance Co., 1981.

5. Gallup G: *Religion in America—50 Years: 1935-1985.* The Gallup Report. Princeton, NJ, Princeton Religious Research Center, 1985.

6. American Psychiatric Association Task Force Report 10: *Psychiatrists' Viewpoints on Religion and Their Services to Religious Institutions and the Ministry.* Washington, DC, APA, 1975.

7. Kadushin C: *Why People Go to Psychiatrists.* New York, Atherton Press, 1969.

8. Tischler GL, Henisz JE, Myers JK, et al.: Utilization of mental health services, I: Patienthood and the prevalence of symptomatology in the community. *Arch Gen Psychiatry* 32:411-415, 1975.

9. Greenley JR, Mechanic D: Social selection in seeking help for psychological problems. *J Health Soc Behav* 17:249-262, 1976.

10. King RR: Evangelical Christians and professional counseling: A conflict of values. *J Psychology and Theology* 6:276-281, 1978.

11. Henry WE, Simms JH, Spray SL: *The Fifth Profession: Becoming a Psychotherapist.* San Francisco, Jossey-Bass, 1971.

12. Marx JH, Spray SL: Psychotherapeutic "birds of a feather": Social class status and religio-cultural value homophily in the mental health field. *J Health Soc Behav* 13:413-428, 1972.

13. Regier DA, Goldberg ID, Taube CA: The de facto U.S. mental health services system. *Arch Gen Psychiatry* 35:685-693, 1978.

14. Shapiro S, Skinner EA, Kessler LG, et al.: Utilization of health and mental health services: Three epidemiologic catchment area sites. *Arch Gen Psychiatry* 41:971-978, 1984.

15. Meissner WW: *Psychoanalysis and Religious Experience.* New Haven, CT, Yale University Press, 1984.

16. Küng H: *Freud and the Problem of God.* New Haven, CT, Yale University Press, 1984.

17. Berger PL: *The Heretical Imperative: Contemporary Possibilities of Religious Affirmation.* Garden City, NY. Anchor Press, 1979.

18. James W: *The Varieties of Religious Experience.* London, Collier Macmillan, 1961.

19. Allport G: *The Individual and His Religion.* New York, Macmillan, 1950.

20. Pattison EM: *Clinical Psychiatry and Religion.* Boston, Little, Brown, 1969.

21. Lindenthal JJ et al.: Mental status and religious behavior. *J for the Scientific Study of Religion* 9:143-149, 1970.

22. Stark R: Psychopathology and religious commitment. *Review of Religious Research* 12:165-176, 1971.

23. Caplow T, Bahr HM, Chadwick BA, et al.: *All Faithful People: Change and Continuity in Middletown's Religion.* Minneapolis, University of Minnesota Press, 1983.

24. Hammond PE (Ed.): *The Sacred in a Secular Age: Toward Revision in the Scientific Study of Religion.* Berkeley, University of California Press, 1985.

25. Houck JB, Moss DM: Pastoral psychotherapy: The fee-for service model and professional identity. *J of Religion and Health* 16:172-182, 1977.

26. Florell JL: After fifty years: Analysis of the national American clinical pastoral education questionnaire 1975. *J Pastoral Care* 19:221-232, 1975.

27. Glock CY, Bellah RN (Eds.): *The New Religious Consciousness.* Berkeley, University of California Press, 1976.

28. Johnston RL: *Religion in Society: A Sociology of Religion,* Second Edition. Englewood Cliffs, NJ, Prentice-Hall, 1983.

29. Shaver P, Lenauer M, Sadd S: Religiousness, conversion, and subjective well-being: The "healthy-minded" religion of modern American women. *Am J Psychiatry* 137:1563-1568, 1980.

30. Hellman RE, Green R, Gray JL, et al.: Childhood sexual identity, childhood religiosity, and "homophobia" as influences in the development of transsexualism, homosexuality, and heterosexuality. *Arch Gen Psychiatry* 38:910-915, 1981.

31. Pattison EM, Pattison ML: "Ex-gays": Religiously mediated change in homosexuals. *Am J Psychiatry* 137:1553-1562, 1980.

32. Harrison MH, Lazerwitz B: Do denominations matter? *AJS* 88:356-377, 1984.

33. Gorsuch RL: Measurement: The boon and bane of investigating religion. *Am Psychol* 39:228-236, 1984.

34. Himmelfarb H: Measuring religious involvement. *Social Forces* 53:606-618, 1975.

35. Silverman W: *Bibliography of Measurement Techniques Used in the Social Scientific Study of Religion.* Psychological Documents 13:7. Washington, DC, American Psychological Association, 1983.

36. Glock CY, Stark R: *Religion and Society in Tension.* Chicago, Rand McNally, 1965.

37. Roof WC: Concepts and indicators of religious commitment: A critical review, in *The Religious Dimension: New Directions in Quantitative Research.* Edited by Wuthnow R. New York, Academic Press, 1979.

38. Davidson JD, Knudsen DD: A new approach to religious commitment. *Sociological Focus* 10:151-172, 1977.

39. Spilka B, Shaver P, Kirkpatrick LA: A general attribution theory for the psychology of religion. *J for the Scientific Study of Religion* 24:1-20, 1985.

40. Spilka B, Hood RW, Gorsuch RL: *The Psychology of Religion: An Empirical Approach.* Englewood Cliffs, NJ, Prentice-Hall, 1985.

41. Buehler C, Hesser G, Weigert A: A study of articles on religion in major sociology journals. *J for the Scientific Study of Religion* 11:165-170,1973.

42. Capps D, Ransohoff P, Rambo L: Publication trends in the psychology of religion to 1974. *J for the Scientific Study of Religion* 15:15-28, 1976.

43. Berkowitz ML, Johnson JE: *Social Scientific Studies of Religion: A Bibliography.* Pittsburgh, University of Pittsburgh Press, 1967.

44. Capps D, Rambo L, Ransohoff P: *Psychology of Religion: An Annotated Bibliography.* Detroit, MI, Gale Research Publications, 1976.

45. Meissner WW: *Annotated Bibliography on Religion and Psychology.* New York, Academy of Religion and Mental Health, 1961.

46. *Religion and Mental Health: A Bibliography.* DHHS Publication No. 80-964. Washington, DC, National Institute of Mental Health, 1980.

47. Pattison EM: Psychiatry and religion circa 1978: Analysis of a decade, part I. *Pastoral Psychology* 27:8-25, 1978.

48. Pattison EM: Psychiatry and religion circa 1978: Analysis of a decade, part II. *Pastoral Psychology* 28:119-141, 1978.

49. Hadaway CK, Roof WC: Religious commitment and the quality of life in American Society. *Review of Religious Research* 12:165-176, 1971.

50. Bergin AE: Religiosity and mental health: A critical re-evaluation and meta-analysis. *Professional Psychology: Research and Practice* 14:170-184, 1983.

51. McCready WC, Greeley AM: *The Ultimate Values of the American Population.* Sage Library of Social Research, Vol. 23. Beverly Hills, CA, Sage Publications, 1976.

52. Rue LD: Our most outrageous blind spot: The academic study of religion. *Chronicle of Higher Education* 29:40, 1985.

Chapter 7

Religious Affiliations in Mental Health Research Samples As Compared with National Samples

David B. Larson
Michael J. Donahue
John S. Lyons
Peter L. Benson
Mansell Pattison
Everett L. Worthington Jr.
Dan G. Blazer

Religious affiliations of patients in research samples in four major psychiatric journals for the years 1978 to 1982 were compared with those reported in national samples. Protestants and the unaffiliated were underrepresented, whereas Jewish persons were overrepresented. Catholics used mental health services in proportions similar to their presence in the population at large. These findings suggest that religious affiliation may influence the use of mental health services.

Inclusion of religion as a variable of study in recent psychiatric research is rare, occurring in about 2 percent of studies, as assessed in a 1986 publication by Larson et al. (1986). The few studies that do include a religious variable generally use religious affiliation as a single measure (Campbell and Coles, 1973). This easy-to-use variable, although far from adequate for capturing the dynamics of religion in a person's emotional life, does have some clinical utility.

Reprinted, with permission, from *Journal of Nervous and Mental Disease* 1989; 177:109-111, copyright Lippincott Williams & Wilkins.

Two findings highlight the importance of religious affiliation in mental health research. First, several studies have shown that people with a religious affiliation suffer fewer psychiatric disorders than do people with no affiliation (Lindenthal et al., 1970; Stark, 1971). Second, different religious groups appear to present somewhat different clinical profiles (MacDonald and Luckett, 1983). That is, Protestants, Catholics, and Jews present different diagnostic profiles, and variations among specific denominational groups have been reported (MacDonald and Luckett, 1983).

There are few data documenting the varying proportions of individuals' different religious denominations in mental health services or psychiatric research. Likewise, there is no information concerning the representativeness of these samples in terms of religious affiliation of the general population of the United States. Therefore, the current review attempts to establish the rate of inclusion of various religious affiliations in psychiatric research published in the last several years.

METHOD

The distribution of four religious groups sampled in studies published in two broad-based psychiatric journals, *The American Journal of Psychiatry* and *The Archives of General Psychiatry,* between 1978 and 1982 was determined. Religious affiliation was categorized as follows: Catholic, Jewish, Protestant, and Other/None. These categories were chosen because they represent the most frequent affiliations found among the studies. This distribution was then compared with distributions established by national surveys.

Similar to what was found in a previous review (Larson et al., 1986), only eighteen, or less than 1 percent of the 2,510 empirical studies published in the two journals from 1978 to 1982, included a measure of religious affiliation. Three of these studies focused on the religious affiliation of psychiatric professionals and were thus excluded. It is the remaining fifteen patient samples that comprise the present population.

Of these fifteen studies, seven sampled directly from the community, whereas eight sampled from either inpatient or outpatient psychiatric populations. Three national surveys done at approximately the same time as the period reviewed were used to provide estimations of the four religious groups in the general population (Gallup, 1985; Connecticut Mutual Life Report, 1981; Veroff, Douvan, and Kulka, 1981).

The distributions were calculated using mean percentages across studies, rather than by decomposing the percentages into their corresponding numerators and denominators and recalculating weighted overall percentages. This is a method consistent with the recommendations of Glass, McGaw, and Smith (1981) for meta-analyses of different datasets. Standard errors were also reported, since they were used in later calculations of statistics (Snedecor and Cochran, 1967).

RESULTS

Data on the distribution of the four religious groups in the fifteen studies are presented in Table 7.1 along with the proportions from the national surveys. In both the psychiatric and the community studies, Protestants are underrepresented, Jews are overrepresented, and Catholics appear in proportion to their distribution in the national surveys. Interestingly, the other/none respondents are overrepresented in the psychiatric population studies, but not in the community studies.

DISCUSSION

The results of the present review indicate that the samples in psychiatric research vary from population norms found in national sur-

TABLE 7.1. Comparison of Psychiatric Patient and Community Population Studies with Three National Surveys Assessing Religious Denomination

Sample	Catholic Percentage		Jewish Percentage		Protestant Percentage		Other/None Percentage	
	Mean	SE	Mean	SE	Mean	SE	Mean	SE
Community	25.5	4.9	13.0[a]	4.0	49.8[a]	7.8	13.5	5.5
Psychiatric	34.5[b]	6.7	14.8[a]	3.4	32.1[b]	3.9	23.4[b]	3.8
National Survey	27.0	1.7	2.5	0.2	62.0	1.9	9.1	0.5

[a]Significantly different from national sample, $z > 3.5$, p. $< .001$.
[b]Significantly different from national sample, $z > 2.0$, p. $< .05$.

veys in regard to religious affiliation. The overrepresentation of Jewish subjects in psychiatric research is not uncommon (Greenley and Mechanic, 1976; Kadushin, 1969; Marx and Spray, 1972). One plausible explanation is that individuals of the Jewish faith are overrepresented as mental health care providers, so that potential Jewish clients may feel greater ease in approaching mental health care professionals than individuals of other religio-ethnic backgrounds (Bergin, 1980; Marx and Spray, 1972). Another plausible explanation is that the studies reviewed were concentrated on populations in urban areas, where the presence of Jewish respondents is disproportionate to their national presence. More recent and representative samples, such as the carefully sampled Epidemiologic Catchment Area studies (Blazer et al., 1985) show higher proportions of Protestants and lower proportions of Jews.

The underrepresentation of Protestants is also a common finding (Kadushin, 1969) and may be related to a perceived lack of congruence between psychotherapeutic and Christian worldviews, especially for the more theological conservatives (Bergin, 1980; Worthington and Gascoyne, 1985). The representative presence of Catholics is a finding that contradicts earlier work (Argyle and Beit-Hallahmi, 1975).

The distribution of the other/none category is less straightforward. This category is highly overrepresented in the psychiatric population, but much less so in the community sample than in the psychiatric sample. Although this finding is congruent with other reports (Greenley and Mechanic, 1976; Marx and Spray, 1972) there are exceptions (Vernon, 1968). Campbell (1972) may shed some light on the large number of other/none subjects in psychiatric patient samples by noting that psychiatric patients are often highly involved in humanistic alternative ideological groups that are religious in function, but not in name.

In a prior study of psychiatric research (Larson et al., 1986), we documented the paucity of religious variables and the use of weak or simplistic measures of religion. In this study, we have documented that the sample of subjects represented in psychiatric research does not generally reflect populations trends. These estimates should be stable, as they are based on fifteen different studies that represent a total of 23,887 subjects. It should be noted that a significant proportion of the total sample of the two studies was included in two studies, one a community population ($N = 7,081$) and one a psychiatric population ($N = 9,024$).

Since there are no differences between the community and psychiatric samples in their distributions of members of the Protestant and Jewish faiths, it is reasonable to assume that these differences from the national surveys represent a sampling bias in psychiatric research. The fact that the psychiatric sample was different from the national sample, but that the community sample was not on the percentage of other/ none, may well relate the relationship of this category to either the etiology of mental illness or the utilization of mental health services.

Future research intended to elucidate the role of religion in mental health and illness must begin by using more sophisticated measures of religious identification than the four-category description presently used. This gross lumping obscures more than it clarifies. Protestants are an obvious melange. The simple label "Catholic" does not reveal the ever-growing theological diversity of people who describe themselves as such. Among those of the Jewish faith, the differences among Orthodox, Conservative, and Reform are substantial (Harrison and Lazerwitz, 1984). Included under the label "other," we find large and devout sects such as those of the Mormons and Jehovah's Witnesses, individuals who have constructed some private belief system, a variety of Eastern religion followers, and many others. Lastly, many who claim no affiliation may endorse a subset of traditional beliefs while professing no formal religious affiliation (Vernon, 1968).

In sum, significant differences in religious affiliation occur between psychiatric samples and national surveys. Although the meaning of these differences is not yet clear to the degree that religious affiliation influences critical variables in any psychiatric research, the generalizability of that research depends on the appropriateness of the sample.

REFERENCES

Argyle M, Beit-Hallahmi B (1975). *The social psychology of religion.* London: Routledge and Kegan Paul.

Bergin AE (1980). Psychotherapy and religious values. *J Consult Clin Psychol* 48:635-639.

Blazer D, George LK, Landerman R, et al. (1985). Psychiatric disorders: A rural/urban comparison. *Arch Gen Psychiatry* 42:65- 656.

Campbell C (1972). *Toward a sociology of irreligion.* New York: Herder and Herder.

Campbell D, Coles RW (1973) Religiosity, religious affiliation, and religious belief: The exploration of a typology. *Rev Religious Res* 14:151-158.

The Connecticut Mutual Life Insurance report on American values in the eighties (1981). Hartford, CT: Connecticut Mutual Life Insurance Company.

Gallup G (1985). *Religion in America—50 years: 1935-1985.* The Gallup Report. Princeton, NJ: Princeton Religious Research Center.

Glass GV, McGaw B, Smith ML (1981). *Meta-analysis in social research.* Beverly Hills, CA: Sage.

Greenley JR, Mechanic D (1976). Social selection in seeking help for psychological problems. *J Health Soc Behav* 13:249-262.

Harrison MI, Lazerwitz B (1984). Do denominations matter? *Am. J Sociol* 88:356-377.

Kadushin C (1969). *Why people go to psychiatrists.* New York: Atherton.

Larson DB, Pattison M, Blazer DG, et al. (1986) Systematic analysis of research on religious variables in four major psychiatric journals, 1978-1982. *Am. J Psychiatry* 143:329-334.

Lindenthal JJ, Myers JK, Pepper MP, et al. (1970). Mental status and religious behavior. *J Scientific Study Religion* 9:143-149.

MacDonald CB, Luckett JB (1983). Religious affiliation and psychiatric diagnosis. *J Scientific Study Religion* 22:15-37.

Marx JH, Spray SL (1972). Psychotherapeutic "birds of a feather": Social class status and religio-cultural value homophily in the mental health field. *J Health Social Behav* 13:413-428.

Snedecor GW, Cochran WG (1967). *Statistical Methods* (Sixth Edition). Ames: The Iowa State University Press.

Stark R (1971). Psychopathology and religious commitment. *Rev Religious Res* 12:165-176.

Vernon GM (1968). The religious "nones." *J Scientific Study Religion* 7:219-229.

Veroff J, Douvan E, Kulka R (1981). *The inner American.* New York: Basic.

Worthington EL Jr, Gascoyne SR (1985). Preferences of Christians and non-Christians for five Christian counselors' treatment plans: A partial replication and extension. *J Psychol Theol* 13:29-41.

Chapter 8

Associations Between Dimensions of Religious Commitment and Mental Health Reported in the *American Journal of Psychiatry* and *Archives of General Psychiatry:* 1978-1989

David B. Larson
Kimberly A. Sherrill
John S. Lyons
Frederic C. Craigie Jr.
Samuel B. Thielman
Mary A. Greenwold
Susan S. Larson

The authors assessed all measures of religious commitment (N = 139) reported in research studies published in the American Journal of Psychiatry *and* Archives of General Psychiatry *in 1978 through 1989 (N < 35). For nearly two-thirds of the measures, the studies either made no hypotheses or reported no results concerning the relationship of religious commitment to mental health status. For the great majority of the measures assessed, the studies reported a positive relationship between religious commitment and mental health.*

Reprinted, with permission, from *American Journal of Psychiatry* 1992; 149:557-559. Presented at the annual meeting of the Southern Psychiatric Association, Fort Lauderdale, Florida, October 2-6, 1991. The views expressed in this article are those of the authors and do not necessarily represent the views of NIMH or the U.S. Department of Health and Human Services.

There is evidence that religious practices and beliefs are under-studied phenomena in clinical fields such as psychiatry[1] and family medicine.[2] When religion has been studied, it has usually been assessed by using a static measure—denominational affiliation. Psychiatric studies seldom contain variables reflecting religious commitment, such as measures of religious experience, belief, attitudes, or practice.[1]

Studies concerning dimensions of religious commitment have emphasized its multidimensional nature,[1-4] including meaning, ceremony and sacramental activities, social support, and relationship with the deity.[5] Each of these religious dimensions might have positive or negative relationships to various aspects of clinical status. For instance, there have been some reports of negative or harmful associations between religious commitment and mental health,[6] but other reports have detailed positive or beneficial effects.[4, 7-10]

A systematic review by Bergin[3] took an important step in clarifying the association between religiousness and mental health. Not only did Bergin find little relationship between religiousness and psychopathology, he also found that religious commitment had a positive association with mental health in nearly half (47 percent) of the study effects tabulated. In contrast, associations with mental health were neutral in 30 percent and negative in less than one-fourth (23 percent) of the tabulated associations.

A recent review by Gartner et al.[8] revealed several interesting trends in research on the relationship between religious commitment and psychopathology or mental health. Most of the studies assessing nonclinical populations (e.g., college students) that used measures of psychopathology not based on psychiatric nosology found religion to have either a neutral or harmful role more often than a positive role. In contrast, studies assessing clinical populations that used measures based on psychiatric nosology found religious commitment to have a beneficial role more often than a harmful role. In addition, studies that included measures of religious practice found religiousness to be associated with mental health benefits more often than did studies including measures of religious attitudes.

Our current study was undertaken to follow up the findings of the review of the field of psychology[3] and the review of the combined mental health field[8] and to provide for psychiatry a state-of-the-art review of associations between religious commitment and mental health. The review entailed the systematic assessment[1, 2] of all religious commitment variables found in research studies published in the two leading psychiatry journals over a twelve-year period. Using the method of Craigie et al.,[10] we determined whether positive, negative, or neutral associations between mental health and religion were found, hypothesized, or reported. We also tabulated the associations and classified them according to the typology of religious dimensions used by Craigie et al.[10]

METHOD

The first step was to locate all quantified religious measures found in research studies published in the *American Journal of Psychiatry* and *Archives of General Psychiatry* in 1978 through 1989. Each religious measure was then categorized into one of the following religious dimensions: (1) ceremony (participation in religious ceremonies, sacraments, or rituals), (2) meaning (personal purpose, values, beliefs, and ethics), (3) social support (use or influence of social support), (4) prayer (prayer or personal religious devotional practices), and (5) relationship with God (issues concerning a personal relationship with God). Because of the ambiguous nature of the remaining measures, a sixth category termed "indeterminate" (e.g., use of the term "religion" or "religiosity" with no further specification) was developed. Measures of denomination were excluded because of their differences with measures of religious commitment.[1, 2, 9, 10] Finally, each religious measure was evaluated to discern whether the research study hypothesized a positive or a negative association between religious commitment and mental health and whether a positive, negative, or neutral result was reported.

Interrater reliability was sufficient across all ratings. Using a kappa coefficient, we found that the reliability of all ratings of the association between religious commitment and mental health was 0.89. The reliability for all hypothesized associations between religious commitment and mental health was 0.82, but it was slightly higher—0.93—for all reported associations between religious commitment and mental health. The reliability kappa for ceremony was 0.82; for meaning, 0.82; for social support, 0.82; for prayer, 0.90; for relationship with God, 0.78; and for the indeterminate dimension, 0.76.

RESULTS

In 1978-1989, all quantified studies in the *American Journal of Psychiatry* and *Archives of General Psychiatry* (N < 35) contained 139 quantified religious commitment measures. Table 8.1 presents the number of measures for which positive or negative associations between mental health and six dimensions of religious commitment were hypothesized, the number of measures for which the hypothesis regarding these associations were not specified, the number of measures for which positive, negative, or neutral associations were reported, and the number of measures for which the association was not tested. Only thirty (22 percent) of the 139 measures were in studies that hypothesized results concerning religion, and only twelve of these were in studies that later tested the given hypothesis. All seven of the twenty-one associations that were expected to be positive and were tested turned out to be positive. Five of the nine associations that were expected to be negative were tested, and four of these turned out to be negative.

Although only twelve of the thirty studies with an a priori hypothesis reported an association between religious commitment and mental health, an additional thirty-eight reported such an association even though no hypothesis was given. Thus, for only fifty (36 percent) of the 139 measures the study reported an association between religious commitment and mental health. Of these fifty, thirty-six (72 percent) of the associations were positive, eight (16 percent) were negative, and six (12 percent) were neutral. As for the dimensional findings, four of the six dimensions (ceremony, social support, prayer, and relationship with God) had uniformly positive, or beneficial, associations (twenty-four of twenty-six, or 92 percent). The remaining two religious dimensions—meaning and the indeterminate dimension—accounted for seven of the eight negative findings and five of the six neutral findings.

DISCUSSION

Consistent with several reviews, the present study found that when a religious variable is studied, it often has a positive association with measures of health[4,10] or mental health.[3, 8] Quite similar to the findings of the family medicine review,[10] the dimensions of ceremony,

TABLE 8.1. Associations Between Dimensions of Religious Commitment and Mental Health Reported in the *American Journal of Psychiatry* and *Archives of General Psychiatry: 1978-1989*

| Dimension of Religious Commitment | Number of Measures Assessing Dimension of Religious Commitment | | | | | | |
| | Hypothesis of Study | | | Results of Study | | | |
	Positive Association	Negative Association	None	Positive Association	Negative Association	Neutral Association	Association Not Tested
Ceremony	2	0	11	4	0	0	9
Meaning	3	5	34	7	4	0	31
Social support	11	1	13	7	0	1	17
Prayer	3	0	13	4	1	0	11
Relationship with God	1	0	14	9	0	0	6
Indeterminate	1	3	24	5	3	5	15
Total	21	9	109	36	8	6	89

social support, prayer, and relationship with God, although seldom assessed, were all found to have positive associations with mental health. More studies clarifying the clinical role of these dimensions, similar to recent studies by Pressman et al.[7] and Williams et al.,[9] are needed.

The dimension of meaning appears to have a greater potential for negative associations. This finding is consistent with the reported research in family medicine,[10] where only one of fifteen studies including this dimension found a positive association with clinical status. Future studies including the dimension of religious meaning need to pay greater attention to precisely defining and accurately measuring religious meaning as well as to evaluating both the negative and the positive effects of this dimension. Given previous research concerning the clinical benefits of religious practices,[4, 7-10] a next step would be to look at the associations between clinical variables and high levels of religious meaning combined with low levels of religious practice. For example, subjects attesting to a high meaningfulness of religion but not attending religious services could experience this incongruity as personal conflict, which would result in a negative mental health effect.

That the indeterminate or ambiguous measurement of religion is associated with most of the neutral findings should not be surprising. Inadequate measurement is generally associated with unreliability and the probability of deflated correlations.[11]

What is perhaps most surprising is that in the majority of cases in which a religious variable was specified, there were no reported efforts either to formulate hypotheses or to test the association between religious measures and mental health. For only thirty (22 percent) of the 139 measures was a hypothesis specified. Of these thirty, only twelve (40 percent) reported the results. For only fifty (36 percent) of the 139 religious measures did the study report findings concerning associations between religious measures and mental health.

Although one can only speculate why the majority of studies neglected to present associations, one possible explanation is that associations were tested, found to be neutral, and, because of their "no effect" status, not reported. Another explanation is that the associations were simply not tested. Unfortunately, in the case of nearly two-thirds of the measures, the studies failed to report any associations whatsoever—whether neutral, positive, or negative—thus leaving important research information for an underdeveloped field of study unaddressed.

In summary, the findings of the present review suggest that religious commitment is a clinically relevant, multidimensional phenomenon with the potential for frequent beneficial and occasional harmful mental health effects. Future research efforts concerning how religious commitment influences mental health status require improvements in research methods. Improvements should include (1) the specification of a priori hypotheses, (2) the accurate measurement of the relevant dimension of religious commitment, and (3) the presentation of the study results concerning the association of religious commitment and mental health status. These improvements are necessary if the next steps are to be taken in this previously neglected but promising area of psychiatric research.

NOTES

1. Larson DB, Pattison EM, Blazer DG, Omran AR, Kaplan BH: Systematic analysis of research on religious variables in four major psychiatric journals, 1978-1982. *Am J Psychiatry* 1986; 143:329-334.

2. Craigie FC Jr, Liu IY, Larson DB, Lyons JS: A systematic analysis of religious variables in *The Journal of Family Practice,* 1976-1986. *J Fam Pract* 1988; 27:509-513.

3. Bergin AE: Religiosity and mental health: A critical reevaluation and meta-analysis. *Professional Psychology: Research and Practice* 1983; 14:170-184.

4. Levin JS, Schiller PL: Is there a religious factor in health? *J Religion and Health* 1987; 26:9-36.

5. Garrett WR: Reference groups and role strain related to spiritual well-being. *Social Analysis* 1979; 40:43-58.

6. Ellis A: Psychotherapy and atheistic values: A response to AE Bergin's "Psychotherapy and Religious Values." *J Consult Clin Psychol* 1980; 48:635-639.

7. Pressman P, Lyons JS, Larson DB, Strain JJ: Religious belief, depression, and ambulation status in elderly women with broken hips. *Am J Psychiatry* 1990; 147:758-760.

8. Gartner J, Larson DB, Allen GO: Religious commitment and mental health: A review of the empirical literarure. *J Psychol Theology* 1991; 19:6-25.

9. Williams DR, Larson DB, Buckler RE, Heckmann RC, Pyle CM: Religion and psychological distress in a community sample. *Soc Sci Med* 1991; 32:1257-1262.

10. Craigie FC, Larson DB, Liu IY: References to religion in *The Journal of Family Practice. J Fam Pract* 1990; 30:477-480.

11. Lipsey MW: A scheme for assessing measurement sensitivity in program evaluation and other applied research. *Psychol Bull* 1983; 94:152-165.

Chapter 9

Religious Content in the DSM-III-R Glossary of Technical Terms

David B. Larson
Samuel B. Thielman
Mary A. Greenwold
John S. Lyons
Stephen G. Post
Kimberly A. Sherrill
Glenn G. Wood
Susan S. Larson

The authors reviewed Appendix C of DSM-III-R, Glossary of Technical Terms, for its references to religion. Religion was referred to more frequently in this glossary than it is in psychiatric research. The authors conclude that although the Glossary uses religion in constructive or cautionary reminders, the high rate of illustrative case examples of psychopathology that involve religion in the Glossary indicates cultural insensitivity in interpreting religion.

Population surveys during the last fifty years consistently show that religious beliefs and practices are common in U.S. society.[1] Beginning with Freud,[2] however, psychiatry's view of religious commitment has been, at best, indifferent. Mental health workers main-

Reprinted, with permission, from *American Journal of Psychiatry* 1993; 150:1884-1885. Presented at the annual meeting of the Southern Psychiatric Association, Fort Lauderdale, Florida, October 2-6, 1991. Points of view or opinions expressed in this paper are those of the authors and should not be construed as representing the official position or policy of the U.S. Department of Health and Human Services or any office therein.

tain beliefs that are generally much less theistic than those of the rest of the U.S. population.[3]

In a systematic review of the leading psychiatric journals,[3] we found that religion variables were often excluded from psychiatric research: less than 1 percent of the studies we reviewed included any quantified measurement of religious commitment. We also found that psychiatry rarely has used state-of-the-art, multidimensional assessments of religion, including measures of religious beliefs, attitudes, and practices. Less than a quarter of the studies assessing religion hypothesized a result, and less than a third with a religious hypothesis included a study result.[3,4] Because religion has remained on the periphery of professional interest, psychiatrists have been unaware of the generally beneficial association religion has with mental health status.[4]

In addition, psychiatry has placed little emphasis on religion in clinical care[3,5,6] and education.[7,8] Given the lack of attention given to religion clinically, educationally, and in psychiatric research, we assessed the presentation and interpretation of religion in the little examined area of psychiatric nosology.

In a letter to the Editor, Post[9] noted possible evidence of bias against religion in Appendix C of DSM-III-R, Glossary of Technical Terms. To more thoroughly examine Post's findings, we systematically reviewed the Glossary to ascertain occurrences for constructive as well as insensitive presentations of religion.[3,4]

METHOD

One hundred major and minor technical terms listed in boldface type in the Glossary were systematically reviewed for (1) the use of religious or demographic (e.g., age, gender, ethnicity) material in case examples to illustrate psychopathology, and (2) the inclusion of reminders concerning the clinical relevance of either religion or a demographic factor. Examples presented as a series of multiple symptoms, as in mood-incongruent psychotic features (p. 402) or psychomotor agitation (p. 404) were excluded, as were case examples presented as an array of additional psychiatric terms, as in the terms "psychotic" (p. 404) and "residual" (p. 405). Case examples consisted of a statement made by a patient or a description of a patient's behavior, thinking, or language.

The 100 definitions of technical terms were also surveyed for "reminders" of clinical relevance—specific issues that clinicians need to be sensitive to, or reminded about, because they might be overlooked or neglected in the diagnostic or treatment process.

Since psychiatry most frequently measures religion as denomination,[3] a demographic factor, demographic factors were chosen for comparison. We systematically reviewed the Glossary for educational status, occupational status, ethnicity, race, age, gender, issues of culture, and marital status.

Given the infrequent attention paid in psychiatry research to religion, we hypothesized that the Glossary would include presentations about religion less frequently than it did each of the eight other demographic factors. Such results would be similar to those found in the research of clinical fields.[10]

RESULTS

Religion in the Case Examples

Twenty-nine of the 100 technical terms included one or more illustrative case examples: eighteen terms contained one example, six terms contained two, and five contained three examples. Thus, we identified forty-five case examples, including fourteen statements made by a patient and thirty-one descriptions of a patient's behavior, thinking, or language.

Of the forty-five case examples, ten (22.2 percent) had substantial religious content, including three verbatim patient statements and seven descriptions of patient behavior, thinking, or language. The three verbatim statements were found in the technical terms "illogical thinking," "incoherence," and "poverty of content and speech," and the seven descriptions were found in "affect," "catatonic posturing," "delusion of being controlled," "hallucinations, tactile I," "hallucinations, tactile II," "magical thinking," and "delusion."

In contrast to the ten case examples with religious content, only three case examples included demographic content—two (4.4 percent) of the forty-five had occupational content and one (2.2 percent) had marital status content. None of the case examples concerned the patient's educational status, ethnicity, race, age, gender, or culture.

Religion in the Clinical Reminders

Thirteen technical terms included reminders that concerned an issue of clinical relevance: seven terms included one reminder, four terms included two, and two terms included three. Thus, we identified twenty-one reminders of clinical relevance. Six (28.6 percent) of the twenty-one reminders had religious content, found in the following technical terms: "delusion," "delusion of being controlled," "delusion," "grandiose," "hallucination," "illogical thinking," and "mental disorder."

In comparison, three (14.3 percent) of the twenty-one reminders concerned educational status, one (4.8 percent) concerned ethnicity, two (9.5 percent) concerned age, and seven (33.3 percent) concerned issues of culture or subculture. There were no reminders of clinical relevance concerning occupational status, race, gender, or marital status. Two of the reminders were neither religious nor demographic in nature.

DISCUSSION

Given the low frequency of studies assessing religion in the psychiatric research literature,[3] the rates of references to religion in both the case examples (22.2 percent) and the reminders of clinical relevance (28.6 percent) in the DSM-III-R Glossary of Technical Terms are surprisingly high. Even more surprising, in view of the beneficial relationship that religion has been found to have with mental health status,[4-6] is the frequent association of religion with psychopathology in the Glossary.

Despite the overrepresentation of religion in case examples of psychopathology, those who developed the Glossary emphasized the need for clinicians to be reminded about the clinical relevance of religion. Six, or nearly 30 percent, of the clinical reminders recognized the need for clinicians to be sensitive to religious issues. In comparison, relatively few of the reminders involved issues of educational status, ethnicity, and age, and none of the reminders involved occupational status, race, gender, or marital status.

These findings highlight the dilemma of those who wrote the Glossary in dealing with religion. On the one hand, the large number of clinical reminders concerning religion illustrates the interest in being sensitive to religious issues. However, the excessive use of religion to illustrate psychopathology in case examples reveals cultural insensitivity—the stereotyping of religion as clinically harmful.

Psychiatry needs to deal with a similar nosologic dilemma. Post[11] has recently started to document troubling consequences of psychiatry's nosologic religious insensitivity. At the same time, other efforts have provided constructive provisions for a more "psychoreligiously" and "psychospiritually" sensitive DSM-IV.[12]

Psychiatry and Religion: Overlapping Concerns[13] was a critical step in beginning to deal with such issues. Providing a V code in DSM-IV for "religious or spiritual problem" is another important step. More steps need to be taken. Psychiatry now has the opportunity to further enhance its religious sensitivities and effectively improve the clinical understanding and interpretation of religion in the Glossary of Technical Terms in the next edition of DSM.

NOTES

1. Gallup G: *Religion in America—Fifty Years: 1935-1985*. Princeton, NJ, Princeton Religious Research Center, 1985.

2. Küng H: *The Terry Lectures: Freud and the Problem of God*. New Haven, CT, Yale University Press, 1979.

3. Larson DB, Pattison EM, Blazer DG, Omran AR, Kaplan BH: Systematic analysis of research on religious variables in four major psychiatric journals, 1978-1982. *Am J Psychiatry* 1986; 143:329-334.

4. Larson DB, Sherrill KA, Lyons JS, Craigie FC Jr, Thielman SB, Greenwold MA, Larson SS: Associations between dimensions of religious commitment and mental health reported in the *American Journal of Psychiatry* and *Archives of General Psychiatry:* 1978-1989. *Am J Psychiatry* 1992; 149:557-559.

5. Andreasen NJC: The role of religion in depression. *J Religion and Health* 1972; 11:153-166.

6. Pressman P, Lyons JS, Larson DB, Strain JJ: Religious belief, depression, and ambulation status in elderly women with broken hips. *Am J Psychiatry* 1990; 147:758-760.

7. Bergin AE: Values and religious issues in psychotherapy and mental health. *Am Psychol* 1991; 46:394-403.

8. Lovinger RJ: *Working with Religious Issues in Therapy*. New York, Jason Aronson, 1984.

9. Post SG: DSM-III-R and religion (letter). *Am J Psychiatry* 1990; 147:813.

10. Orr RD, Isaac G: Religious variables are infrequently reported in clinical research. *Fam Med* 1992; 24:602-606.

11. Post SG: DSM-III-R and religion. *Soc Sci Med* 1992; 35:81-90.

12. Lukoff D, Lu F, Turner R: Toward a more culturally sensitive DSM-IV: Psychoreligious and psychospiritual problems. *J Nerv Ment Dis* 1992; 180:673-682.

13. Robinson LH (Ed.): *Psychiatry and Religion: Overlapping Concerns.* Washington, DC, American Psychiatric Press, 1986.

Chapter 10

The Couch and the Cloth: The Need for Linkage

David B. Larson
Ann A. Hohmann
Larry G. Kessler
Keith G. Meador
Jeffrey H. Boyd
Elisabeth McSherry

Data from the Epidemiologic Catchment Area study were used to compare the demographic characteristics and psychiatric symptomatology of persons classified into four groups based on source of

Reprinted, with permission, from *Hospital and Community Psychiatry* 1988; 39: 1064-1069. The views expressed in this paper are the authors'. No official endorsement by NIMH is intended nor should be inferred. The Epidemiologic Catchment Area Program is a series of five epidemiologic research studies performed by independent research teams in collaboration with staff of the Division of Clinical Research of the National Institute of Mental Health. The NIMH principal collaborators are Darrel A. Regier, MD, MPH, Ben Z. Locke, MSPH, and Jack D. Burke Jr., MD, MPH; William J. Huber is NIMH project officer. The principal investigators and coinvestigators from the five sites are Jerome K. Myers, PhD, Myrna M. Weissman, PhD, and Gary Tischler, MD, Yale University, New Haven, Connecticut; Morton Kramer, ScD, Sam Shapiro, and Shephard Kellam, PhD, Johns Hopkins University, Baltimore; Lee N. Robins, PhD, and John Helzer, MD, Washington University, St. Louis; Linda George, PhD, and Dan Blazer, MD, PhD, Duke University, Durham, North Carolina; and Marvin Karno, MD, Richard L. Hough, PhD, Javier Escobar, MD, Audrey Burnam, PhD, and Diane Timbers, PhD, University of California, Los Angeles. The authors are most grateful to Barbara Burns, Kim Sherrill, Peter Benson, Jack D. Burke, Dan Blazer, Marvin Karno, Lee Robins, and Sam Shapiro for their helpful comments, and to Donald S. Rae for assistance with the data.

145

mental health services: clergy only, mental health specialists only, both clergy and mental health specialists, and neither source. Those receiving services from both clergy and mental health specialists were more likely to have major affective and panic disorders than those who sought services from clergy or mental health specialists only or who sought services from neither. Those in the care of mental health specialists were more likely to have substance abuse disorders. Those in the care of clergy only were as likely as those seeing mental health specialists only to have serious mental disorders. The data make clear the need for formal linkages between clergy and mental health professionals.

The 1961 mental health initiative issued by the Joint Commission on Mental Illness and Health recognized the importance of clergy in the provision of mental health services and encouraged their participation in the mental health service system.[1] More than fifteen years later, in 1978, linkages between clergy and mental health professionals were still largely nonexistent. The continuation of the gap was acknowledged in the report on the country's mental health needs published that year by the President's Commission on Mental Health.[2]

In the section on community support, the commission recommended improved linkages between formal mental health services and community support networks, including clergy; the development of demonstration programs to identify effective ways to create links between mental health professionals and community support networks; and the development of research on the efficacy of community support networks as adjuncts to mental health professionals.

The 1978 commission report implicitly acknowledged years of research documenting the importance of nonmental health specialists in the identification and treatment of the mentally ill.[3-7] Estimates from data on use of mental health services indicate that on an annual basis, of the 15 to 20 percent of the U.S. population suffering from mental disorders, only 21 percent are served by mental health professionals (psychiatrists, psychologists, psychiatric nurses, and social workers). The majority (54 percent) are served by the primary medical care sector, 3 percent by general hospitals or nursing homes, and the remaining 22 percent by the clergy and other nonmedical therapists and therapy groups.[5]

When individuals were asked directly in a community survey whom they sought help from for personal problems (problems that may or may not have been associated with a diagnosable mental illness), the relative percentages were somewhat altered but the importance of nonmental health professionals was not. Of the 26 percent of Americans who reported seeking help for personal problems, 57 percent reported seeking help from a mental health professional, 21 percent from a primary care physician, and 39 percent from clergy.[7]

Thus, regardless of the data source, the evidence points to an important role for clergy in the provision of mental health services. This role is one that is not likely to diminish given the discrepancy between the religious orientation of most Americans and that of most mental health professionals. In fifty years of Gallup Poll results, the average percentage of Americans who reported a belief in God was 96 percent.[8] The percentage of mental health professionals who have reported a belief in God ranges from 43 to 61 percent,[9-11] a substantial difference. In addition, depending on specialty, from 26 to 40 percent of mental health specialists report that they have discarded the faith of their family of origin and have become either agnostic or atheistic.[12,13]

Clearly, a discrepancy exists between the secular orientation of the providers of mental health services and the religious beliefs of those seeking help. Problems in the interactions between therapists and clients are most likely to occur between religiously conservative clients and secular therapists. Religious conservatives are concerned that nonreligious therapists will ignore religious issues, will treat religious beliefs and experiences as pathological, will fail to comprehend religious language and concepts, will assume clients' values coincide or should coincide with theirs, and will recommend therapeutic steps considered inappropriate or unacceptable by religious conservatives.[14,15]

Given these concerns, if a religious conservative considers seeking care from a mental health professional, one or more of the following is likely to occur: he or she may be uncooperative in therapy, may drop out of therapy once it is initiated, or may decide to avoid the mental health system altogether.[16-18] Regardless of which event occurs, the religiously conservative client is likely to return to seek help from the clergy and to resist referral.

The ideological discrepancy also exists between the beliefs of the clergy, who have a clear public commitment to a religious ideology, and those of mental health professionals. This is most apparent in the referral patterns of clergy and mental health professionals.[19] Conservative clergy, those most likely to see religiously conservative parishioners who are in need of psychiatric assistance, are least likely among clergy to refer these parishioners to mental health professionals.[20-25] And even among all clergy, whether religiously liberal or conservative, fewer than 10 percent of the parishioners seeking their help are referred to mental health professionals.[21,23,25,26] Mental health specialists are at least as reluctant to refer patients to mental health professionals who recognize the importance of religious beliefs, and those who do refer patients to religiously oriented therapists are themselves active participants in religious activities.[9,13,27,28]

In the ten years since the commission's report, an alliance between mental health professionals and clergy has appeared to be just as distant as it was more than twenty-five years ago. While the clergy themselves have acknowledged that they lack training in the diagnosis and treatment of mental disorders,[29-31] it might be argued that the problems parishioners bring clergy are not serious mental health problems and therefore do not require skilled diagnosticians or therapists. There is evidence to the contrary.[25,32,33]

The purpose of this paper is to explore the demographic and diagnostic characteristics of individuals who have sought help for mental health problems from clergy and from mental health professionals. These individuals will then be contrasted with those who did not seek help from any source and those who sought help from both clergy and mental health professionals. This information will help clarify the needs of the clergy and the need for an alliance between mental health professionals and clergy.

METHODS

Data for these analyses came from the combined five-site, first wave of the Epidemiologic Catchment Area (ECA) study, the contents and methods of which have been described in detail elsewhere.[34-38] The core data set includes responses from a multistage probability sample of adults in New Haven, Connecticut (N = 5,034); eastern Baltimore (N = 3,281); St. Louis (N = 3,004); five counties in the Durham, North Carolina, area (N = 3,921); and the Venice and East Los Angeles areas of Los Angeles County (N = 3,255). Information on demographic variables, health and mental health services utilization, and psychiatric diagnosis was obtained in interviews with the respondents. All analyses were weighted to the original demographics of the areas sampled.

Measures

Psychiatric status was determined through use of the Diagnostic Interview Schedule (DIS), a diagnostic algorithm based on DSM-III criteria.[39,40] To be compatible with the services questions that ask for lifetime use of clergy or outpatient mental health specialists, lifetime DIS diagnoses and symptom counts were used.

Data on the diagnosis of generalized anxiety disorder were not collected until wave 2 of the ECA study and thus were not available for use in the analysis. That is unfortunate, since anxiety and adjustment disorders may be far more common among persons seeking help from clergy.

The analysis focused on four mutually exclusive ECA subgroups: individuals who reported paving sought help from clergy for problems with emotions, nerves, drugs, alcohol, or mental health at any time in their lives but not from outpatient mental health specialists (N = 526); individuals who reported having sought help from outpatient mental health specialists at any time in their lives but not from clergy (N = 2,059); individuals who reported having contacted both (N = 519); and individuals who reported seeking help from neither (N = 15,461).

Treatment by an outpatient mental health specialist was defined as that received from outpatient public or private psychiatrists, mental health centers, psychiatric outpatient clinics in general or psychiatric hospitals, Veterans Administration outpatient clinics, and drug or alcohol clinics. A caveat in interpreting the results is important. Because we are using lifetime diagnoses and lifetime service-use estimates, there is no way of knowing if symptoms preceded service use, how close in time use followed an individual's recognition of symptoms (if indeed that was the time sequence), how often a source of care was used, or to what degree individuals forgot or concealed certain types of service use. Thus these results should be considered as indicative of trends, not definitive patterns.

Statistical Methods

The complex, nonrandom sampling of the ECA project requires sophisticated variance estimation. Standard statistical packages assume random sampling and can greatly underestimate the variance and overestimate the statistical significance of variables included in the analyses. Thus SESUDAAN[41] was used to obtain appropriate standard errors for determination of statistical significance.

RESULTS

Table 10.1 shows the percentages of ECA respondents in each of the five sites who sought help from clergy, mental health specialists, both, or neither for problems with emotions, nerves, drugs, alcohol, or mental health. In general, the groups did not differ significantly across sites. The major exception was in Los Angeles, where respondents were significantly more likely than those at other sites to have sought services from mental health specialists and were significantly less likely to have chosen neither mental health specialists nor clergy as a source of care. However, there were no significant differences

TABLE 10.1. Weighted Percentage of Persons Who Did and Did Not Seek Help from Mental Health Professionals and Clergy, by Epidemiologic Catchment Area Site

Site	Clergy only		Mental health specialist only		Both		Neither	
	%	SE	%	SE	%	SE	%	SE
New Haven	2.5	0.3	13.4	0.6	2.8	0.3	81.4	0.7
Baltimore	3.1	0.3	10.9	0.6	2.2	0.3	83.8	0.7
St. Louis	2.8	0.3	10.6	0.7	3.0	0.4	83.6	0.8
Durham	3.0	0.4	9.1	0.7	2.9	0.3	85.0	0.9
Los Angeles[1]	2.7	0.4	15.3	0.9	2.8	0.3	79.1	1.0
Five-site total	2.8	0.2	12.1	0.3	2.8	0.2	82.4	0.4

[1]Compared with respondents at other sites, Los Angeles respondents were significantly more likely (p < .001) to seek services from mental health specialists and were significantly less likely (p < .05) to choose neither source of care.

across sites in the percentage of respondents who chose clergy or both clergy and mental health specialists. Thus, since Los Angeles was the only unusual site and the sites were generally homogeneous otherwise, subsequent analyses used the combined five-site data.

Table 10.2 presents demographic information on the respondents' gender, age, race, and socioeconomic status. Those who sought help from clergy and those who sought help from both clergy and mental health professionals were more likely to be female than those who sought help from both or neither. Those who chose not to seek help from any of these sources were significantly older than those who sought help from clergy, mental health specialists, or both. A significantly higher proportion of nonwhites chose to avoid both clergy and mental health specialists when in need of help for emotional problems. Finally, as could be predicted from the literature on use of psychiatrists,[3,10,27] those who sought help from mental health specialists or both clergy and mental health specialists were significantly more likely to belong to the highest socioeconomic quartile.

Table 10.3 presents the lifetime prevalence estimates for various disorders for each of the four groups. Here many significant differences, both statistically and substantively, emerge. First, those who chose to seek help from both clergy and mental health specialists were significantly more likely to have received a DIS diagnosis of bipolar disorder, major depression, major depression associated with grief, panic disorder, and any lifetime diagnosis.

Second, those who chose to seek help from neither source were significantly less likely to have received a diagnosis of major depression, major depression associated with grief, dysthymia, single depression, recurrent depression, schizophrenia, obsessive compulsive disorder, phobia, and any lifetime diagnosis. Third, those who sought help from clergy or from neither source were significantly less likely than those who visited a mental health professional to have received a DIS diagnosis of alcohol or drug abuse.

DISCUSSION

The ECA data provide a unique opportunity to begin an exploration of the role of clergy in the treatment of mental illness. The data show a remarkably similar pattern of help-seeking from clergy across

TABLE 10.2. Demographic Characteristics of ECA Respondents Who Sought Help for Problems with Emotions, Nerves, Drugs, Alcohol, or Mental Health, by Source of Help Sought

Characteristic	Clergy only %	SE	Mental health specialist only %	SE	Both %	SE	Neither %	SE
Female[1]	65.6	2.4	54.0	1.4	65.0	2.6	52.5	0.5
Age[2]								
18 to 44	63.4	2.6	68.2	1.4	68.70	2.7	54.9	0.5
45 to 64	26.7	2.4	25.9	1.4	27.09	3.0	28.1	0.5
65 and over	9.9	1.2	5.8	0.5	4.3	0.9	17.0	0.4
Race[3]								
White	72.2	2.2	75.9	1.0	76.6	2.0	66.0	0.6
Black	15.5	1.7	13.8	0.8	13.5	1.9	19.6	0.5
Hispanic	9.9	1.7	6.7	0.7	6.6	1.3	9.7	0.3
Other	2.3	0.7	3.6	0.5	3.3	0.9	4.7	0.2
Socioeconomic quartile[4]								
First	12.7	1.4	12.3	1.1	12.9	1.4	18.2	0.5
Second	35.2	2.9	27.9	1.1	25.9	2.7	34.1	0.5
Third	35.5	2.5	34.7	1.2	40.1	2.7	31.7	0.5
Fourth	16.6	1.8	25.2	1.3	21.1	2.4	16.0	0.5

[1]Females were significantly more likely ($p < .01$) to seek help from clergy only and from both clergy and mental health specialists.
[2]Older respondents were significantly more likely ($p < .001$) to seek help from neither source.
[3]Nonwhites were significantly more likely ($p < .001$) to seek help from neither source.
[4]Respondents in the fourth (highest) economic quartile were significantly more likely ($p < .01$) to seek help from mental health specialists or from both mental health specialists and clergy.

the five sites. Even those who live in southern rural counties of North Carolina are no more likely to seek out clergy for assistance with mental health problems than are those in urban New Haven. And while those who seek out clergy are more likely to be female and of lower socioeconomic status than those seeking out mental health professionals, they are of similar age and racial distributions.

TABLE 10.3. Lifetime Prevalence of Disorders in ECA Respondents Who Sought Help for Problems with Emotions, Nerves, Drugs, Alcohol, or Mental Health, by Source of Help Sought

Type of Disorder	Clergy only		Mental health specialist only		Both		Neither	
	%	SE	%	SE	%	SE	%	SE
Cognitive disorder	1.9	0.7	2.6	0.4	1.0	0.4	2.7	0.1
Bipolar disorder[1]	2.4	0.8	3.1	0.5	7.3	1.3	1.7	0.1
Major depression[2,3]	15.7	2.1	18.2	1.1	34.0	2.5	3.7	0.2
Major depression associated with grief[2,3]	17.5	2.1	19.3	1.1	36.0	2.7	4.1	0.2
Dysthymia[3]	10.7	1.9	10.4	0.9	15.1	2.0	3.0	0.2
Single depression[3]	5.7	1.2	5.2	0.5	7.7	1.3	2.0	0.1
Recurrent depression[3]	9.2	1.7	12.0	0.9	22.2	2.1	2.8	0.1
Abnormal bipolar disorder	1.7	0.6	1.9	0.3	3.5	0.9	1.5	0.1
Alcohol abuse[4]	12.6	1.9	28.0	1.2	23.3	2.3	12.4	0.3
Drug abuse[4]	6.6	1.5	17.6	1.0	19.3	2.2	5.2	0.2
Schizophrenia[3]	5.0	1.8	5.3	0.6	10.6	1.9	2.0	0.1
Schizophreniform	2.8	1.6	1.2	0.3	1.7	0.6	1.6	0.1
Obsessive-compulsive[3]	7.7	1.4	7.5	0.7	14.9	2.5	3.2	0.2
Phobia[3]	25.7	2.7	23.6	1.0	30.5	2.1	12.4	0.4

TABLE 10.3 (continued)

Type of Disorder	Clergy only		Mental health specialist only		Both		Neither	
	%	SE	%	SE	%	SE	%	SE
Somatization	0.4	0.2	1.1	0.3	2.0	1.0	1.5	0.1
Panic disorder[1]	1.7	1.0	5.9	1.0	16.8	2.2	2.2	0.1
Antisocial personality	5.0	1.2	8.8	1.0	10.4	1.6	3.7	0.2
Any lifetime disorder[3,5]	54.5	2.9	62.5	1.2	71.8	26.2	26.2	0.5

[1]Significantly higher (p < .01) for respondents seeking help from both clergy and mental health specialists.
[2]Significantly higher (p < .001) for respondents seeking help from both clergy and mental health specialists.
[3]Significantly lower (p < .05) for respondents seeking help from neither source.
[4]Significantly lower (p < .05) for respondents seeking help from neither source or from clergy only.
[5]Significantly higher (p < .05) for respondents seeking help from both clergy and mental health specialists.

Important differences do emerge in the lifetime prevalence estimates of mental health disorders for the four groups. The most striking differences are not those between users of clergy and users of mental health specialists. Instead, they are the prevalence differences between those who seek care from both clergy and mental health specialists and the rest of the ECA respondents.

Those who seek care from both sources are individuals with major, life-altering affective and anxiety disorders. Major depression, the depression associated with bipolar disorder, and panic disorders are conditions that not only severely alter an individual's ability to function in everyday life but also make the individual acutely aware of his or her impaired functioning. In contrast, several of the diagnostic groups who less frequently seek care from both sources (for example, schizophrenics or alcohol or drug abusers) tend to be less aware of their impaired functioning. More information is needed before it can be said with certainty, but it appears that individuals who use both clergy and mental health specialists are in a desperate search for someone to help them and may be high users of other public and private sources of support.

Those who choose neither clergy nor mental health specialists as sources of care are less likely to have a major mental disorder than are those who seek care from either or both of these sources. However, those who choose neither clergy nor mental health professionals are as likely as those who choose either or both of them to have cognitive, abnormal bipolar, schizophreniform, or somatization disorders and as likely as those seeking care from mental health professionals to have bipolar disorder. Thus individuals with these disorders do not have rates of service use above those of the general population.

The most important finding from these data is not one that stands out because of its statistical significance; it is the lack of statistical significance that is important. Among those in a community population who seek help for emotional problems either from clergy or from mental health professionals, the prevalence of major psychiatric disorders is very similar for all psychiatric diagnostic categories except alcohol abuse, drug abuse, and panic disorder. Thus the clergy are as likely as mental health professionals to be sought out by individuals from the community who have serious psychiatric disorders.

In fact, because of the way the question on use of services by clergy is asked in the ECA survey, the clergy-only prevalence estimate may be low. Respondents were asked about use of services as a result of problems with "emotions, nerves, drugs, alcohol, or mental health." If the respondent had marital or job problems and did not define those problems as belonging to any of the ECA categories, then the respondent's use of clergy would not be counted. If the problem was a diagnosable mental disorder, the respondent and the disorder would be counted for the mental health specialist only or for both groups. Thus the prevalence of disorder may be underestimated for those seeking help from the clergy only and for the subgroup seeking help from both clergy and mental health professionals.

Whether this underestimate occurred, the conclusion is clear: the clergy are coping, with or without the assistance of mental health professionals, with parishioners who have a broad spectrum of psychiatric disorders. Clergy feel isolated from mental health professionals and are afraid or unwilling[42,43] to ask for assistance, in part because they know they are deficient in diagnostic and treatment skills.[29-31] Therefore it is incumbent on mental health professionals to make a concerted and diplomatic effort to reach out to them.

A first step could be made by individual clinicians. In light of the findings about the group who seek help from both clergy and mental health professionals, mental health professionals should be particularly sensitive to a patient's past use of mental health services and attempt, with the permission of the patient, to contact the clergyman or clergywoman who helped the patient initially. The clinician could probably learn much from the clergy about a patient's symptomatology and past life stresses and about how the patient has coped with those stresses.

A second step would be for the professional organizations of mental health specialists to make formal efforts to create linkages with schools of theology and departments of pastoral counseling. Formal agreements offering consultation and liaison services to faculty and students in these educational settings would provide a foundation for future cooperation. Then mental health professionals could become involved in actually designing and teaching courses in recognition, diagnosis, treatment, and referral of those suffering from mental illness.

With these gradual steps, all would benefit. Clergy would be relieved of the terrible burden of trying, alone, to counsel parishioners with serious mental disorders; those with the disorders would be given a chance to obtain more appropriate mental health services; and mental health professionals would have another source to identify individuals in need of care. Since the need for this collaboration has been known for over twenty-five years with little progress made, it would seem time for the national associations of mental health professionals to put this item on their agendas.

NOTES

1. *The Final Report of the Joint Commission on Mental Illness and Health: Action for Mental Health.* New York, Basic Books. 1961.

2. *Report to the President from the President's Commission on Mental Health,* volume 1. Washington, DC, U.S. Government Printing Office, 1978.

3. Gurin G, Veroff J, Feld S: *Americans View Their Mental Health.* New York, Basic Books, 1960.

4. Kulka RA, Veroff J, Douvan E: Social class and the use of professional help for personal problems: 1957 and 1976. *Journal of Health and Social Behavior* 20: 2-17, 1979.

5. Regier DA, Goldberg ID, Taube CA: The de facto U.S. mental health services system: A public health perspective. *Archives of General Psychiatry* 35:685-693, 1978.

6. Veroff J, Douvan E, Kulka RA: *The Inner American.* New York, Basic Books, 1981.

7. Veroff J, Kulka RA, Douvan E: *Mental Health in America: Patterns of Help-Seeking from 1957 to 1976.* New York, Basic Books, 1981.

8. Gallup G: *Religion in America—50 Years: 1935-1985.* Princeton, NJ, Gallup Report, 1985.

9. *Psychiatrists' Viewpoints on Religion and Their Services to Religious Institutions and the Ministry,* task force report no. 10. Washington, DC, American Psychiatric Association, 1975.

10. Marx JH, Spray SL: Psychotherapeutic "birds of a feather": Social-class status and religio-cultural value homophily in the mental health field. *Journal of Health and Social Behavior* 13:413-428, 1973.

11. Ragan C, Malony HN, Beit-Hallahmi B: Psychologists and religion: Professional factors associated with personal belief. *Review of Religious Research* 21:208-217, 1980.

12. Henry WE, Simms JH, Spray SL: *The Fifth Profession: Becoming a Psychotherapist.* San Francisco, Jossey-Bass, 1971.

13. Larson DB, Pattison EM, Blazer DG, Omran AR, and Kaplan BH: Systematic analysis of research on religious variables in four major psychiatric journals, 1978-1982. *American Journal of Psychiatry* 143:329-334, 1986.

14. Worthington EL, Scott GG: Goal selection for counseling with potentially religious clients by professional and student counselors in explicitly Christian or secular settings. *Journal of Psychology and Theology* 11:318-329, 1983.

15. Worthington EL, Gascoyne SR: Preferences of Christians and non-Christians for five Christian counselors' treatment plans: A partial replication and extension. *Journal of Psychology and Theology* 13:20-41, 1985.

16. Bergin AE: Psychotherapy and religious values. *Journal of Consulting and Clinical Psychology* 48:95-105, 1980.

17. Dougherty SG, Worthington EL: Preferences of conservative and moderate Christians for four counselors' treatment plans for a troubled client. *Journal of Psychology and Theology* 10:346-354, 1982.

18. Pattison EM: Psychiatry and religion circa 1978: Analysis of a decade, part I. *Pastoral Psychology* 27:8-25, 1978.

19. Gottlieb JF, Olfson M: Current referral practices of mental health care providers. *Hospital and Community Psychiatry* 38:1171-1181, 1987.

20. Cole JD, Costanzo PR, Cox G: Behavioral determinants of mental illness concerns: A comparison of gatekeeper professions. *Journal of Consulting and Clinical Psychiatry* 43:626-636, 1975.

21. Gilbert MG: Characteristics of pastors related to pastoral counseling and referral. *Journal of Pastoral Counseling* 16:30-38, 1981.

22. Larson RF: The clergyman's role in the therapeutic process: Disagreement between clergymen and psychiatrists. *Psychiatry* 31:250-260, 1968.

23. Lowe DW: Counseling activities and referral practices of ministers. *Journal of Psychology and Christianity* 5:22-29, 1986.

24. Meylink WD, Gorsuch RL: Relationship between clergy and psychologists: The empirical data. *Journal of Psychology and Christianity* 7:56-72, 1988.

25. Mollica RF, Streets FJ, Boscarino J, et al.: A community study of formal pastoral counseling activities of the clergy. *American Journal of Psychiatry* 143:323-328, 1986.

26. Virkler HA: Counseling demands, procedures, and preparation of parish ministers: A descriptive study. *Journal of Psychology and Theology* 7:271-280, 1979.

27. Kadushin C: *Why People Go to Psychiatrists,* New York, Atherton, 1969.

28. Preston C: Meaning and organization of religious experience: An exploratory study. *Review of Religious Research* 28:252-267, 1987.

29. Arnold JD, Schick C: Counseling by clergy: A review of empirical research. *Journal of Pastoral Counseling* 14:76-101, 1979.

30. Linebaugh DE, Devivo P: The growing emphasis on training pastor-counselors in Protestant seminaries. *Journal of Psychology and Theology* 9:266-268, 1981.

31. Wylie WE: Health counseling competencies needed by the minister. *Journal of Religion and Health* 23:237-249, 1984.

32. Lieberman MA, Mullan JT: Does help help?: The adaptive consequences of obtaining help from professionals and social networks. *American Journal of Community Psychology* 6:499-517, 1978.

33. Wagner EE, Dobbins RD: MMPI profiles of parishioners seeking pastoral counseling. *Journal of Consulting Psychology* 31:83-84, 1967.

34. Burnam MA, Hough RL, Escobar JI, et al.: Six-month prevalence of specific psychiatric disorders among Mexican Americans and non-Hispanic whites in Los Angeles. *Archives of General Psychiatry* 44:687-694, 1987.

35. Eaton WW, Holzer CE, Von Korff M, et al.: The design of the epidemiologic catchment area surveys: The control and measurement of error. *Archives of General Psychiatry* 41:942-948, 1984.

36. Eaton WW, Kessler LG (Eds.): *Epidemiologic Field Methods in Psychiatry: The NIMH Epidemiologic Catchment Area Program.* New York, Academic Press, 1985.

37. Regier DA, Hyers JK, Kramer M, et al.: The NIMH epidemiologic catchment area program. *Archives of General Psychiatry* 41:934-941, 1984.

38. Robins LN, Helzer JE, Weissman MM, et al.: Lifetime prevalence of specific psychiatric disorders in three sites. *Archives of General Psychiatry* 41:949-958, 1984.

39. Robins LN, Helzer JE, Croughan J, et al.: The NIMH Diagnostic Interview Schedule: Its history, characteristics, and validity. *Archives of General Psychiatry* 38:381-389, 1981.

40. Robins LN, Helzer JE, Ratcliff KS, et al.: Validity of the Diagnostic Interview Schedule, Version II: DSM-III diagnoses. *Psychological Medicine* 12:855-870, 1982.

41. Shah BV: *SESUDAAN: Standard Errors Program for Computing of Standardized Rates from Sample Survey Data.* Research Triangle Park, NC, Research Triangle Institute, 1981.

42. King RR: Evangelical Christians and professional counselors: A conflict of values? *Journal of Psychology and Theology* 6:276-281, 1978.

43. Worthington EL: Religious counseling: A review of published empirical research. *Journal of Counseling and Development* 64:421-431, 1986.

Chapter 11

The Impact of Religion
on Men's Blood Pressure

David B. Larson
Harold G. Koenig
Berton H. Kaplan
Raymond S. Greenberg
Everett Logue
Herman A. Tyroler

Most clinical studies examining the relation between religion and blood pressure status have focused on church attendance, finding lower pressures among frequent attenders. The present study examines the effect on blood pressure status of a religious meaning variable, importance of religion, both by itself and together with frequency of church attendance. The relation between blood pressure, self-perceived importance of religion, and frequency of church attendance was examined among a rural sample of 407 white men free from hypertension or cardiovascular disease. The data confirmed an interaction between the effects of both religious variables on blood pressure status, with importance of religion having an even greater association with lower pressures than church attendance. Diastolic blood pressures of persons with high church attendance and high reli-

Reprinted, with permission, from *Journal of Religion and Health* 1989; 28:265-278. Funding for this study was provided by the Department of Public Health, University of North Carolina, Chapel Hill; the Center for the Study of Aging and Human Development, Duke University Medical Center; and the Geriatric Research Education and Clinical Center, Durham, North Carolina. The authors thank Dan Blazer for his advice, assistance, and encouragement. They are also grateful to Dana Anne Mlekush for her help with manuscript preparation and her thoughtful input to this project.

gious importance were significantly lower than those in the low attendance, low importance group. These differences persisted after adjusting the analyses for age, socioeconomic status, smoking, and
weight-height ratio (Quetelet Index). The difference in mean diastolic pressures based on response to the religious importance variable alone was statistically and clinically significant, particularly
among men aged fifty-five and over (6 mm) and among smokers
(5 mm). These findings suggest that both religious attitudes and
involvement may interact favorably in their effects on cardiovascular
hemodynamics.

INTRODUCTION

Jenkins, in his classic review of psychological and social risk factors for coronary disease, encouraged further research to evaluate the
suggested association between religious variables and reduced coronary risk.[1] In the twelve years since this publication, there have been
few efforts either to confirm or refute that protective association, despite the fact that at least five separate prospective studies have shown
lower mortality rates among the more actively religious.[2]
Systematic analyses of studies published in psychiatric journals
and in the family practice literature have only rarely found the inclusion of religious variables.[3] Among 2,348 psychiatric articles reviewed between 1978 and 1982, Larson and his co-authors found a
religious variable in only 2.5 percent of these studies.[4] Craigie and his
co-authors, reviewing 1,086 studies published in the *Journal of Family Practice* from 1976 to 1986, found a religious variable included in
only 1.9 percent of these.[5] In both of these reviews, religious denomination was commonly the religious variable used (63 percent of psychiatric and 41 percent of family practice studies). Kaplan noted earlier that many studies have used denomination as representative of
one's religious practices, despite the fact that denomination poorly
discriminates for such practices which may vary widely among individual members.[6] Kaplan infers research should move away from denominational variables as religious behavior indicators and move
toward scaling and measuring the essence of religious behavior, that
is, the beliefs and practices.

The present effort extends previous work done on a similar sample of Evans County, Georgia, white males.[7] In that work Graham and his co-authors found a consistent association between frequent church attendance and lowered mean age-standardized systolic and diastolic blood pressure levels. This association maintained itself for the two smoking levels, the three levels of socioeconomic status, and two of four quartiles of the Quetelet Index. In addition to evaluating the effect that church attendance has on blood pressure, the present study examined the effect of importance of religion, with and without the attendance variable, on blood pressure levels. The foundation for this work lies on a probable association between blood pressure and social and psychological processes, which may in turn be influenced by powerful cultural forces such as religion.

Support for the hypothesis that importance of religion, a subjective religiosity variable, may have an impact on physiological processes and cardiovascular status comes from the work of Moberg, who notes that a "meaningful and purposeful relationship with God" will improve the nature of one's relationship both with one's self and with one's fellow persons.[8] Moberg notes that beneficial religious behavior may include: (1) coming to terms with forgiving oneself; (2) developing emotionally healthier self-concepts; (3) giving unselfishly to others; and (4) coming to terms with forgiving others. Any of these behaviors, acting through psycho-physiologically mediated processes, might influence blood pressure and other cardiovascular processes.

This is not a new conceptualization. William James with his "religion of healthy-mindedness" and Gordon Allport with his "mature religious sentiment" both discuss healthy or mature religion as one that may benefit social and psychological dimensions of one's life.[9] Hence, there is ample justification for examining how perceived importance of religion affects blood pressure levels in a community-dwelling population. The authors are not aware of any other community study where a subjective religiosity variable has been tested to see what effect it has on cardiovascular status. More specifically, is religious importance (either alone or with church attendance) protective against higher blood pressure?

Support for using the combination of perceived importance of one's religion and frequency of church attendance together as indicators of religious behavior comes from two sources. The first source is Campbell and his co-authors' *Quality of American Life*.[10] In

McNamara and St. George's re-analysis of Campbell's original results, they found that the variables, "importance of a strong religious faith" and "frequency of church attendance," were two of the four strongest religious correlates of four of the five main dependent variables measures.[11]These dependent variables were indices of: personal life satisfaction, marriage satisfaction, family life satisfaction, and personal competence.[12] High scores on these variables would seem to be conducive to lower blood pressures, given a psycho-physiologically mediate influence on blood pressure levels. Hence, it is reasonable to use a combination of religious importance and frequency of attendance as an index of one's religious beliefs and practices to compare with mean blood pressure levels.

Because of the potential impact of a number of other variables besides religion on blood pressure, an examination of the religion-blood pressure relationship would be incomplete without accounting for their confounding effects. The systolic blood pressure increases linearly with age, while the diastolic blood pressure increases until middle age, plateaus, and then decreases in the later ages.[13] Socioeconomic status has also been implicated as a potential confounder owing to evidence that increased hypertension[14] or increased hypertension-related deaths[15] occur in the lower social classes. A sizeable correlation has also been demonstrated between blood pressure and the relation of body weight to height in children and adults, suggesting the need to control for this variable.[16] Smoking had been felt for years to influence blood pressure adversely, although recent studies have called this association into question.[17] There is ample evidence that smoking and socioeconomic status are variables that might influence or be influenced by religion; age may also be related to religiosity.[18]

In the current study, the answers to four major questions were sought:

1. Do those who attend church frequently or view their religion as very important experience lower systolic and diastolic blood pressures?
2. Do those who both attend church frequently and view their religion as very important experience lower systolic and diastolic blood pressures? Do these differences hold up after controlling for age, socioeconomic status, smoking, and the Quetelet Index (height to weight comparison)?

3. What is the impact of age on the relation between religious attendance, religious importance, and mean systolic and diastolic blood pressures?
4. What influence does smoking status have on the relation between blood pressure and religious factors? All questions were asked prior to the analysis of the data (a priori) with the exception of question #4, which was asked after the analysis was completed (a posteriori).

METHODS

Sample

The sample for this study was those white males who were re-examined during the 1967-1969 follow-up of the Evans County (Georgia) Cardiovascular Epidemiologic Study. Previous studies have discussed the initial 1960-1962 prevalence study and its results.[19] The total population originally sampled was 771 white males. In order to eliminate possible confounding effects of diagnosed cardiovascular disorders, 246 participants were excluded from the analysis owing to a present or past history of hypertension or cardiovascular disease (persons with diagnosable heart disease from 1960-1962 through 1967-1969 or taking medicines for either their heart or circulation). An additional 118 persons were excluded for not responding to or giving an invalid response to the religious portion of the sociological questionnaire (n = 109) or for being less than twenty-four years of age (n = 9). The final sample size upon which these analyses are reported, then, was 401. The participants were all white males over the age of twenty-five and were free of diagnosed hypertension or any cardiovascular diseases; 13 percent were over the age of sixty-five. A more detailed description of participants in this rural sample has been reported elsewhere.[20]

Procedure

Three blood pressure readings were taken of the left arm with the respondent seated. The second reading was taken between thirty and sixty minutes after the first, while the third reading was taken some fifteen to twenty minutes following the second. To determine the diastolic blood pressure, the fifth Korotkoff component was used.[21]

The religious variables were abstracted from a sociological questionnaire, not used in the initial 1960-1962 prevalence study.[22] The main items to be used from the sociological questionnaire are related to the frequency of one's church attendance and the importance of one's religion: (1) "Are you a church-goer?" If yes, "How often do you generally attend?" (with nine response options ranging from daily to never) and (2) "Quite aside from churchgoing, how important in general would you say religion is to you: very important, somewhat important, or not important at all?" Church attendance was then dichotomized into those who attended church at least weekly (64.6 percent), and those who attended church on a less than weekly basis. Two categories were used for the importance question: those who view their religion as very important to them (75.5 percent), and those who view their religion either as somewhat important or not important at all to them.

The four covariates were measured and analyzed in the following fashion. Socioeconomic status was measured using the McGuire-White Scale, a scale found especially useful in rural settings.[23] As a covariate in the adjusted analyses, this was treated as a continuous variable. Height to weight comparison was calculated using the Quetelet Index, which is calculated by dividing the weight (pounds) by the height (inches) and multiplying the result by 100.[24] Socioeconomic status and the Quetelet Index, as covariates, were treated as continuous variables in the adjusted analyses. For smoking, there were three different levels consisting of those who smoked (29.0 percent), those who were ex-smokers (21.6 percent), and those who were nonsmokers (49.4 percent). For smoking, there were three different levels consisting of those who smoked (29.0 percent), those who were ex-smokers (21.6 percent), and those who were nonsmokers (49.4 percent). For the analyses stratified by smoking status, only smokers and nonsmokers were considered. The age variable was used as a continuous variable in the adjusted analyses, or else it was dichotomized into those less than or equal to fifty-four (64.1 percent) and those fifty-five or older.

Statistical Methods

For the unadjusted analyses, mean systolic and diastolic blood pressures were compared using the Student T-test. For the adjusted analyses, analysis of covariance was employed using the SAS General Linear Model procedure.[25] Because of the a posteriori nature of the evaluation concerning the effect of smoking status on the religion-blood pressure relationship, the unadjusted analysis was performed using the Scheffe's method, a multiple comparisons method permitting the investigator to make postanalytical comparison of means;[26] likewise, for the adjusted analysis, the Bonferroni method was used to account for multiple comparisons.[27]

RESULTS

Do those who attend church frequently or view their religion as very important experience lower blood pressures? Comparison of mean systolic and diastolic blood pressures between frequent and infrequent church attenders revealed a nonsignificant trend toward lower pressures among frequent attenders (Table 11.1). Both mean systolic and diastolic pressures were also lower for those with high religious importance, with the difference becoming statistically significant for diastolic pressure. For the adjusted analysis (not shown), these trends remained but failed to reach statistical significance ($.10 < p < .20$) for either the church attendance or the religious importance.

Do those who both attend church frequently and view their religion as very important experience lower blood pressures? When importance of religion and frequency of attendance were combined in a two-item index, more notable differences in blood pressures were found (Table 11.2). For those with high importance and high attendance (high-high), mean systolic and diastolic pressures were significantly lower than those of the low importance and low attendance group (low-low). The differences here were substantially greater than for either religious variable examined alone. While the differences did not reach statistical significance for systolic pressure, diastolic pressure was almost 5 mm lower among the high-high group compared with the low-low group. Intermediate diastolic pressures were noted for the high-low and low-high groups. Adjusting for covariates

TABLE 11.1. Unadjusted Mean Systolic and Diastolic Blood Pressure Levels for Religious Attendance and Religious Importance

	Systolic			Diastolic		
	BP	N	SD	BP	N	SD
Religious Attendance[1]						
High	134.1	263	18.6	83.9	263	10.2
Low	136.3	144	11.8	86.4	144	11.8
p-value		ns			ns	
Religious Importance[2]						
High	134.0	308	18.3	84.0	308	10.5
Low	137.3	99	20.2	87.2	99	11.7
p-value		.09			.01	

SD = Standard Deviation
[1]High indicates high religious attendance (at least weekly); low indicates low religious attendance (less than weekly).
[2]High indicates high religious importance (very important); low indicates low religious importance (somewhat important or not important at all).

did decrease the magnitude of these differences; however, statistical significance was retained for diastolic pressures. These findings are indicative of an interaction between religious meaning and activity variables in their association with blood pressure.

What is the impact of age on the relation between religious importance and mean blood pressures? Stratification of the sample by age, with fifty-five years as the cutoff, demonstrated that only in the older age group did the differences in blood pressures between high and low importance groups reach statistical significance (Table 11.3). In those under the age of fifty-five, little difference was seen. For those fifty-five and over, mean systolic pressure was almost 9 mm lower and mean diastolic pressure over 6 mm lower among the high importance group. Once adjusted for smoking, socioeconomic status, and weight to height ratio, the differences lessened and dropped just below statistical significance ($.05 < p < .10$); differences still remained in the 6 mm range, a clinically significant quantity.

What is the impact of smoking status on the relation between religious importance and mean blood pressures? As with age,

TABLE 11.2. Unadjusted and Adjusted Mean Systolic and Diastolic Blood Pressure Levels for Religious Importance by Religious Attendance

Religious Category[1]	Unadjusted						Adjusted			
	Systolic			Diastolic			Systolic		Diastolic	
	BP	N	SD	BP	N	SD	BP	SE	BP	SE
High-High	133.5	232	18.2	83.8	232	10.0	133.5	1.1	83.9	0.6
High-Low	135.6	76	18.4	84.8	76	11.8	135.1	2.1	85.4	1.1
Low-High	138.8	31	20.9	85.0	31	11.5	139.9	3.0	85.0	1.6
Low-Low	137.2	68	20.0	88.2	68	11.7	135.0	2.1	86.8	1.3
p-value[2]	ns			< .005			ns		< .05	

SD = Standard Deviation
SE = Standard Error
[1]High-high indicates high religious importance (very important) and high church attendance (at least weekly); low-low means low importance (somewhat important or not important at all) and low church attendance (less than weekly); high-low means high importance, low attendance; low-high means low importance, high attendance.
[2]For difference between mean blood pressures in high-high and low-low categories.

TABLE 11.3. Unadjusted and Adjusted Mean Systolic and Diastolic Blood Pressure Levels for Religious Importance Stratified by Age

Religious Importance[1]	Unadjusted						Adjusted			
	Systolic			Diastolic			Systolic		Diastolic	
	BP	N	SD	BP	N	SD	BP	SE	BP	SE
Under 55										
High	131.2	195	17.4	84.1	195	10.7	134.3	1.6	85.3	0.9
Low	133.0	66	18.9	85.6	66	11.6	131.7	2.0	85.2	1.2
p-value		ns			ns		ns		ns	
55 and Over										
High	138.9	113	18.8	83.9	113	10.1	139.7	1.7	82.6	1.3
Low	147.2	33	19.6	90.3	33	11.5	146.2	3.2	88.5	1.7
p-value		<.05			<.005		.07		.08	

SD = Standard Deviation
SE = Standard Error
[1]High indicates high importance (very important); low indicates low importance (somewhat or not important at all).

stratification of the sample between smokers and nonsmokers revealed notable differences (Table 11.4). For the nonsmoker, there was almost no difference in blood pressures between high and low religious importance groups, with or without adjustment for covariates. For the smoker, on the other hand, substantial differences were observed. For the latter group, diastolic pressure was 7 mm lower (adjusting to 5.3 mm) for the high religious importance group, a significant difference, even in the adjusted analysis using the Bonferroni correction (requiring p < .005 for significance). Although an even larger difference between groups was observed for systolic pressure (10.3 mm adjusting to 8.9 mm), this was not statistically significant using the conservative Scheffe's method of analysis.

Odds ratios were calculated for the likelihood of having an elevated blood pressure (defined as 140 for systolic and 90 for diastolic) based on importance of religion. Among smokers, those with *low* religious importance had a 4.3 times greater likelihood of having an abnormal systolic and 7.1 times greater likelihood of having an abnormal diastolic pressure than did those with *low* religious importance (p < .001 for both ratios, unadjusted). For church attendance, odds ratios neared unity for nonsmokers; for smokers, however, risk of an abnormal diastolic pressure for low attenders was almost four times higher (OR = 3.97, p < .001, unadjusted) and abnormal systolic twice as high (OR = 2.0, p = .06, unadjusted) as for high attenders.

DISCUSSION

This is the first community-based cardiovascular study where first a religious meaning variable, the importance of religion, and then the same meaning variable and another religious variable, frequency of attendance, were both used to evaluate the association between religion and cardiovascular status. All other studies evaluating the effects of religion in the community context have used what was found in this study to be the less powerful predictor, frequency of (church) attendance as the single religious independent variable.[28] None of them included a religious meaning factor, as has this effort. The unadjusted results provided confirmation that the single meaning variable alone and together with the frequency of attendance variable had significant protective effects for the blood pressures of the rural, white male

TABLE 11.4. Unadjusted and Adjusted Mean Systolic and Diastolic Blood Pressure Levels for Religious Importance Stratified by Smoking

Religious Importance[1]	Unadjusted						Adjusted			
	Systolic			Diastolic			Systolic		Diastolic	
	BP	N	SD	BP	N	SD	BP	SE	BP	SE
Smoker										
High	131.4	95	16.9	83.8	95	9.0	131.8	1.6	84.0	0.9
Low	142.1	23	19.0	90.8	23	10.2	140.7	3.3	89.3	2.0
p-value	ns			< .05			< .05		< .005	
Nonsmoker										
High	134.7	147	19.3	83.6	147	11.2	134.7	1.4	84.3	0.8
Low	134.0	54	20.4	84.5	54	12.2	133.6	2.3	84.3	1.3
p-value	ns			ns			ns		ns	

SD = Standard Deviation
SE = Standard Error
[1]High indicates high importance (religion very important); low indicates low importance (religion somewhat or not important at all).

samples studied. When the religious meaning variable was dichotomized and the four covariables, the Quetelet Index, age, smoking status, and socioeconomic status were adjusted for, the very important group was still found to have lower blood pressures than the less important group though the resulting p-values were no longer at levels less than .10 as they were for the crude analyses.

A comparison of the unadjusted and adjusted results obtained from considering the importance and attendance variables together as a "single" exposure variable showed little difference and suggested an interaction between the effects of these religious variables on blood pressure. For both unadjusted and adjusted analyses, a dose-response relationship was observed with the high importance-attendance groups having the lowest blood pressures, the low importance-attendance groups having the highest blood pressures, and the low-high and high-low importance-attendance groups having intermediate blood pressure levels. For the systolic blood pressure, similar trends were observed, but these did not achieve statistical significance. These blood pressure findings support the hypothesis that both religious importance and attendance could be considered as different individual forms of social support that can be accumulated (similar to the conclusion reached by Berkman and Syme).[29]

The well-established link between psychological and physiological processes provides the basis upon which hypothesized religious effects may be explained. As Weiner describes in his *Psychobiology of Essential Hypertension,* most of the early studies of patients with hypertension focused on the psychological status or personalities of patients. Some cases emphasized the patients' anxieties, while others focused on their repressed hostility. Some noted their depressive personalities, while others noted their perfectionism.[30] Indirect support for anxiety playing a role in the etiology of hypertension comes from two more recent works.[31] In both reports, a significantly greater reduction in blood pressure was experienced with the relaxation intervention when compared to placebo or other controls. Increasing the stress level experienced by subjects has been shown to increase the resistance to lowering blood pressure levels.[32] Blood pressure levels have also been shown to vary directly with certain stressful conditions and inversely with socioeconomic status.[33] Likewise, death rates from hypertension have been found to be higher in persons from lower socioeconomic groups and in persons with marital instability or involved in crime.[34] Several studies have demonstrated hypertensives to have difficulty in coping with and expressing feelings, especially anger in interpersonal situations.[35]

Other investigators, examining coping style and blood pressure levels, noted that as a result of hypertensives' inability to cope with social stresses, they have little confidence in their interpersonal styles and deficient skills to cope adequately with their interpersonal social stresses.[36] Religion has been found to be a commonly reported coping behavior among persons of all ages, but especially among the elderly.[37] Because many religious communities often have well-established rules for relating to one another and place a heavy emphasis on positive relationships,[38] religiously motivated persons may suffer less stress, anxiety, and conflict in this area, and thus experience lower blood pressure levels. While this effect might seem to be more prominent among frequent church attenders, the actual implementation of such religious prescriptions may be more highly associated with the *meaning* that religion has to the individuals, that is, the importance of their religion to them.

Only recently have investigators explored the effects of age on the relation between blood pressure and religious attitudes and activities. Higher well-being, morale, and coping levels have been associated with religious attitudes and activities in later life.[39] Successful adaptation and ability to handle stress might confer protection from increases in blood pressure commonly seen at this time, though admittedly the link between psychosocial stress and hypertension is weak. In a study of older patients attending a geriatric clinic, significantly lower levels of intrinsic religiosity (a subjective religiosity variable akin to importance of religion) was found among older women with depression or anxiety disorders.[40] While similar differences existed for older men, these did not reach statistical significance. In that study, however, there were no differences in intrinsic religiosity between older women with or without hypertension. In older men, on the other hand, intrinsic religiosity was higher among those who did not have hypertension compared with those who did ($.05 > p > .10$). Both that study (among medical patients) and the present one (among males without diagnosable cardiovascular disease) have found an association between lower blood pressure levels and subjective religiosity among men—older men, in particular.

Turning to the smoking findings, even after adjusting for the confounding effects of other variables and employment of the Bonferroni correction for multiple comparisons, blood pressures were significantly lower among smokers reporting high religious importance compared to smokers with low religious importance. In fact, the risk of diastolic hypertension among smokers who did not see their religion as important to them was greater than 4.3 times that of smokers with high religious importance. No difference, however, was seen among nonsmokers. These findings are particularly notable given the prevalent presumption that the positive effects of religion on health are mediated through health care practices resulting from religious proscriptions against cigarette smoking, alcohol consumption, and harmful dietary practices.[41] In the present study, however, it was among those who smoked that religious importance made the biggest difference in blood pressure. This may reflect a preferentially greater moderating effect for religion on blood pressure among more tense or nervous individuals who may also be more likely to smoke.

CONCLUSION

This is the first community-based cardiovascular study where a religious meaning variable, the importance of one's religion, and another religious variable, frequency of attendance, were used separately and then together to evaluate the association between religion and blood pressure. The unadjusted results indicated that the single meaning variable, when examined alone and together with frequency of church attendance, had an inverse association with the blood pressures of rural, white males. The differences were most notable for diastolic blood pressures, for persons over the age of fifty-five, and among those who smoked. Lower blood pressure found among smokers who considered religion very important to them also challenges the widespread presumption that the health effects of religion are due primarily to lifestyle alterations.

What is the clinical significance for the difference in blood pressures noted between the groups in this study? A difference of 5-10 mm of either systolic or diastolic blood pressure may make the difference between blood pressure control and failure of control, and thereby affect the decision of whether or not to add an antihypertensive medication whose side effects may include depression and diminished quality of life. Furthermore, cardiovascular risk increases with even small increases in blood pressure, and the majority of deaths resulting from higher blood pressures occur at pressures below treatment thresholds.[42] In fact, a reduction of a population's mean blood pressure by as little as 2 to 4 mm Hg could reduce cardiovascular disease by nearly 10 percent to 20 percent.[43] Awareness by clinicians of the positive association between religion and blood pressure status should engender positive attitudes toward and respect for religious behaviors and attitudes in patients.

NOTES

1. Jenkins, C.D., "Recent Evidence Supporting Psychological and Social Risk Factors for Coronary Disease," *New England J. Medicine,* 1976, 294, 987-994.

2. Larson, D.B., "Religious Involvement." In Rekers, G.A., Ed., *Family Building.* Ventura, CA., Regal Books, 1985, pp. 121-148.

3. Larson, D.B., Pattison, E.M., Blazer, D.B., Omran, A.R., and Kaplan, B.H., "Systematic Analysis on Research of Religious Variables in Four Major Psychiatric Journals, 1978-82," *Amer. J. Psychiatry,* 1986, 143, 329-334.

4. Craigie, F.C., Liu, I.Y., and Larson, D.B., "A Systematic Analysis of Religious Variables, 1976-1986," *J. Family Practice,* 1988, 27, 509-513.

5. Ibid.

6. Kaplan, B.H., "A Note on Religious Belief and Coronary Heart Disease," *J. South Carolina Medical Association,* Supplement, February 1976, 60-64.

7. Graham, T.W., "Socioeconomic Status, Church Attendance and Blood Pressure Elevation," A Master's Thesis presented to the School of Public Health, University of North Carolina, Chapel Hill, NC, 1976; Graham, T.W., et al., "Frequency of Church Attendance and Blood Pressure Elevation," *J. Behavioral Medicine,* 1978, 1, 37-43.

8. Moberg, D.O., "The Development of Social Indicators of Spiritual Well-Being for Quality of Life Research," in *Spiritual Well-Being: Sociological Perspectives,* Moberg, D.O. (Ed.), University Press of America: Washington, DC, 1979, pp. 1-14.

9. James, W., *The Varieties of Religious Experience.* London, Collier Macmillan Publishers, 1961; Allport, G., *The Individual and His Religion.* New York, The Macmillan Company, 1950.

10. Campbell, A., Converse, P.E., and Rodgers, W.L., *The Quality of American Life.* New York, Russell Sage Foundation, 1976.

11. McNamara, P.H., and St. George, A., "Measures of Religiosity and the Quality of Life: A Critical Analysis." In Moberg, D.O., Ed., *Spiritual Well-Being: Sociological Perspectives.* Washington, DC, University Press of America, 1979, pp. 229-236.

12. Campbell, A., Converse, P.E., and Rodgers, W.L., *The Quality of American Life.*

13. Tyroler, H.A., "Hypertension." In Last, J.M., Ed., *Public Health and Preventive Medicine,* Eleventh Edition. New York, Appleton-Century-Crofts, 1980; Stamler, J., et al., *The Epidemiology of Hypertension.* New York, Grune and Stratton, 1967.

14. Syme, S.L., et al., "Social Class and Racial Differences in Blood Pressure," *Amer. J. Public Health,* 1974, 64, 619-630.

15. James, S.A., and Kleinbaum, D.G., "Socioecologic Stress and Hypertension Related Mortality Rates in North Carolina," *Amer. J. Public Health,* 1976, 66, 354-358.

16. Chiang, B.W., Perlman, L.V., and Epstein, F.H., "Overweight and Hypertension: A Review," *Circulation,* 1969, 39, 403-421; Tyroler, H., Heyden, S., and Hames, C., "Weight and Hypertension: Evans County Studies of Blacks and Whites." In Oglesby, P., Ed., *Epidemiology and Control of Hypertension.* New York, Stratton Intercontinental Medical Book Association 1975, pp. 177-204.

17. Greene, S.B., et al., "Smoking Habits and Blood Pressure Change: A Seven Year Follow-Up," *J. Chronic Diseases,* 1977, 30, 401-413.

18. Princeton Religion Research Center. *Religion in America.* Princeton, NJ, The Gallup Poll, 1982.

19. Cassel, J.C., "Summary of Major Findings of the Evans County Cardiovascular Studies," *Archives of Internal Medicine,* 1971, 128, 887-889; "Review of 1960 Through 1962 Cardiovascular Disease Prevalence Study," *Archives of Internal Medicine,* 1971, 128, 890-895.

20. Ibid. p. 893.

21. Tyroler, H.A., et al., "Blood Pressure and Cholesterol As Coronary Heart Disease Risk Factors," *Archives of Internal Medicine,* 1971, 128, 907-914.

22. Kaplan, B.H., et al., "Occupational Mobility and Coronary Heart Disease," *Archives of Internal Medicine,* 1971, 128, 938-942.

23. McGuire, C., and White, G.D., "The Measurement of Social Status," Research Paper in Human Development, No. 3 (Revised), Department of Educational Psychology, University of Texas.

24. Tyroler, H., Heyden, S., and Hames, C., "Weight and Hypertension: Evans County Studies of Blacks and Whites," p. 180.

25. *Statistical Analysis Systems,* 1979 edition, Cary, NC.

26. Kleinbaum, D.G., and Kupper, L.L., *Applied Regression Analysis and Other Multivariable Methods.* N. Scituate, MA., Duxbury Press, 1978; Neter, J., and Wasserman, W. *Applied Linear Statistical Models.* Homewood, IL, Richard D. Irwin, Inc., 1974.

27. Ibid.

28. Nuckolls, K., Cassel, J.C., and Kaplan, B.H., "Psychosocial Assets, Life Crises and the Prognosis of Pregnancy." *Amer. J. Epidemiology,* 1972, 95, 431-441; Berkman, L. and Syme, S.L., "Social Networks, Host Resistance and Mortality," *Amer. J. Epidemiology,* 1979, 109, 186-204.

29. Berkman, L., and Syme, S.L., "Social Networks, Host Resistance and Mortality," pp. 186-204.

30. Weiner, H., *The Psychobiology of Essential Hypertension.* New York, Elsevier, 1979.

31. Jacob, R.G., Kramer, H.C., and Agras, W.S., "Relaxation Therapy in the Treatment of Hypertension," *Archives of General Psychiatry,* 1977, 34, 1417-1427; Blanchard, E.B., and Miller, S.T., "Psychological Treatment of Cardiovascular Disease," *Archives of General Psychiatry,* 1977, 34, 1402-1416.

32. Brody, S.D., "Psychological Distress and Hypertension Control," *J. Human Stress,* March 1980, 2-6.

33. Harburg, E., et al., "Socioecological Stressor Areas and Black-White Blood Pressure, Detroit," *J. Chronic Disease,* 1973, 26, 596-611.

34. James, S.A., and Kleinbaum, D.G., "Socioecologic Stress and Hypertension Related Mortality Rates in North Carolina." pp. 354-358.

35. Taylor, C.B., and Fortman, S.P., "Psychosomatic Illness Review: Hypertension," *Psychosomatics,* 1983, 24, 433-448; Harburg, E., Blakelock, E.H., and Roeper, P.J., "Resentful and Reflective Coping with Arbitrary Authority and Blood Pressure, Detroit," *Psychosomatic Medicine,* 1979, 41, 189-202, Sapira, J.D., Scheib, E.T., et al., "Differences in Perception Between Hypertensive and Normotensive Populations," *Psychosomatic Medicine,* 1971, 33, 239-250; Pilowski, I., et al., "Hypertension and Personality," *Psychosomatic Medicine,* 1973, 35, 50-56.

36. Linden W., and Feuerstein, M., "Essential Hypertension and Social Coping Behavior," *J. Human Stress,* March 1981, 28-34; Harburg, E., Blakelock, E.H., and Roeper, P.J., "Resentful and Reflective Coping with Arbitrary Authority and Blood Pressure," pp. 189-202.

37. Koenig, H.G., George, L.K., and Siegler, I.C., "The Use of Religion and Other Emotion-Regulating Coping Strategies Among Older Adults," *The Gerontologist,* 1988, 28, 303-310.

38. Koenig, H.G., Kvale, H.N., and Ferrel, C., "Religion and Well-Being in Later Life," *The Gerontologist,* 1988, 28, 18-28.

39. Koenig, H.G., Smiley, M., and Gonzales, J. *Religion, Health and Aging.* Westport, CT, Greenwood Press, 1988.

40. Koenig, H.G., Moberg, D.O., and Kvale, J.N., "Religious Activities and Attitudes of Older Adults in a Geriatric Assessment Clinic," *J. Amer. Geriatric Society,* 1988, 36, 362-374.

41. Larson, D.B., "Religious Involvement," pp. 121-148.

42. Rose G., "Strategy of Prevention: Lessons from Cardiovascular Disease," *British Medical J.,* 1981, 282, 1847-1855.

43. Marmot, M.G., "Diet, Hypertension and Stroke." In Turner, M.R., Ed., *Nutrition and Health.* New York, Alan R. Liss, 1982, p. 243.

Chapter 12

A Systematic Review of Nursing Home Research in Three Psychiatric Journals: 1966-1985

David B. Larson
John S. Lyons
Ann A. Hohmann
Robert S. Beardsley
Wendy M. Huckeba
Peter V. Rabins
Barry D. Lebowitz

This article presents the results of a systematic review of two decades of research on nursing home populations in three major psychiatric journals. The review indicates that very little psychiatric research has been undertaken in nursing home settings. The work that has been done is more often qualitative: case studies, program reports or reviews of the research rather than quantitative research studies. The small amount of empirical research that has been published has suffered from sampling, design, and analytic shortcomings. Until recently, there has been little funded psychiatric research in nursing home settings, reflected in a worse than average disap-

Reprinted, with permission, from *International Journal of Geriatric Psychiatry* 1989; 4(3):129-134, copyright John Wiley & Sons Limited. The authors thank the members of the American Psychiatric Association Task Force on Nursing Homes, including Drs. Benjamin Liptzin (Chair), Soo Borson, James Nininger, and Peter Rabins. The views expressed in this article are those of the authors, and do not necessarily reflect those of NIMH. Portions of this article were presented at the American Psychiatric Association meeting, Washington, DC, May 10-16, 1986.

*proval rate for NIMH grant submissions involving nursing home pop-
ulations. The implications of this review are discussed and recommendations are made for advancing this area of study among health
professionals.*

Nursing homes represent the largest and perhaps most costly component of the health care system for the elderly (Rango, 1982;
Freedland and Schendler, 1983; Levit, 1985). As of 1985, an esti-
mated 1.2 million Americans lived in nursing homes (General Accounting Office, 1986), nearly 90 percent of whom were over the age
of sixty-five (Burns et al., 1988). Roughly the same proportion of all
nursing home patients have diagnosable psychiatric conditions. Though
the recent psychiatric Epidemiological Catchment Area studies indicate
that for the elderly population in the community psychiatric morbidity is lower than that of the general population (Weissman et al., 1985;
Robins et al., 1984; Myers et al., 1984), this is not the case for the elderly in nursing homes. Rovner et al. (1986) found that of the nursing
home patients sampled, 94 percent had a DSM-III diagnosable condi-
tion, with the majority having organic impairment. Earlier work reported nursing home prevalence rates of psychiatric conditions to be
over 80 percent (Goldfarb, 1962; Teeter et al., 1976). In addition,
nursing homes have become service alternatives for the management
of chronically mentally ill patients discharged from psychiatric hospitals (Goldman et al., 1986; Linn et al., 1985).

Thus approximately one million Americans are living in nursing
homes and are in need of psychiatric care. However, there is evidence
that psychiatric problems in nursing home patients often go unde-
tected by nursing home staff (Sabin et al., 1982). When detected, they
are frequently misdiagnosed (Ernst et al., 1977) or inappropriately
treated (National Institute on Aging Consensus Task Force, 1980);
Burns and Kamerow, 1988; Burns et al., 1988). Most disconcerting is
the evidence suggesting the inappropriate, inadequate, or excessive
use of psychotropics in nursing homes (Beers et al., 1988; Burns and
Kamerow, 1988; Burns et al., 1988). At this time, although so expen-
sive to consumers and federal government, there is yet little empirical
data on effective means of treating the mental health needs of the
elderly in nursing home settings (Beardsley et al., 1989).

Clearly a need exists for systematic, policy-relevant research in the
area of psychiatric services for nursing home patients. In order to determine the quality and quantity of the existing research and to ascer-

tain where deficiencies exist, a systematic review of articles in three broad-based U.S. psychiatric journals that pertain to nursing home patients was undertaken.

Assessing publications alone does not tell the complete story. The quantity, and more importantly the quality, of publications may be limited by the availability of funds to conduct studies in a particular field. Thus, a second review was conducted. This review was undertaken to determine the quantity and quality of mental health research focusing on nursing home patients with psychiatric disorders. To be more specific, a systematic review of all grant applications submitted to the National Institute of Mental Health (NIMH) over a ten-year period was also undertaken.*

METHODS

Journals

A systematic review seeks to determine both the quantity and quality of research published in specific journals of a certain field. The journals to be reviewed are selected based on the particular field and the area of interest, in this case psychiatry and nursing homes. The journals are reviewed over a defined time period, only those articles dealing with the area of interest (Beardsley et al., 1989, Light and Pillemer, 1984; Mulrow, 1987; Morgan, 1986; Larson et al., 1986; Rabins et al., 1987) being selected.

The journals chosen for this review were *The American Journal of Psychiatry, The Archives of General Psychiatry,* and *Hospital and Community Psychiatry.* These three journals were chosen because each addresses a broad spectrum of issues in psychiatry (specialty journals were excluded), is representative of state-of-the-art psychiatric research, and targets the psychiatric community as its audience. Articles published in the 1966 to 1985 volumes were reviewed.

---

*It is recognized that other sectors of the federal and the private sectors have encouraged research in nursing home settings. These analyses are restricted to the federal sector alone and could have included: National Institute of Aging, National Center for Health Services Research, or the Health Care Financing Administration. The National Institute of Mental Health (NIMH) was chosen because of its specific mental health and mental health services emphases.

Two major dimensions of the articles reviewed were assessed. First, we categorized the articles into two crude groups based on whether the authors had attempted to quantify any of their assertions. The first category, qualitative studies, included review of the literature, studies of case series, descriptions of new programs or therapeutic approaches and editorials. The second category, quantitative, included studies that analyzed data. Quantitative studies analyzed data using either descriptive (e.g., means, standard deviations) and/or inferential statistics (e.g., *t*-tests, ANOVA) (Remington and Schork, 1970). Using a liberal approach, if a study employed at least one inferential statistic, it was classified as inferential.

Second, we assessed the degree of external and internal validity of the quantitative studies by examining the sampling, measures, and statistical procedures (Campbell and Stanley, 1963). External validity was evaluated based on five criteria: (1) the number of persons in the sample; (2) the number of nursing homes included in the study; (3) the sampling method (whether it was specified, and if so, whether it was random); (4) the similarity of the study sample to nursing home populations; and (5) the extent of nonresponse.

Internal validity of the qualitative studies was evaluated based on three criteria: (1) the presence or absence of a control group in the research design; (2) the presentation of reliability statistics on measures used; and (3) the type of statistics (descriptive versus inferential) used. Reports of reliability statistics were considered essential for scales measuring patient status, including physical, cognitive, and psychiatric status, social functioning, and life satisfaction. Reports of interrater reliability were considered essential in diagnostic classifications.

Finally, focusing again on all the articles published on nursing homes in the twenty-year period, we classified the central themes of the articles into three groups: (1) placement, relocation, and adjustment to moves; (2) prevalence of psychiatric disorders; and (3) therapeutic services or treatments.

Grant Proposals

As described previously in our study of nursing home research in clinical geriatric journals (Beardsley et al., 1989) in order to assess the interest in mental health research focusing on the nursing home population, nursing home research proposals submitted to the NIMH were counted and analyzed. Proposals submitted in fiscal years 1975-1986 were classified into three categories: (1) disapproved, (2) approved but not funded, and (3) approved and funded. Nursing home proposal submissions were compared to all other submissions made during the same time period.

RESULTS

In the twenty-year review of articles in the *American Journal of Psychiatry* (AJP), *Archives of General Psychiatry* (AGP), and *Hospital and Community Psychiatry* (HCP), only eighteen qualitative and fifteen quantitative articles were found that focused on a nursing home population. One-third of the quantitative articles used only descriptive statistics; two-thirds included at least one inferential statistic. These thirty-three articles represent 0.25 percent of the total number of articles published in the three journals in a twenty-year period.

Of the thirty-three articles published in twenty years, *AJP* published eight (0.11 percent of the *AJP* total), *AGP* five (0.17 percent of the *AGP* total), and *HCP* 20 (0.64 percent of the *HCP* total). The *HCP* rate of publication of nursing home articles was found to be significantly higher than that of either *AJP* ($Z = 4.65, p < 0.0001$) or *AGP* ($Z = 2.87, p < 0.005$) (Table 12.1).

External Validity

The five external validity criteria to be evaluated were the sample size, the number of nursing homes sampled, the sampling method, the similarity of the sample to the nursing home population, and the

TABLE 12.1. Number of Nursing Home Related Articles Published in Three Psychiatric Journals: 1966-1985

	HCP	AJP	AGP	Totals
Nursing home articles	8	5	20	33
Non-nursing home articles	6,976	2,957	3,100	13,033
Totals	6,984	2,962	3,120	13,066

degree of nonresponse. The results from each evaluation are presented separately. First, in the fifteen quantitative studies, five had samples of fifty to seventy-five, four had 100-200, four had 300-500, and two had more than 1,000 respondents. Second, only seven of the fifteen studies specified the number of nursing homes studied. Of these, three drew their samples from one nursing home, three drew from two or three homes, and one drew from twelve homes.

Third, the method of sampling was specified in only nine of the fifteen quantitative studies. Of those that specified a method, three sampled randomly and the remaining six entered all cases meeting entry criteria within a specified time frame.

Fourth, five studies drew their samples from all patients in the nursing home; ten drew their sample from psychiatric patients only. Among those ten focusing on psychiatric patients, eight selected psychiatric patients who were eventually admitted to nursing homes and two selected psychiatric patients who were already in nursing homes. Of the eight studies with patients eventually admitted to nursing homes, five selected patients from state hospitals, two from Veterans Administration psychiatric units, and one from a psychiatric outpatient unit.

Fifth, the majority of the studies (nine) did not identify the response rate. Of those that did, two had a response rate greater than 80 percent, three had a rate of 60 to 80 percent, and one had a rate of less than 60 percent (Eaton et al., 1984).

Internal Validity

The three internal validity criteria were: presence of a control group, report of reliability statistics, and type of statistics used. Each evaluation is reported separately. First, fourteen of the fifteen studies included control groups. Second, only six of the fifteen reported reliability statistics. In those six studies, reliabilities were never reported on measures of physical status or life satisfaction, once on a measure of cognitive status, twice on measures of social functioning, and three times for psychiatric diagnosis. Third, ten of the fifteen studies used inferential statistics, six of which included analysis of variance. Five studies used descriptive statistics only.

Central Themes

The central theme of the studies varied by whether the article was initially classified as qualitative or quantitative. Sixty-seven percent of the qualitative articles focused on therapeutic services; only 13 percent of the quantitative did ($Z = 1.84$, $p = 0.06$). Twenty-two percent of the qualitative articles focused on issues relating to placement, relocation, and adjustment to moves; 53 percent of the quantitative did ($Z = 1.38$, $p = 0.16$). Finally, 11 percent of the qualitative articles sought to determine the prevalence of psychiatric disorder; 33 percent of the quantitative articles did so ($Z = 3.09$, $p = < 0.01$). Clearly, mental health services research in nursing homes lacks investigators who bring rigorous empirical methods to their investigations.

NIMH Grant Submissions

As reported in our previous study (Beardsley et al., 1989) between fiscal year 1975 and 1986, 20,904 proposals were submitted to the NIMH. Of these 49 percent were disapproved, 25 percent were approved but not funded, and 26 percent were approved and funded. During this time, only sixty-one (0.29 of one percent) submissions involved either the study of nursing homes or nursing home populations. This low proportion of NIMH nursing home grant applications is similar to the low frequency of nursing home publications presented above.

Of the sixty-one nursing home studies, 67 percent were disapproved, 21 percent were approved but not funded, and 12 percent were approved and funded. The proportion of nursing home proposals approved is significantly less than that of all other proposals submitted to NIMH ($Z = 2.74$, $p < 0.01$). Clearly, nursing home proposals were significantly less likely to receive fundable priority scores. Presumably this difference is due to differences in quality, not reviewer bias.

DISCUSSION

In summary, our review of nursing home research found in three psychiatric journals and in proposal submissions to NIMH demonstrates the paucity of quality research being conducted that focuses on nursing home patients in need of psychiatric services. The proportion of articles published in the three major psychiatric journals is very small. The quality and empirical rigor of these articles is low: fewer than half quantify their assertions and even fewer make use of inferential statistics; response rate reporting is poor and presumably these unreported rates reflect a low response; sampling is only adequate; and report of reliability statistics is poor. The area of nursing home research that suffers most neglect is mental health services. The picture is no brighter when proposal funding decisions at NIMH are examined. If an investigator submits a proposal focusing on a nursing home related area, he or she is less than half as likely to receive a fundable priority score than if the proposal focused on another mental health area.

We propose four possible explanations for this situation. First, our choice of journals may be a poor representation of the research published in this field. Our own sense of the journals publishing research in this area suggests that this is not the case. Our presumption is supported by the low rate of funding by NIMH of nursing home research proposals.

Second, practical and methodological barriers may exist in doing research in a nursing home setting which are limiting the number of studies conducted. The majority of nursing homes are proprietary and administrators may object to the scrutiny that empirical research entails. In addition, nursing homes seldom have resources for in-house evaluators with behavioral science backgrounds. It is also clearly difficult to obtain informed consent for clinical trials from many patients who would be the focus of any study of psychiatric illness in nursing homes (Warren et al., 1985). A methodological barrier impeding research is the paucity of psychiatric and psychosocial measures whose validity and reliability have been established for a nursing home population (Shadish et al., 1981).

Third, investigators who have an interest in studying psychiatric morbidity may ignore the nursing home population because other populations are more accessible and easier to study.

Fourth, investigators may be avoiding the entire area of study because it lacks prestige. It has traditionally been difficult to attract the best clinicians, and for that matter any clinicians, into geriatrics and treatment of the severely mentally ill (Committee on Leadership for

Academic Geriatric Medicine, 1987; Mechanic and Aiken, 1987). Since many nursing home patients fall into both categories, the problem of attracting first-rate clinicians to treat nursing home patient populations is compounded. Clinicians, feeling that such patients are neither exciting nor curable, typically avoid geriatrics and seek to treat the least ill psychiatric patients. This aversion to the "hopeless" may also be operating among research investigators. The small proportion of submitted and funded nursing home research proposals at NIMH lends credence to this argument.

The problems we have enumerated are not all equally difficult to remedy and point to the apparent source of the problem. The practical and methodological barriers to nursing home research can be addressed by those currently conducting research in this area. Problems of access, informed consent, and reliability and validity testing are standard features of experimental design that have been addressed by experienced investigators in other fields with patients who also pose unique research challenges. Clinical fields facing similar research barriers that have made significant strides include psychotherapy (American Psychiatric Association, 1982), child psychiatry (Rutter, 1986), and consultation-liaison psychiatry (Larson et al., 1987).

Problems of convenience are usually solved by enticing investigators into an area with public or private grant money. However, NIMH tried to do just that by supporting a program to encourage nursing home research (Harper and Lebowitz, 1986). Although the initiative did increase the number of nursing home submissions to NIMH, it did not alter the quality issue since very few of the submissions were funded.

Thus it would appear that the fourth explanation may be the most credible: nursing home research lacks the prestige of other fields. Problems of perception are considerably more serious and difficult to remedy, if indeed they do exist. Changes in attitudes of medical school faculty toward care of the severely mentally ill and geriatric patient populations are critical. Since interest typically follows funding, clinical and research training programs focusing on this patient population would be one mechanism to improve the image of this area of patient care and research. Others need to be explored.

The cost of nursing home care exceeds $20 billion each year and will continue to grow as the population ages. Vladeck (1983) characterizes the issues surrounding nursing homes and nursing home policy as "among the most complex and troubling in the entire arena of social welfare policy" (p. 352). Given the trend of our country's demographics plus what we have found in this review, it would seem imperative to take steps to stimulate interest in psychiatric nursing home research. This recommendation is not a new one; others have sounded a similar chord (Butler, 1983; Williams and Retchin, 1984; Cassel, 1985; Palumbo et al., 1987). It is the responsibility of the clinical and research community to address these issues, and address them with sound research methodology.

REFERENCES

American Psychiatric Association Commission on Psychotherapies (1982). *Psychotherapy Research*. American Psychiatric Association Press, Washington, DC.

Beardsley, R. S., Larson, D. B., Lyons, J. S. et al. (1989). Health services research in nursing homes: A systematic review of three clinical geriatric journals. *J. of Geront: Med. Sci.* 44, 30-35.

Beers, M., Avorn, J., Soumerai, S. B. et al. (1988). Psychoactive medication use in Intermediate Care Facility residents. *J. Am. Med. Assoc.* 260, 3016-3020.

Burns, B. J. and Kamerow, D. B. (1988). Psychotrophic drug prescriptions for nursing home patients. *J. Fam. Pract.* 26, 155-160.

Burns, B., Larson, D., Goldstrom, I. et al. (1988). Mental disorders among nursing home patients: Preliminary findings from the National Nursing Home Survey Pretest. *Int. J. Geriat. Psychiat.* 3, 27-35.

Butler, R. N. (1983). An overview of research in aging and the status of gerontology today. *Milbank Memorial Fund Quart.* 61, 351-361.

Campbell, D. T. and Stanley, J. C. (1963). *Experimental and Quasi-Experimental Designs for Research*. Rand McNally, Chicago.

Cassel, L. K. (1985). Research in nursing homes. *J. Am. Geriat. Soc.* 33, 795-799.

Committee on Leadership for Academic Geriatric Medicine (1987). Report of the Institute of Medicine: Academic geriatrics for the year 2000. *J. Am. Geriat. Soc.* 35, 773-791.

Eaton, W. W., Holzer, C. E. III, Von Korff, M. et al. (1984). The design of Epidemiologic Catchment Area surveys. *Arch. Gen. Psychiat.* 41, 942-948.

Ernst, P. E., Badash, D., and Beran, B. (1977). Incidence of mental illness in the aged: Unmasking the effects of a diagnosis of chronic brain syndrome. *J. Am. Geriat. Soc.* 25, 371-375.

Freedland, M. S. and Schendler, C. E. (1983). National health expenditure in the 1980s: An aging population, new technologies, and increasing competition. *Health Care Financing Rev.* 4(1), 1-58.

General Accounting Office (1986). *An Aging Society: Meeting the Needs of the Elderly While Responding to Rising Federal Costs.* GAO-HRD-86-135. Washington, DC: U.S. Government Printing Office.

Goldfarb, A. (1962). Prevalence of psychiatric disorders in metropolitan old age and nursing homes. *J. Am. Geriat. Soc.* 10, 77-84.

Goldman, H. H., Feder, J., and Scanlon, W. (1986). Chronic mental patients in nursing homes: Reexamining data from the National Nursing Home Survey. *Hosp. Com. Psychiat.* 37, 269-272.

Harper, M. S. and Lebowitz, D. B. (1986). *Mental Illness in Nursing Homes: Agenda for Research.* U.S. Department of Health and Human Services. Publication No (ADM) 86-1459. Rockville, MD: National Institute for Mental Health.

Larson, D. B., Kessler, L. C., Burns, B. J. et al. (1987). A research development workshop to stimulate outcome research in consultation-liaison psychiatry. *Hosp. Commun. Psychiat.* 38, 1106-1109.

Larson, D. B., Pattison, M., Blazer, D. G. et al. (1986). Systematic analysis of research on religious variables in four major psychiatric journals, 1978-1982. *Am. J. Psychiat.* 143, 329-334.

Levit, K. R. (1985). Personal health care expenditures by state: 1962-82. *Health Care Financing Rev.* 6(4), 1-39.

Light, R. J. and Pillemer, D. B. (1984). *Summing Up: The Science of Reviewing Research.* Harvard University Press, Cambridge, MA.

Linn, M. W., Gurel, L., Williford, W. O. et al. (1985). Nursing home care as an alternative to psychiatric hospitalization. *Arch. Gen. Psychiat.* 42, 544-551.

Mechanic, D. and Aiken, L. H. (1987). Improving the care of patients with chronic mental illness. *New Eng. J. Med.* 317, 1634-1638.

Morgan, P. P. (1986). Review articles: 2. The literature jungle. *Can. Med. Assoc. J.* 134, 98,99.

Mulrow, C. D. (1987). The medical review article: State of the science. *Ann Intern. Med.* 106, 485-488.

Myers, J. K., Weissman, M. M., Tischler, G. L. et al. (1984). Six-month prevalence of psychiatric disorders in three communities. *Arch. Gen. Psychiat.* 41, 959-967.

National Institute on Aging Consensus Task Force (1980). Senility reconsidered: Treatment possibilities for mental impairment in the elderly. *J. Am. Med. Assoc.* 244, 259-263.

Palumbo, F. B., Magaziner, J. S., Tenney, J. H. et al. (1987). Recruitment of long-term care facilities for research. *J. Am. Geriat. Soc.* 35, 154-158.

Rabins, P. V., Rovner, B. W., Larson, D. B. et al. (1987). The use of mental health measures in nursing home research. *J. Am. Geriat. Soc.* 35, 431-434.

Rango, N. (1982). Nursing home care in the U.S.: Prevailing conditions and policy implications. *New Eng. J. Med.* 370, 883-889.

Remington, R. R. and Schork, M. A. (1970). *Statistics with Applications to the Biological and Health Sciences.* Prentice-Hall, Englewood Cliffs, NJ.

Robins, L. N., Helzer, J. E., Weissman, M. M. et al. (1984). Lifetime prevalence of specific psychiatric disorders in three sites. *Arch. Gen. Psychiat.* 41, 949-958.

Rovner, B., Kafonek, S., Fillipp, L., et al. (1986). Prevalence of mental illness in a community nursing home. *Am. J. Psychiat.* 143, 1446-1449.

Rutter, M. L. (1986). Child psychiatry: The interface between clinical and development research. *Psychol. Med.* 16, 151-169.

Sabin, T. D., Vitug, A. J., and Mark, V. H. (1982). Are nursing home diagnosis and treatment inadequate? *J. Am. Med. Assoc.* 248, 321-322.

Shadish, W. R., Bootzin, R. R., Koller, D. et al. (1981). Psychometric instability of measures in novel settings: Use of psychometric rating scales in nursing homes. *J. Behav. Assess.* 3, 221-232.

Teeter, R. B., Garetz, F. K., Miller, W. R. et al. (1976). Psychiatric disturbances of aged patients in skilled nursing homes. *Am. J. Psychiat.* 133, 1430-1434.

Vladeck, B. C. (1983). Nursing homes. In *The Handbook of Health, Health Care and the Health Professions* (D. Mechanic, Ed.). Free Press, New York, pp. 352-364.

Warren, J. W., Sobal, J., Tenney, J. H. et al. (1985). Informed consent by proxy: An issue in research with elderly patients. *New Eng. J. Med.* 315, 1124-1128.

Weissman, M. M., Myers, J. K., Tischler, G.L. et al. (1985). Psychiatric disorders (DSM-III) and cognitive impairment among the elderly in a U.S. urban community. *Acta Psychiatr. Scand.* 71, 366-379.

Williams, M. E. and Retchin, S. M. (1984). Clinical geriatric research: Still in adolescence. *J. Am. Geriat. Soc.* 32, 851-856.

Chapter 13

Mortality and Religion/Spirituality: A Brief Review of the Research

David B. Larson
Susan S. Larson
Harold G. Koenig

Factors that either help reduce risk of earlier death or potentially improve quality of life when dealing with serious illness stand out as important to recognize clinically in various fields of medical treatment. Over the past decades, quantitative research has increasingly studied potential links between religious/spiritual involvement and mortality among various types of study populations, including regional, national, and international community samples, as well as patient populations in the United States. This article provides an overview of findings regarding these various study populations and the potential relevance of religious/spiritual involvement to longevity.

More specifically, recent studies[1-3] of community-dwelling samples in the United States have found a consistent link between frequent religious attendance and increased chances of living longer, which ranged from 23 percent to 29 percent after controlling for demographic, biomedical, and psychosocial factors that might also contribute to living longer. The odds of living longer increased by 29 percent among the religiously involved in a meta-analysis[4] of forty-two study populations totaling nearly 126,000 people. The meta-analysis found that the protective effects were greater for women than for men

Reprinted, with permission, from *Annals of Pharmacotherapy* 2002; 36: 1090-1098. Support for the writing of this article was provided by Monarch Pharmaceuticals, a wholly owned subsidary of King Pharmaceuticals, Inc., Bristol, Tennessee, and the John Templeton Foundation, Radnor, Pennsylvania.

and also greater when religious practices were measured as public involvement compared with private practices. Two longitudinal community studies in Israel[5,6] have found similar positive links between religious involvement and living longer.

Among seriously medically ill populations, a study[7] of hospitalized patients did not find increased survival rates, but did find protection from depression and increased social support among the religiously involved. Another study[8] of medically ill patients found that religious distress, such as feeling abandoned by God, could increase the risk of earlier death by as much as 28 percent, about the same effect size, but in the opposite direction as that found in the mortality meta-analysis.[4] Furthermore, another study (a case series)[9] found that parents' refusal of medical care for their children for religious reasons led to fatalities from treatable diseases, pointing to negative outcomes of religious beliefs for mortality in this context.

However, among U.S. community samples, whether regional or national, frequent religious practices such as attending religious services emerges as a factor linked with living longer even when confounding variables are statistically controlled for. How frequently one attends religious services is a measure of religious participation and may not necessarily indicate spiritual commitment. Nevertheless, in longitudinal studies[10] of community populations, the association between religious/spiritual involvement and longevity generally appears to be positive and statistically significant.

When examining longitudinal studies conducted in the United States, the religious demographics of the United States are important to identify. According to Gallup Poll data,[11] 95 percent of U.S. respondents believe in God or a universal spirit, and 5 percent are atheist or agnostic. Among those who believe in God, 64 percent are Protestant, 28 percent Roman Catholic, 2 percent Jewish, 1 percent Eastern Orthodox, 1 percent Mormon, and 4 percent are of other faith traditions, such as Muslim, Buddhist, or Hindu. Furthermore, approximately 40 percent attend at least weekly one of the 500,000 places of worship in the United States, including churches, synagogues, and mosques.[12] Another 20 percent attend places of worship at least monthly. In a number of mortality studies, "frequent attendance" is often defined as attending religious services weekly or more often.

It is also noteworthy that these mortality findings generally reflect large samples of people statistically analyzed over time. The associations are not meant to be interpreted as an assured health outcome for any one individual. Many individuals who actively practice a strong spiritual or religious faith die of terminal illnesses at an early age. Furthermore, a spiritual motivation to care for, assist, or protect others may propel individuals into life-threatening situations, shortening their lives.

Also, stark lessons from history point to not only adverse but potentially fatal effects of religious beliefs and practices, especially when fanatical motivations are taken to extremes. The mass suicide of more than 900 followers of cult leader Jim Jones in Jonestown, Guyana, or the slaughter and suicide in the September 11, 2001, attacks on the World Trade Center in New York and the Pentagon in Washington, DC, vividly demonstrated disciples employing religious fanaticism for destructive ends. Religion has been misappropriated to justify aggression, hatred, anger, violence, and prejudice, and, at times, encouraged unquestioning devotion to single religious leaders with agendas of power and hate. In contrast, religious beliefs focusing on compassion, caring, and forgiveness can be life-enhancing and provide an optimistic, hope-empowering worldview. Religious beliefs and activities that promote thankfulness, kindness, understanding, generosity, compassion, forgiveness, and hope are more likely to be associated with coping strength[13] and mental health benefits that may contribute to longevity.[14]

MORTALITY FINDINGS IN COMMUNITY-DWELLING STUDY POPULATIONS

Early Study Findings of Regional Samples

Early studies published from 1972 to 1984 revealed some significant findings between religious involvement and mortality, with most published in the leading epidemiology journals. In a ground-breaking study,[15] deaths from a number of causes among adults in Washington County, Maryland, were studied by Comstock and Partridge, who assessed whether frequency of attendance at religious services had any link with living longer. The community study of more than 54,800 people found that the risk of dying from arteriosclerotic heart disease was 40 percent less for men who attended church weekly or more often, after controlling for smoking, socioeconomic status, and water hardness. Among women, the risk of dying from arteriosclerotic heart disease was about twice as high among infrequent attenders compared with those who attended religious services weekly or more often. Death rates from pulmonary emphysema and suicide were also more than twice as high for infrequent attenders. Death by cirrhosis of the liver was nearly four times as high, possibly from high alcohol use among women who were less frequent attenders. The researchers concluded that even if the mechanism behind the association of less frequent religious attendance with greater incidence of disease and earlier death was unknown, this behavior, like that of smoking, could still prove useful in identifying groups at increased risk of developing a number of important diseases.

Importantly, in this pioneering effort, which stated "it is possible that the observed associations came about because health can affect church attendance," the authors called for further investigation. They noted that this could take either or both of two directions: ill people may not be able to attend church frequently, on the one hand; on the other hand, "Ill people, anxious to make peace with their Creator" may start to attend services frequently. Thus, the uncontrolled relationship between health status and religious participation, once controlled, could either: (1) lessen religious participation's beneficial impact on mortality if people go to church more when they become ill, or (2) appear to increase religious participation's beneficial impact by eliminating sicker people if they stop coming to church once disabled or too sick to attend.[15] These concerns paved the way for future studies to control for functional and health status and also assess it over time when looking at the relationship between religious attendance and mortality.

In discussing their findings for increased incidence of certain diseases among those who did not attend religious services, Comstock and Partridge[15] raised the issue of religiously motivated health behaviors. Increased mortality among nonattenders from cirrhosis of the liver suggests alcoholism, they noted, and higher rates of cervical cancer among nonattenders were consistent with Kinsey's observation[16] that religious attendance and extramarital contacts are inversely related. They commented:

> This discussion is intended primarily to stimulate interest in various aspects of religious behavior as potential determinants of health and health behavior. Possibly other investigators will be encouraged to include frequency of church attendance and other measures of religious behavior in their battery of personal characteristics.[15]

Strawbridge et al.[17] in a twenty-eight-year longitudinal study, found that religious attendance increased survival by improving and maintaining good health behaviors over time (Table 13.1).

In a second study,[18] published five years after the pioneering 1972 study focusing on the relationship between education level and mortality, Comstock and Tonascia again noted that the strong protective effect of religious attendance remained as they tracked Washington County death rates, this time controlling for race, age, gender, marital status, cigarette smoking, years of schooling completed, and whether the dwelling unit had a complete bathroom. "Over the entire 8-year period, there was a strong association of usual frequency of church attendance and mortality risk," they noted, as found in Comstock and Partridge's earlier 1972 study. Comstock and Tonascia observed, "Persons who went to church at least once a week had the lowest mortality and those who never attended church had the highest mortality."

During the last two years of the nine-year 1977 study, the inverse relationship between frequent religious attendance and lowered mortality weakened. Since the study did not control for initial health sta-

TABLE 13.1. Improved Health Behaviors Linked with Religious Participation

Behavior	Odds Ratio
Stopped being depressed	2.31
Quit smoking	1.78
Increased social relationships	1.62
Became married and did not divorce	1.57
Became frequently physically active	1.54
Stopped heavy drinking	1.39

tus, the authors wondered whether the inverse association of religious attendance with earlier mortality could be that chronically ill persons were attending church less frequently.[18] However, later studies that did control for initial health status and physical functioning found that the disabled may be even more likely to attend religious services, perhaps to enhance their sense of well-being despite their disabilities.[19,20] Also, as people become sick, they are more likely to turn to their religious faith and practices in coping.[21]

Other authors[22] have implied that the findings of the 1977 study lessened the findings of the 1972 study. Yet the correlation between frequent religious attendance and mortality remained, although decreasing in the last two years of the study. In discussing what might contribute to this, Comstock and Tonascia[18] pointed to the importance of future research needing to control for initial health status and physical functioning to determine whether these factors were accountable for the mortality-religion relationship. Yet in their 1977 study, they continued to point to the relevance of including religious measures such as frequency of attendance as independent variables, as they again documented an inverse relationship between religious attendance and mortality.

Other researchers[23,24] continued the investigation of religious/spiritual involvement and mortality. In a study of older adults published in 1984,[25] the more religious were found to be twice as likely to be alive two years later than their less religious counterparts. In this case-controlled study of an elderly population living near New Haven, Connecticut, 225 study subjects and 173 controls were selected according to certain criteria to provide more stringent comparisons. Religious/spiritual commitment was assessed using three items: frequency of attendance at religious services, how religious one saw oneself, and how important religion was as a personal source of strength or comfort. Marital status, education, income, race, gender, blood pressure, and history of cardiovascular disease, as well as subjective health ratings and previous hospitalizations, were all controlled for. The less religious had mortality levels double those of the more religious.

Interestingly, the protective mortality effect of religious involvement was not found among the healthy elderly in this sample, but "only among the elderly in poorer health" for both genders.[25]

LONGITUDINAL MORTALITY STUDIES IN ISRAEL

In 1993, researchers in Israel reported predictors of mortality from coronary heart disease in a sample of > 10,000 male Israeli government workers followed for twenty-three years.[5] They found increased religiousness to be linked with greater chances of living longer. The study employed a 3-item measure for "orthodoxy" including: (1) type of education (religious or secular); (2) whether the respondent indicated "orthodox," "traditional," or "secular"; and (3) frequency of synagogue attendance. Each standard unit increase in orthodoxy was associated with a 16 percent rise in odds of survival during the twenty-three years. The data were adjusted for age, but not demographic, biomedical, or psychosocial factors.

In another study conducted in Israel,[6] a sixteen-year follow-up found lower rates of early death among those living in religious kibbutzim compared with those living in secular kibbutzim, evident in both genders, at all ages, and with remarkable consistency over all causes of death. The magnitude of the protective religious effect wiped out the usual gender advantage for women: secular women did not live longer than religious men.

RECENT MORTALITY STUDIES
OF U.S. REGIONAL COMMUNITY SAMPLES

These earlier findings led to research critique and improvement. Results of studies on mortality and religious/spiritual involvement were questioned based on methodologic concerns such as failure to adjust for potentially confounding variables including health conditions and educational status.[26] Longitudinal mortality studies published in recent years have become more rigorous in design. Studies in the United States published since 1997 with either regional or national samples have controlled for more potential confounders and possible mediating factors, such as social supports and healthier lifestyles. Of the ten studies published since 1997, only one study had as few as seven factors that were controlled for, and all others had >10, with a mean of 11.3 factors. By controlling for numerous demographic, biomedical, and health behavior variables, these studies address the concern that the link between religious/spiritual involvement and odds of living longer may merely reflect the effect of one, or a combination, of these confounding or mediating factors such as socioeconomic status, social support, or healthier lifestyles. Findings of some of these recent studies are highlighted below.

Findings in Alameda County, California

A twenty-eight-year longitudinal study[1] of 5,286 residents of Alameda County, California, which investigated associations between religious attendance and mortality, found that those who attended religious services weekly or more often were 23 percent more likely to survive during the study period after numerous factors were controlled for. The randomly selected study sample was from a large urban county including the cities of Oakland and Berkeley. Methodologic difficulties of earlier studies were addressed by including potential confounding variables such as age, education level, and functional health; and potential mediating or explanatory factors including social support, social activities, and healthy and unhealthy lifestyle practices.

Associations between frequent attendance and lowered mortality during the study period were stronger for women than for men, possibly since religious organizations might fulfill needs for social support among the high proportion of widows among older women, and since women are more prone to seek and use social interaction to cope with illness, the researchers suggested.[27]

The researchers[1] also investigated the progression of health practices and social connections to see whether frequent religious attendance may help spur the adoption of better health practices and stronger social connections over time during the nearly three decades from 1965 to 1994.

The study demonstrated lower mortality rates for frequent attenders compared with infrequent attenders during the twenty-eight years, with chance of survival 33 percent greater after controlling for age, gender, ethnicity, education, and physical and mental health variables, using time-dependent covariate survival models. Adjusting for social connections effected a slight reduction to 31 percent. When adjusting for health practices, including cigarette smoking, level of alcohol consumption, level of exercise, and body mass index, the effect was reduced to 23 percent, yet still remained significant.

The researchers noted that health practices and social connections could either confound the relationship between attendance and mortality—by persons with good health practices and strong social connections also being frequent attenders at religious services—or act as intervening variables on a causal pathway between attendance and mortality. The researchers found stronger evidence for the latter, intervening model. For instance, at baseline, frequent attenders were much less likely to smoke cigarettes or drink heavily. However, frequent attenders who did smoke at baseline were twice as likely as infrequent attenders to stop. Frequent attenders also were more likely to discontinue heavy drinking. Also, frequent attenders in 1965 who exercised never or only sometimes were > 33 percent more likely to increase frequency of exercise. There were no differences in marital status at baseline for frequent attenders compared with less frequent or nonattenders. But those who were married were more likely to stay married over time to the same person if they were frequent attenders. Also, frequent attenders increased in social memberships of nonreligious organizations and increased close contacts.[1,27]

Consequently, frequent attendance may have lower mortality rates partly because attendance over time facilitates the adoption of better health practices, increased social connections, and marital stability. Also, the fact that many frequent attenders did not drink heavily or smoke at baseline might possibly be due to religious attendance influencing health practices before the study began, the researchers suggested.[1,27]

To investigate the connection between religious attendance and health practices in more depth, in 2001 the same research team[17] analyzed the longitudinal data further for the 2,676 participants who survived from 1965 to 1994. Religious attendance appeared to have a link with initiating and maintaining protective health behaviors over time.

The study examined the association between religious attendance and exercise, smoking, excessive alcohol consumption, depression, medical checkups, social interactions, and marital status. This important analysis found that those reporting weekly attendance were both likely to improve health behaviors and maintain good ones than were those whose attendance was less or none.[17]

For both genders, weekly attendance was associated with a statistically significant improvement in (1) quitting smoking, (2) becoming frequently physically active, (3) alleviation of depression, (4) increasing the number of individual personal relationships, and (5) initiating and sustaining stable marriages (Table 13.1). In addition, women were more likely to stop heavy drinking. Notably, attenders did not all start with such healthy lifestyle behaviors. Improved health behaviors and more extensive social relationships occurred in conjunction with their becoming frequent attenders at religious services. Persons who either stopped going to religious services or never or infrequently attended were more at risk for (1) stopping annual medical checkups, (2) decreasing social relationships, and (3) becoming divorced or separated.

The researchers stated:

> The analyses here indicate that attenders did not all start off with such good behaviors; to some extent, their good health behaviors and more extensive social relationships occurred in conjunction with their attendance. If this is so, the commonly employed strategy in analyses focusing on associations between religious attendance and mortality of adjusting for health behaviors and social relationships over the follow-up period may actually underestimate the impact of attendance.[17]

Even baseline adjustments for these variables are subject to the same error because attendance at religious services could have influenced health behaviors and social relationships before the analyses began, the authors added.[17]

The researchers suggested further investigations of mechanisms that might contribute to impacting healthy lifestyle behaviors. These might include religious/spiritual/philosophical tenets, such as viewing one's body with respect; relational aspects, such as supportive friendships and community; cognitive aspects, such as a stronger sense of coherence, meaning, or sense of control; and psychological, such as enhanced coping skills or potentially increased self-esteem stemming from religious beliefs or practices.

Koenig et al.[21] have noted the frequent role of positive religious coping in reducing psychological distress and reducing the risk of depression. In addition, in > 800 studies that have examined the relationship between religious involvement and some indicator of mental health, the large majority find that religious involvement is associated with greater well-being and life-satisfaction, more self-esteem, greater purpose and meaning in life, greater hope and optimism, less anxiety and depression, more stable marriages, and lower rates of alcohol or drug abuse.[14]

Findings in Marin County, California

In another longitudinal study in California,[2] 2,025 residents of Marin County aged ≥ 55 years were followed for five years. A wide range of factors that could contribute to health and living longer were assessed to see what might contribute to longer life. During the study period, 454 of these people died. One of the most significant factors predicting survival was attendance of religious services. Weekly attenders had the lowest mortality and nonattenders had the highest mortality for both genders.

Further analyses examined a range of activities to evaluate whether it was activities in general that explained the protective factor; these analyses showed that attending religious services was significantly associated with mortality, while attending museums or art galleries was marginally protective.[2]

When analyzing other social support and types of meeting attendance, they found that although attending other clubs rather than religious services failed to help people live longer, a "complementary" effect appeared between attendance and volunteer work. Persons who engaged in volunteer work along with attending religious services were even more likely to live longer than those who did neither or only attended religious services.[2]

As with the previous Alameda County study, the researchers comprehensively analyzed an extensive range of factors that could affect health that might instead explain why those attending religious services might live longer. These included age, gender, race, ethnic group, income, education, and employment; chronic diseases such as stroke, heart disease, cancer, diabetes, and other illness; physical functioning and driving status; health habits such as exercise, drinking, smoking, body fat, and seeking medical care; social participation, activities, marital status, health of spouse, and having confidants; and psychological status such as depression and fearfulness.[2]

Even after controlling for six classes of potential confounding and intervening variables, the researchers were unable to explain the protection against mortality offered by religious attendance. They noted that their findings supported other research that showed attending religious services was linked with lower blood pressure, lower risk of death from cardiovascular disease, less depression, and reduced mortality from all causes studied.

Findings in Piedmont, North Carolina

A random sample[3] of nearly 4,000 seniors aged ≥ 64 years living in the Piedmont region, North Carolina, was interviewed annually for up to six years. The study found chances to live longer increased by 28 percent for those attending religious services each week, after controlling for demographic, health, and psychosocial factors. The study, supported by the National Institute on Aging, found that older adults, particularly women, who attended religious services at least once a week appeared to have a survival advantage over those attending services less frequently.

Age, race, gender, education, marital status, ability to perform daily-living tasks, subjective feelings of health, chronic health conditions, depression, negative life events, social support, and attendance at religious meetings, as well as health practices such as cigarette smoking and alcohol use, were taken into account. Death rates of 30 percent among this sample were relatively high during the study's six years of follow-up, which provided substantial power for examining predictors of survival.[3]

Analyses revealed that the risk of dying for those attending religious services at least weekly was 46 percent lower than for those attending less often. At the study's start, and similar to the Alameda County study noted above, the researchers found that religious attenders had more social support and lived healthier lifestyles than did less frequent attenders.[3]

After adjusting for these explanatory factors of social support and health behaviors (as opposed to confounding factors such as age, education level, income, or initial health status) that could explain why religion helped to foster longer lives, frequent attenders were still 28 percent less likely to have died during the six years. As in the Alameda County study, the protective mortality link was strongest for women. After controlling for other factors, women had a 35 percent lower risk of death, compared with a 17 percent lower risk for men in this study. The authors noted that other studies have found women are more likely than men to pray, to rate religion as important in their lives, and to depend on religion to cope with stress, which in turn perhaps conveys greater health benefits than merely attending religious services.[3]

Commenting on the results, the researchers stated that religious attendance is related to lower rates of depression, anxiety, and stress. A strong religious faith reinforced by active religious participation may help persons to cope with life stressors, particularly physical health problems later in life. Lower rates of depression, as well as higher social support, may also translate into stronger immune systems and better defenses against disease.[3]

Findings in a National Community Sample

In a national sample[28] of > 21,000 U.S. adults, researchers examined rates of religious attendance and death rates by any cause during a nine-year period. Analyses showed that attending religious services more than once a week predicted a seven-year longer life span for the overall population and a fourteen-year longer life for African Americans.

For the overall population, the > 7-year gap in life expectancy between those who attended religious services more than once a week compared with those who never attended was similar to the female-male and white–African American gaps in U.S. life expectancy.[28]

The study controlled for the demographics of age, gender, race, education, family income, and geographical region; for baseline health status measured by self-reported health status, activity limitations, and sick-bed days; for the lifestyle choices of smoking and level of alcohol use; and for social ties in terms of marital status, numbers of social activities, and numbers of friends and relatives to call on in times of need, in order to see to what degree these factors might account for the mortality-religion relationship. When controlling for age, gender, race, and region, compared with those who attended more than once a week, those who never attended exhibited an 87 percent higher risk of dying in the follow-up period.[28]

Regarding income and education, the researchers found little evidence that religious attendance was associated with lower mortality rates only because of socioeconomic factors. In fact, somewhat surprisingly, religious attendance in this national study outweighed socioeconomic factors in helping to prevent earlier death:

Religious involvement, however, has received far less attention in the mortality literature than socioeconomic status. Moreover, there is still a sense among much of the scientific community that religious effects are minor at best or are even irrelevant. Our findings help to dispel such a notion. [28]

Both social ties and health behaviors mediated the association between religious attendance and mortality to some degree, but did not account for the full association. Control persons who never attended religious services exhibited a 50 percent higher risk of mortality over the follow-up period than those who attended more than once a week. Furthermore, the authors found intermediate mortality effects for intermediate levels of religious attendance. Those who attended weekly or less than once a week displayed about a 20 percent higher risk of mortality than those who attended more than once a week. [28]

Certain causes of death appeared more frequently among nonattenders. Persons who never attended were about four times as likely to die from respiratory disease, diabetes, or infectious diseases. However, adjusting for stronger social ties also helped reduce the risk of diabetes. In addition, healthier lifestyle choices, such as not smoking, lowered the risk of death from respiratory and circulatory diseases. But these factors did not fully account for the gap between very high attenders and nonattenders in risk of death from these diseases. Consequently, the study found frequent religious attendance was consistently protective across all causes of death analyzed, but to different magnitudes, depending on the disease.[28]

Since religious involvement was related to a reduction in mortality from numerous diseases, the researchers suggested that religious involvement might be a "fundamental cause" of longevity. In other words, that it works through such a multitude of pathways and mechanisms that controlling for any single mechanism or cause of death does not bring about the disappearance of the association.[28]

META-ANALYSIS OF MORTALITY STUDIES

In a meta-analysis[4] summing the results of forty-two study samples totaling nearly 126,000 people, active religious involvement increased odds of living longer by 29 percent. Based on this effect size, the lack of religious belief or practices stood out as a risk factor for earlier death to the same degree as heavy alcohol consumption, exposure to organic solvents in the workplace, or hostility.

This review, published in May 2000, included all published and unpublished studies through 1999 examining religious involvement and death by any cause. It was the first review to address this topic using analytic tools for aggregating and making sense of the results of many different empirical studies. The study populations included both community samples, including the ones cited above, as well as study populations of medical patients.[4]

This meta-analysis found that religious involvement was associated with higher odds of survival, or conversely, lower odds of death, during any specified follow-up period. The relationship was so strong it would take 1,418 new studies showing no association between religious involvement and living longer to overturn the significance of the findings.[4]

When summing studies, the review excluded mortality studies that investigated only specific religious affiliation—such as Muslim, Jewish, or Christian—and instead focused on studies that included some measure of religious involvement. For instance, the measures included how often one attends religious services, how personally important one ranks one's religious faith, or the degree to which one finds strength or comfort from one's relationship with God.[4]

Interestingly, the review found a stronger link between living longer and factors of participation in religious organizations such as attending religious services, increasing the odds of living longer by 43 percent, rather than from private religious practices such as prayer, attitudes, or beliefs alone, which increased the odds by only 4 percent. Also, the meta-analysis found that the relationship between religious involvement and mortality for women was considerably stronger than for men, increasing the odds of living longer for women by 59 percent, compared with 33 percent for men (Table 13.2). The gender difference might be due to differences in the psychosocial resources that men and women receive from religion, the researchers suggested. Because women live longer than men and are generally more religious than men in most cultures, the research team recommended that researchers consider controlling for gender when looking at the link between religion and mortality.[4]

Since other variables might predict longer lives (e.g., explanatory factors, such as living healthier lifestyles or increased social support,

TABLE 13.2. Religious Involvement and Mortality[a]

Study Results	Odds Ratio
Omnibus analysis	1.29
Controlled for sociodemographic status, gender, race, income, education	1.30
Controlled for above and functional status, and clinical-biomedical measures of physical health	1.26
Controlled for above and health practices, social support, social connections, and marital status	1.23
Private measures of religious involvement	1.04
Public measures of religious involvement	1.43
For a 100 percent male sample	1.33
For a 100 percent female sample	1.59

[a]Meta-analysis from forty-two independent samples examining the association of religious involvement and all-cause mortality.

or confounders, such as age, education, income level, or better overall initial health), the review closely examined studies that controlled for up to fifteen variables that also might play some role in contributing to living longer to assess what role they might play in explaining the religious effect found in the lower odds of early death among the more religious. These factors accounted for part of the link, reducing the chances of living longer among the more religious from 29 percent to 26 percent when adjusting for the confounders of sociodemographic and physical health status factors, and reducing it further to 23 percent when explanatory variables such as health practices, social support, social connections, and marital status, were controlled for (Table 13.2).[4]

These fifteen variables included race, income, education, employment status, functional health, global health appraisals, clinical or biomedical measures of physical health, social support, social activities, marital status, smoking, alcohol use, obesity/body mass index, mental health or affective distress, and exercise. Of all these factors, the only one that appeared to approach the protective affect of religious involvement was lack of obesity, although the p value was not significant ($p = 0.12$).[4]

Surprisingly, studies that did control for the health practices of smoking and alcohol use found an even stronger link between religious involvement and living longer than studies that did not control for alcohol and smoking, a somewhat unexpected finding.[4]

FINDINGS AMONG PATIENT POPULATIONS

Recovery from Heart Surgery

A Dartmouth Medical School study of elderly patients[29] undergoing elective heart surgery found that the patients were less likely to die in the six months following surgery if they found strength and comfort in their religious faith and were also socially involved in some type of organization. Among the 232 patients, those who said they derived no strength or comfort from their religious faith had almost three times the risk of death at the six-month follow-up as patients who found at least some strength. Somewhat surprisingly, none of those who saw themselves as deeply religious prior to surgery had died six months later, compared with 12 percent of those who rarely or never went to religious services.

After controlling for biomedical indices, the lack of participation in an organized regular social activity was associated with a four times greater risk of death after surgery than those who had been actively participating in groups, whether the group might be a historical society, local government, a church supper club, or senior center, or other type of organized group. None of the other social support variables, including presence of confidants, monthly network contacts, support received, or adequacy of support, showed a trend of a relationship to risk of death.[29]

The effect of lack of group participation and the absence of strength and comfort from religion had independent effects, evidenced in patients with one risk factor and not the other. Additive effects also emerged. When adjusted for biomedical risk factors, patients who did not participate in an organized social group nor found strength or comfort from their religious faith were fourteen times more likely to die during the six-month follow-up.[29]

To assess for levels of social support, the researchers used three different instruments to measure frequency of contact with different types of relationships, such as a spouse, confidant, relative, friend, or group; the type and amount of support provided by their network; and whether patients rated the support they received as enhancing their well-being. The researchers also assessed psychological factors that might influence mortality, including personality characteristics, depressive symptoms, or history of psychiatric disorder, to examine whether social support and religion characteristics were surrogate measures for these emotional and personality factors or independent factors.[29]

No significant relationship was found between past or current psychiatric disorder and death. Although people who are depressed or have other psychiatric problems are often less likely to participate in regular social groups, the researchers noted, controlling for these psychiatric factors did not affect the prospective, predictive relationship with mortality.[29]

Findings Among Seriously Ill Patients

A nine-year longitudinal mortality study[1] of > 1,000 seriously ill, hospitalized men found that religious coping did not increase chances of longevity but did enhance mental health status and social support. The study found that those who most strongly relied on their religious faith to cope had lower rates of depression and a wider network of supportive friends, yet they lived no longer than patients who did not draw on religious/spiritual resources to cope. The researchers commented that dependence on a strong personal religious/spiritual faith, while not always adding years to life "may add life to years."

Approximately 68 percent of all these patients died within the nine years, whether they drew on their religious faith for strength or comfort to a great degree, somewhat, or not at all. About one-fifth of these hospitalized patients indicated at the start of the study that "religion was the most important coping factor that kept them going."[7]

Unlike in community samples, the fact that many of these hospitalized men were seriously ill at the start of the study may partly explain why no differences were found in survival rates among the strong religious copers and others, the researchers suggested. Physical illness may have limited the clinical effects of religious coping and other psychosocial predictors of mortality. Neither marital status, education, income level, social support, nor depression had any effect on survival in this study, despite the fact they are recognized psycho-social predictors of mortality in community-dwelling populations.[7]

Many of these patients may have sought comfort in spirituality/religion as they became sicker and required acute hospitalization, the researchers added, supporting in part Comstock and Partridge's 1972 supposition[15] that as patients become sicker they might turn to religion, thus affecting the religion-mortality relationship. Consequently, an association between nearness to death and religious coping could have arisen, canceling out any protective effect that long-term or life-long religious participation may have afforded.[7]

Spiritual Distress and Mortality Among Medical Inpatients

A two-year study[8] of 600 hospitalized patients aged > 55 years found that spiritual distress such as feeling abandoned by God increased the risk of dying by as much as 28 percent. As noted earlier,[4] this was almost the same-size effect, but in the opposite direction as found in the meta-analytic mortality review. Conducted at Duke University Medical Center, this study[8] controlled for physical health—including eighteen illness categories and their severity—and cognitive and mental health status, physical functioning, and demographic factors such as age, education, race, and gender.

Frequent worship attendance was linked with a reduced risk of dying in the two-year follow-up,[8] consistent with the findings of the meta-analytic review.[4] Yet patients who reported they felt alienated from or unloved by God or attributed their illness to the devil were associated with a 19 to 28 percent increase in risk of dying during the two-year follow-up.[8]

In this first study to investigate the potential impact of religious distress on mortality risk, the researchers used a fourteen-item questionnaire to assess the extent the patient used specific types of religious coping. Items identified positive religious coping such as seeking spiritual support, seeking a spiritual connection, collaboration with God in problem solving, religious forgiveness, and benevolent religious appraisals of one's illness. Religious distress was measured by items that assessed spiritual discontent, interpersonal religious discontent, demonic appraisals, and assessing God as punishing, powerless, or abandoning.[8]

Higher religious distress scores at the beginning of the study predicted a significantly greater risk of mortality ($p < 0.05$) that increased by 6 percent for every one-point increase on the twenty-one-point distress scale. Three religious distress items pointed to a particularly elevated risk: (1) "Wondered whether God had abandoned me," a 28 percent increased risk of dying; (2) "Questioned God's love for me," a 22 percent increased risk; and (3) "Decided the devil made this happen," a 19 percent increased risk. A patient feeling "punished by God for the lack of their devotion," predicted a slightly increased risk of death after demographic factors were controlled for, but not after physical and mental health status had been factored in.[8]

In discussing the findings' implications, the researchers suggested that religious distress could contribute to poorer physical health outcomes. Further analyses revealed that religious distress did predict declines in independence in daily activities among the survivors in this study. Similarly, a study of medical rehabilitation patients found anger at God by the patients predicted poorer physical recovery four months later.[30]

Although religious distress was predictive of greater risk of earlier mortality even after depressed mood and quality of life were controlled for, other emotions such as fear, anxiety, guilt, and anger (not specifically measured, but emotions possibly connected with feeling abandoned or alienated from God) could have contributed to the earlier mortality risk.[8] Another possibility was that those elderly who voiced religious dissatisfaction may have alienated themselves from support by friends and family, resulting in social isolation. The researchers commented that further research is needed to determine whether interventions that reduce religious distress might also improve medical prognosis. Given findings such as these, spiritual assessment in clinical settings is warranted, particularly to screen for spiritual distress.[31,32]

Refusal of Medical Treatment and Mortality from Treatable Diseases

In looking at other religious/spiritual factors linked with increased risk of earlier mortality, religious groups' rejection of medical interventions for "faith healing" can lead to earlier death from often treatable diseases. A study in *Pediatrics*[9] found that when faith healing was used to the exclusion of medical treatment, the number of preventable child fatalities and the associated suffering was substantial. A case series of 172 children who died in the setting of their parents refusing medical treatment on religious grounds found that 80 percent of those would have had a 90 percent chance to live if their parents had sought medical care. Another 18 percent had medical conditions that had a > 50 percent chance of responding positively to medical care. Only three of the 172 died of ailments that would not have responded to medical care. Although this report has potential methodologic weaknesses (e.g., a single pediatrician, the study's lead author, determined whether the refusal of treatment was the cause of the child's death), these results are similar to other studies[33,34] finding excess child or adult mortality among religious groups that refuse standard medical care.

SUMMARY

Longitudinal studies published during the past thirty years have found significant associations between frequent attendance at religious services and reduced risk of early mortality among community populations and in some patient populations such as those undergoing surgery.

Since 1997, studies investigating the relationship between religious attendance and mortality have substantially improved methodologically. These studies control for a wide range of confounding variables such as sociodemographics and initial physical and mental health status and physical functioning and also adjust for potentially explanatory factors such as various types of social connections and health behaviors. Since some health behaviors and certain types of social support may have religious/spiritual motivations, adjusting for these explanatory factors may actually be underestimating the impact of religious attendance to the extent that the adjustments involve intervening variables rather than confounders.[17]

The findings in these mortality studies are notable. A meta-analysis[4] summing the results of forty-two study samples totaling nearly 126,000 people found active religious involvement increased the odds of living longer by 29 percent. The relationship was so strong it would take 1,418 new studies showing no association between religious involvement and living longer to overturn the significance of the findings.

In other studies, religious distress such as feeling abandoned by God put seriously ill patients at increased risk for earlier death,[8] and refusal of medical treatment for treatable diseases for religious reasons also led to higher mortality.[9]

Whether finding that frequent religious attendance was linked with a longer life span of seven years in a national community sample,[28] or that religious distress was linked with risk of earlier death among patients, mortality research shows that assessing for religious factors finds significant correlations. The beneficial and neutral aspects, as well as potential negative clinical aspects of religious beliefs and practices need to be further clarified. Given the high prevalence of religious factors in the U.S. population, religious/spiritual factors are important to recognize and incorporate as independent clinical variables in future health research and health care.

NOTES

1. Strawbridge WJ, Cohen RD, Shema MS, Kaplan GA. Frequent attendance at religious services and mortality over 28 years. *Am J Pub Health* 1997;87:957-961.

2. Oman D., Reed D. Religion and mortality among the community-dwelling elderly. *Am J Pub Health* 1998;88:1469-1475.

3. Koenig HG, Hays JC, Larson DB, George LK, Cohen HJ, McCullough ME, et al. Does religious attendance prolong survival?: A six-year follow-up study of 3,968 older adults. *J Gerontol Med Sci* 1999;54A(4): M370-M376.

4. McCullough ME, Larson DB, Hoyt WT, Koenig HG, Thoresen C. Religious involvement and mortality: A meta-analytic review. *Health Psychology* 2000;19: 211-222.

5. Goldbourt U, Yaari S, Medalie JH. Factors predictive of long-term coronary heart disease mortality among 10,059 male Israeli civil servants and municipal employees. *Cardiology* 1993;82:100-121.

6. Kark JD, Shemi G, Friedlander Y, Martin O, Manor O, Blondheim SH. Does religious observance promote health?: Mortality in secular vs. religious kibbutzim in Israel. *Am J Pub Health* 1996;86:341-346.

7. Koenig HG, Larson DB, Hays JC, McCullough ME, George LK, Branch PS, et al. Religion and survival of 1010 male veterans hospitalized with medical illness. *J Religion Health* 1998;37:15-29.

8. Pargament KL, Koenig HG, Tarakeshwar N, Hahn J. Religious struggle as a predictor of mortality among medically ill elderly patients: A two-year longitudinal study. *Arch Intern Med* 2001;161:1881-1885.

9. Asser SM, Swan R. Child fatalities from religion-motivated medical neglect. *Pediatrics* 1998;101:625-629.

10. McCullough ME. Religious involvement and mortality: Answers and more questions. In Plante TG, Sherman AC, Eds., *Faith and health: Psychological perspectives* (pp. 53-74). New York: Guilford Press, 2001.

11. Gallup GH. *Religion in America: 1992-1993.* Princeton, NJ: The Gallup Organization, 1993.

12. Gallup GH. *Religion in America: 1996.* Princeton, NJ: The Gallup Organization, 1996.

13. McCullough ME, Snyder CR, Eds. Classical sources of human strength. *J Soc Clin Psychology* 2000;19:1-159.

14. Koenig HG, McCullough ME, Larson DB. *Handbook of religion and health.* Oxford: Oxford University Press, 2001.

15. Comstock GW, Partridge KB. Church attendance and health. *J Chronic Dis* 1972;25:665-672.

16. Kinsey AC, Pomeroy WB, Martin CE, Gebhard PH. *Sexual behavior in the human female.* Philadelphia: Saunders, 1953.

17. Strawbridge WJ, Shema SJ, Cohen RD, Kaplan GA. Religious attendance increases survival by improving and maintaining good health behaviors, mental health, and social relationships. *Ann Behavioral Med* 2001;23:68-74.

18. Comstock GW, Tonascia JA. Education and mortality in Washington County, Maryland. *J Health Social Behav* 1977;18:54-61.

19. Idler EL, Kasl SV. Religion among disabled and nondisabled persons I: Cross-sectional patterns in health practices, social activities, and well-being. *J Gerontol Soc Sci* 1997;52B:S294-S305.

20. Idler EL, Kasl SV. Religion among disabled and nondisabled persons II: Attendance at religious services as a predictor of the course of disability. *J Gerontol Soc Sci* 1997;52B:S306-316.

21. Koenig HG, Larson DB, Larson SS. Religion and coping with serious medical illness. *Ann Pharmocother* 2001;35:352-358.

22. Sloan RP, Bagiella E, Powell T. Without a prayer. In Plante TG, Sherman AC, Eds., *Faith and health: Psychological perspectives,* New York: Guilford Press, 2001:343.

23. Berkman L, Syme L. Social networks, host resistance, and mortality: A nine-year follow-up study of Alameda County residents. *Am J Epidemiol* 1979;109:186-204.

24. House JS, Robbins C, Metzner HL. The association of social relationships and activities with mortality: Prospective evidence from the Tecumseh Community Health Study. *Am J Epidemiol* 1982;116:123-140.

25. Zuckerman DM, Kasl SV, Ostfeld AM. Psychosocial predictors of mortality among the elderly poor. *Am J Epidemiol* 1984;119:410-423.

26. Sloan RP, Bagiella E, Powell T. Religion, spirituality, and medicine. *Lancet* 1999;353:664-667.

27. Idler EL. *Cohesiveness and coherence: Religion and the health of the elderly.* New York: Garland Publishing, 1994.

28. Hummer RA, Rogers RG, Nam CB, Ellison CG. Religious involvement and U.S. adult mortality. *Demography* 1999;36:273-285.

29. Oxman TE, Freeman DH, Manheimer ED. Lack of social participation or religious strength and comfort as risk factors for death after cardiac surgery in the elderly. *Psychosom Med* 1995;57:5-15.

30. Fitchett G, Rybarczyk BD, DeMarco GA, Nichols JJ. The role of religion in medical rehabilitation outcomes: A longitudinal study. *Rehab Psychol* 1999;44:1-22.

31. Lo B, Quill T, Tulsky J, for the American College of Physicians—American Society of Internal Medicine End-of-Life Care Consensus Panel. Discussing palliative care with patients. *Ann Intern Med* 1999;130:744-749.

32. Post SG, Puchalski CM, Larson DB. Physicians and patient spirituality: Professional boundaries, competency, and ethics. *Ann Intern Med* 2000;132:578-83.

33. Simpson WF. Comparative longevity in a college cohort of Christian scientists. *JAMA* 1989;262:1657-1658.

34. Kaunitz AM, Spence C, Danielson TS, Rochat RW, Grimes DA. Perinatal and maternal mortality in a religious group avoiding obstetric care. *Am J Obstet Gynecol* 1984;150:826-831.

Chapter 14

Have Faith:
Religion Can Heal Mental Ills

David B. Larson

If a new health treatment were discovered that helped to reduce the rate of teenage suicide, prevent drug and alcohol abuse, improve treatment for depression, reduce recovery time from surgery, lower divorce rates and enhance a sense of well-being, one would think that every physician in the country would be scrambling to try it. Yet, what if critics denounced this treatment as harmful, despite research findings that showed it to be effective more than 80 percent of the time? Which would you be more ready to believe—the assertions of the critics based on their opinions or the results of the clinical trials based upon research?

As a research epidemiologist and board-certified psychiatrist, I have encountered this situation time and again during the last fifteen years of my practice. The hypothetical medical treatment really does exist, but it is not a new drug: It is spirituality. While medical professionals have been privately assuming and publicly stating for years that religion is detrimental to mental health, when I actually looked at the available empirical research on the relationship between religion and health, the findings were overwhelmingly positive.

Just what are the correlations that exist between religion and mental health? First, religion has been found to be associated with a de-

---

crease in destructive behavior such as suicide. A 1991 review of the published research on the relationship between religious commitment and suicide rates conducted by my colleagues and I found that religious commitment produced lower rates of suicide in nearly every published study located. In fact, Stephen Stack, now of Wayne State University, showed that nonchurch attenders were four times more likely to kill themselves than were frequent attenders and that church attendance predicted suicide rates more effectively than any other factor, including unemployment.

What scientific findings could explain these lower rates of suicide? First, several researchers have noted that the religiously committed report experiencing fewer suicidal impulses and have a more negative attitude toward suicidal behavior than do the nonreligious. In addition, suicide is a less-acceptable alternative for the religiously committed because of their belief in a moral accountability to God, thus making them less susceptible than the nonreligious to this life-ending alternative. Finally, the foundational religious beliefs in an afterlife, divine justice, and the possibility of eternal condemnation all help to reduce the appeal of potentially self-destructive behavior.

If religion can reduce the appeal of potentially self-destructive behavior such as suicide, could it also play a role in decreasing other self-destructive behavior such as drug abuse? When this question has been examined empirically, the overwhelming response is yes. When Richard Gorsuch conducted a review of the relationship between religious commitment and drug abuse nearly twenty years ago, he noted that religious commitment "predicts those who have not used an illicit drug regardless of whether the religious variable is defined in terms of membership, active participation, religious upbringing or the meaningfulness of religion as viewed by the person himself."

More recent reviews have substantiated the earlier findings of Gorsuch, demonstrating that even when employing varying measures of religion, religious commitment predicted curtailed drug abuse. Interestingly, a national survey of 14,000 adolescents found the lowest rates of adolescent drug abuse in the most "politically incorrect" religious group—theologically conservative teens. The drug-abuse rates of teens from more liberal religious groups rose a little higher but still sank below rates of drug abuse among nonreligious teens. The correlations between the six measures of religion employed in the survey and the eight measures of substance abuse all were consistently negative. These findings lead the authors of the study to conclude that the amount of importance individuals place on religion in their lives is the best predictor of a lack of substance abuse, implying that "the (internal) controls operating here are a result of deeply internalized norms and values rather than fear . . . or peer pressure." For teens living in a society in which drug rates continue to spiral, religion may not be so bad after all.

Just as religious commitment seems to be negatively correlated with drug abuse, similar results are found when examining the relationship between religious commitment and alcohol abuse. When I investigated this area myself, I found that those who abuse alcohol rarely have a strong religious commitment. Indeed, when my colleagues and I surveyed a group of alcoholics, we found that almost 90 percent had lost interest in religion during their teenage years, whereas among the general population, nearly that same percentage reported no change or even a slight increase in their religious practices during adolescence. Furthermore, a relationship between religious commitment and the nonuse or moderate use of alcohol has been extensively documented in the research literature. Some of the most intriguing results have been obtained by Acheampong Amoateng and Stephen Bahr of Brigham Young University, who found that whether or not a religion specifically proscribed alcohol use, those who were active in a religious group consumed substantially less than those who were not active.

Not only does religion protect against clinical problems such as suicide and drug and alcohol abuse, but religious commitment also has been shown to enhance positive life experiences such as marital satisfaction and personal well-being. When I reviewed the published studies on divorce and religious commitment, I found a negative relationship between church attendance and divorce in nearly every study that I located.

To what can these lower rates of divorce be attributed? Some critics argue that the religiously committed stay in unsatisfactory marriages due to religious prohibitions against divorce. However, research has found little if any support for this view. In my review, I found that, as a group, the religiously committed report a higher rate of marital satisfaction than the nonreligious. In fact, people from long-lasting marriages rank religion as one of the most important components of a happy marriage, with church attendance being strongly associated with the hypothetical willingness to remarry a spouse—a very strong indicator of marital satisfaction. Could these findings be skewed because, as is believed by some in the mental-health field, religious people falsify their response to such questions to make themselves look better? When the studies were controlled for such a factor, the researchers found that the religiously committed were not falsifying their responses or answering in a socially accept-able manner and truly were more satisfied in their marriages.

Although the religiously committed are satisfied with their mar-riages, is this level of satisfaction also found in the sexual fulfillment of married couples? Though the prevailing public opinion is that reli-gious individuals are prudish or even sexually repressed, empirical evidence has shown otherwise. Using data from *Redbook* magazine's survey of 100,000 women in 1975, Carole Tavris and Susan Sadd contradicted the longstanding assumption that religious commitment fosters sexual dysfunction. Tavris and Sadd found that it is the most religious women who report the greatest happiness and satisfaction with marital sex—more so than either moderately religious or non-religious women. Religious women also report reaching orgasm more frequently than nonreligious women and are more satisfied with the frequency of their sexual activity than the less pious. Thus, while surprising to many, research suggests that religious commitment may play a role in improving rather than hindering sexual expression and satisfaction in marriage.

Not only has religious commitment been found to enhance sexual satisfaction, but overall life satisfaction as well. For example, David Myers of Hope College reviewed well-being literature and found that the religiously committed have a greater sense of overall life satisfac-tion than the nonreligious. Religion not only seems to foster a sense of well-being and life satisfaction but also may play a role in protect-ing against stress, with religiously committed respondents reporting much lower stress levels than the less committed. Even when the reli-giously committed have stress levels that are similar to the nonreli-gious, the more committed report experiencing fewer mental illness problems than do the less committed.

Mental health status has been found to improve for those attending religious services on a regular basis. Indeed, several studies have found a significant reduction in diverse psychiatric symptomatology following increased religious involvement. Chung-Chou Chu and colleagues at the Nebraska Psychiatric Institute in Omaha found lower rates of rehospitalization among schizophrenics who attended church or were given supportive aftercare by religious homemakers and ministers. One of my own studies confirmed that religious commitment can improve recovery rates as well. When my colleagues and I examined elderly women recovering from hip fractures, we found that those women with stronger religious beliefs suffered less from depression and thus were more likely to walk sooner and farther than their nonreligious counterparts.

Yet, despite the abundance of studies demonstrating the beneficial effects of religious commitment on physical and mental health, many members of the medical community seem immune to this evidence. This resistance to empirical findings on the mental health benefits of religious commitment may stem from the antireligious views espoused by significant mental health theorists. For example, Sigmund Freud called religion a "universal obsessional neurosis" and regarded mystical experience as "infantile helplessness" and a "regression to primary narcissism." More recently, Albert Ellis, the originator of rational-emotive therapy, has argued that "unbelief, humanism, skepticism and even thoroughgoing atheism not only abet but are practically synonymous with mental health; and that devout belief, dogmatism and religiosity distinctly contribute to, and in some ways are equal to, mental or emotional disturbance." Other clinicians have continued to perpetuate the misconception that religion is associated with psychopathology by labeling spiritual experiences as, among other things, borderline psychosis, a psychotic episode, or the result of temporal-lobe dysfunction. Even the consensus report, "Mysticism: Spiritual Quest or Psychological Disturbance," by the Group for the Advancement of Psychiatry supported the long-standing view of religion as psychopathology, calling religious and mystical experiences "a regression, an escape, a projection upon the world of a primitive infantile state."

What is perhaps most surprising about these negative opinions of religion's effect on mental health is the startling absence of empirical evidence to support these views. Indeed, the same scientists who were trained to accept or reject a hypothesis based on hard data seem to rely solely on their own opinions and biases when assessing the effect of religion on health. When I conducted a systematic review of all articles published in the two leading journals of psychiatry, the

American Journal of Psychiatry and the *Archives of General Psychiatry,* which assessed the association between religious commitment and mental health, I found that more than 80 percent of the religious-mental health associations located were clinically beneficial while only 15 percent of the associations were harmful—findings that run counter to the heavily publicized opinion of mental-health professionals. Thus, even though the vast majority of published research studies show religion as having a positive influence on mental health, religious commitment remains at best ignored or, at worst, maligned by the professional community.

The question then begs to be asked: Why do medical professionals seem to ignore such positive evidence about religion's beneficial effect on mental health? One possible source of this tension could lie in clinicians' unfamiliarity with or rejection of traditional religious expression. For example, no only do mental health professionals generally hold levels of religious commitment that diverge significantly from the general population, but they have much higher rates of atheism and agnosticism as well. The most recent survey of the belief systems of mental health professionals found that less then 45 percent of the members of the American Psychiatric Association and the American Psychological Association believed in God—a percentage less than half that of the general population. When asked whether they agreed with the statement, "My whole approach to life is based on my religion," only one-third of clinical psychologists and two-fifths of psychiatrists agreed with that statement—again, a percentage that is nearly half that of the U.S. population. Indeed, more then 25 percent of psychiatrists and clinical psychologists and more than 40 percent of psychoanalysts claimed that they had abandoned a theistic belief system, compared with just less than 5 percent of the general population reporting the same feelings.

Science is assumed to be a domain that progresses through the gradual accumulation of new data or study findings, yet the mental health community seems to be stalled in its understanding of the interface between religion and mental health. If a field is to progress in its knowledge and understanding of a controversial issue such as religion, empirical data and research must be relied upon more than personal opinions and biases. At a time when the rising cost of health care is causing so much discussion in our country, no factor that may be so beneficial to health can be ignored. The continuing neglect of published research on religion prevents clinicians and policymakers from fully understanding the important role of religion in health care and deprives patients as well as themselves of improved skills and methods in clinical prevention, coping with illness, and quality of care. The mental health establishment needs to begin to recognize that it is treating a whole person—mind, body and, yes, even spirit.

PART III:
THE LIFE OF DR. DAVID B. LARSON

Dave Larson, the scholar and scientist, was known for many things: his pioneering essays and reviews of research findings linking religion and mental health; his development of the systematic review as a tool for summarizing empirical study results; his career-long efforts to bring about a rapprochement between religion and psychiatry; his successes in promoting religion as a vital topic for medical education; and, perhaps most important, his years of work, within academia and within both the government and nonprofit sectors, to reverse decades-long biases against proreligious and profamily values as somehow antithetical to the deliberations of social policymakers and social scientists. Dave achieved unprecedented success in all of these endeavors. We honor and salute him, accordingly.

Throughout his career, the past two decades of which were conducted outside of academia, Dave also left a legacy of scholarly work, including peer-reviewed publications and conference presentations, that is nothing short of astonishing. A little context: the two of us, Jeff Levin and Harold Koenig, are generally recognized as the most published researchers in the relatively brief history of the religion and health field. Yet only if one added together the entire contents of each of our curricula vitae would one end up with anything exceeding the length and fullness of Dave Larson's record—and not by much. In preparing his curriculum vitae for publication in this book, we received a computer file version which, when printed out, exceeded sixty pages!

In Part III of *Faith, Medicine, and Science,* Dave Larson's jaw-dropping curriculum vitae (CV) is included in full (Chapter 16). Some vital statistics (as Dave always liked quantifying things): at the time of his passing, Dave had published 274 scholarly papers, had made 174 conference presentations, and served on sixty-seven professional task forces or committees. These numbers, moreover, are not entirely complete: When Dave passed away, he had many other works in progress, including an additional sixteen scholarly papers that are not yet published at the time of this writing. It is thus likely that in the "final" version of Dave's CV, whenever it may be compiled, his publication numbers will be closer to 300.

What needs to be kept in mind when reading this remarkable document is that Dave's CV is not the accumulated record of a lengthy career spent in the ivory towers of academia leading a large lab or research team comprising dozens of hungry young scientists who over the years built their mentor's résumé. Dave, instead, spent nearly all of his postgraduate career working, first, as a commissioned officer in the U.S. Public Health Service and, later, to build and run his own 501(c)(3) institute. Outside of academic medicine, in the "real world" where Dave labored, scholarly productivity is not generally required or expected, nor is it typically encouraged or facilitated, perhaps unless one is, say, a laboratory scientist at a big pharmaceutical company or a researcher at the CDC. For Dave, maintaining a scholarly presence was not due to pressures that he "publish or perish"; it was simply a labor of love. Keep that in mind when perusing the contents of his CV, and also remember that all of this work was accomplished by the age of fifty-four.

Preceding Dave's CV is a beautiful essay penned by his wife, Susan (Chapter 15). This ultimate tribute describes the private Dave that his family knew best. This Dave Larson was much more than a brilliant scholar and an important and trailblazing medical scientist and educator. To Susan and Chad and Kristen Larson, Dave was a loving and devoted husband and father who, in Susan's words, was a "daring jester" characterized by "dauntless drive," "pervasive integrity," "wiley insight," and "indelible devotion." This could just as well describe Dave the public figure, as his drive, integrity, insight, and devotion touched all aspects of his life, personal and professional, and were plain to everyone who knew him.

Chapter 15

David: My Daring, Dauntless, Devoted White Knight

Susan S. Larson

Rarely do little girls say, "When I grow up I hope to marry a psychiatrist." Neither did I. Yet Dave demolished the stereotype of a withdrawn, beard-stroking man in black. He radiated warmth. He exuded exuberance. He lived with the drive, energy, and tenacity of a racehorse released from the starting gate. He also wore strikingly bright ties.

Dave strode six feet three inches tall, with deep-set blue eyes, and a friendly demeanor. He emanated boyish enthusiasm. Once when Dave flew to Yale for a research site visit, the person picking him up at the airport inquired how she might recognize him. One of Dave's colleagues at the National Institute of Mental Health (NIMH) told her, "Just look for a big Boy Scout." With only that description, she found him.

Dave abounded with zest, sustained by a profound, ebullient faith. He had a compassionate and generous heart overflowing with gratitude. He wielded a wacky sense of humor that cut through pretense. And under that affable exterior dwelt an astoundingly strategic mind.

I gained a glimpse of his ingenuity the first time we met.

At a small study group connected with Duke Medical Center, Dave, a first-year psychiatry resident, sat among us. At one point Dave glanced at his watch and commented, "It's eight o'clock Chicago time." Since Duke is in Durham, North Carolina, this startled me. I was all the more intrigued because I grew up in the Chicago area, and had just spent the summer there before starting my next semester of English graduate work. So after the meeting I made a beeline to Dave.

I later discovered he had made that comment as a way to entice me to come talk to him. He had just completed a rotating internship in Chicago, having picked that city in order to spend time with his ninety-year-old Swedish immigrant grandparents. Fresh from the Midwest, he had picked up my Chicago accent. So he embedded his comment as a potential conversation starter. His lure worked beautifully.

Little did I realize then the life adventure that I would soon embark on with this man of wacky wit. He had weathered an early loss and tackled life with an unflagging faith, dauntless drive, pervasive integrity, wiley insight, indelible devotion, and a playful love of numbers. A year and a half later I married him: David—my daring, dauntless, devoted white knight.

DARING JESTER

Dave's zany humor emerged some weeks after our initial meeting. He first presented himself in our study group as a pondering, curious intellectual, grappling with the finer points. Not until I saw him arrive at a friend's birthday gathering dressed in a 1930s tuxedo and flippers did I begin to fully appreciate the wild and wacky side of him. For someone like me, immersed in "preponderant propriety," a delayed introduction was probably a good thing. Yet here was a smart man who dared to have fun.

Dave's life-giving sense of humor magnetized me. As our daughter Kristen asked me at age five, "Aren't you glad you married that funny man?" His ability to make jokes about himself and to tease in comical, disarming ways gave us a legacy of laughter. Humor helped us maintain emotional honesty with ourselves and with each other.

Professionally, Dave's humor helped him handle discouraging situations. When he submitted research studies for peer review that discovered findings that went against conventional assumptions, he would sometimes receive rejections with comments that made no sense based on the study itself. Rejection was painful, but he made a game out of it, calling these ungrounded critiques "FLRs"—Funny-Looking Reviews.

Dave skillfully developed how to wield humor. Often serving as a consultant in medical research and education, Dave masterfully employed humor as a Heimlich maneuver to dislodge tension. When a log jam of contention occurred, a little humor dislodged the antagonism and allowed more open discussion to flow.

Dave traveled the country presenting research at medical schools and medical conferences. Since a research presentation usually falls short of a gripping adventure story, Dave interjected jokes to keep listeners engaged.

Humor furthermore helped him shake off ridicule. When a university dean once called him a "charlatan" and accused him of "making up" the findings of beneficial links between religious faith and physical and mental health, he was soon able to shrug it off as funny.

His humor was well honed both from a gift for picking out the comical along with dispensing it as an antidote to deal with difficult times. He loved to tip people off balance into laughter with a surprise turn of phrase.

As an able leader he was able to laugh at himself. He refused to overdose on a sense of his own importance, but saw himself as a team member with foibles like anyone. His humor-heightened humility made him a fun person to work with and to live with, a fact I can attest to, having undertaken dozens of writing projects with him as co-author as well as enjoying life as his wife.

One of Dave's favorite jester ploys to protect our family from taking ourselves too seriously involved calling us by various names. Occasionally he would introduce me, Susan, as his wife "Barbara." Our son Chad he would call "Bob." Our daughter Kristen—first "Wonder Woman" as she toddled in diapers—became "Bernice."

Not long after Dave died, a lady mistakenly called me Barbara. I felt like Dave was winking at me. Kristen remarked in the weeks after Dave's memorial service, "Thank you, Lord. Dad taught Mom how to laugh."

EARLY SHATTERED WORLD

Dave's childhood world ruptured early. His dad died of melanoma when Dave was only six. He was the third of three sons with a little sister. The devastating loss encountered by John Larson's death marked a hard road emotionally and financially.

Knowing as a child what it is like to grow up without a dad and sometimes with no gifts under the Christmas tree, Dave never took blessings for granted. As one close colleague remarked about Dave at his memorial service, he had "never met a more grateful man."

Dave wrestled early with questions of life and death, pain and coping. Spiritual strength that delved deeper than circumstances helped catalyze his joyful living and dauntless drive. He celebrated each year he lived past the age his dad died as an unexpected gift.

DAUNTLESS DRIVE

Dave's tenacious persistence to wholeheartedly pursue career choices fraught with controversy astounded me. Yet, when tackling challenges, he sought mentors to guide him and colleagues to collaborate with in order to gain wisdom and teamwork for the task. He also gave an all-out commitment to his work, developing a new methodology, founding a research institute, and tirelessly pursuing his goals.

Dave's exuberance and strengthening faith did make for stormy sailing across the Freudian-controlled waters of psychiatry in the 1970s.

Historically, psychiatry had sometimes taken a less than neutral stance toward the spiritual/religious dimension of people's lives. Sigmund Freud[1] had proclaimed religion as "a universal obsessional neurosis . . . infantile helplessness . . . a regression to primary narcissism." Other psychiatrists echoed these assertions. Religion had been labeled a "borderline psychosis . . . a regression, an escape, a projection on the world of a primitive infantile state" in the middle 1970s by the Group for the Advancement of Psychiatry.[2]

Such pronouncements by field leaders prevailed at the time of Dave's psychiatry training. When Dave, as a psychiatrist and epidemiologist, decided to quantitatively investigate the potential benefits as well as harms of religious/spiritual commitment, he was not only going against the current, he paddled against the entire flow of the mainstream.

When presenting published, peer-reviewed findings, Dave was sometimes asked if he was religious. The question implied that if he was, no matter how excellent his research methods, he would be biased and that would undermine the validity of his research. Dave would jest and say, "No, I'm not religious. I'm Episcopalian."

Yet he would also comment that no one precluded African Americans from pursuing African-American studies or women from focusing on women's studies. An individual interested in the religious/ spiritual dimension would perhaps be more sensitive to the nuances of religious culture than someone totally unfamiliar with it who might be more apt to misinterpret it.

Dave wanted to discover what the data showed regarding both potential harms or benefits, and move beyond unsubstantiated theories. But calling into question psychiatry's prevailing theory of religion's harm or lack of relevance was less than popular. In fact, Dave called studying the potential relevance of religion and spirituality to mental health "the anti-tenure factor."[3] It took dauntless drive to persist in the face of flack. Part of this drive was fueled by helpful mentors.

Having grown up without a dad, Dave avidly sought mentors to guide him. He also truly listened to them. He did not just seek people to affirm him in doing what he had already decided to do. He took action on what they told him, even if it required making difficult changes. Once he was convinced of the need to pursue a course of action, he would do so with fervor.

Dave's first medical mentor, Dr. William P. Wilson, now emeritus professor of psychiatry at Duke University Medical Center, had graciously invited Dave to undertake a rotation with him his fourth year in medical school. This led to Dave's psychiatry residency at Duke. In time, Dr. Wilson encouraged Dave to pursue research.

To tackle research meant pursuing another degree, a Master of Science in Public Health in epidemiology. Dave decided to invest this time and energy. In so doing, he discovered the career that he loved. He adored quantitative research.

His mentor at the University of North Carolina School of Public Health, Dr. Berton H. Kaplan, encouraged Dave to investigate what truly fascinated him: the potential relevance of religious/spiritual commitment to physical and mental health. That led to Dave's first published paper developed from his master's thesis.[4] The significance of the findings even surprised some of Dave's collaborators. Among men who smoked, those who rated religion as very important to them were seven times less likely to have an abnormal diastolic pressure than those smokers who gave a low rating for the personal importance of religion. The article launched Dave's research pursuits.

Dave also sought out other mentors at the National Institutes of Health (NIH). He was told by one that he really needed to improve his writing skills. So Dave took courses in writing. He also read the classic *Elements of Style*[5] nine times. One of Dave's former high school teachers later commented that not even she had read it that often.

At Dave's death at age fifty-four, he had more than 270 professional articles published and had served as a co-author of the Oxford University Press' landmark *Handbook of Religion and Health*.[6] *Elements of Style* authors Strunk and White would be proud.

Having known the importance of mentors in his life, Dave also greatly enjoyed mentoring others. At Duke, he loved teaching medical students and residents. While at NIH and as president of the non-profit research institute he founded, he loved to help young researchers approach a project and learn how to write papers acceptable for publication. Just weeks before he died he told me he wanted to cut back on his high-stress presentation schedule of more than fifty trips a year: "I want to take more time to mentor."

Dave's drive involved an all-out commitment to investigating the potential relevance of religion and spirituality in the various fields of physical and mental health. Dave committed himself to conducting objective quantitative research. He devised a new research review methodology to avoid selection bias: the Systematic Review. As a psychiatrist who had been taught that religious faith and practice were harmful to mental health, he decided to discover what research studies had found to date in psychiatry's own journals. He decided to systematically examine all quantitative articles in specified journals published over a certain time period and to count the number of findings that showed any links with harm, with benefit, or that were neutral to mental health.

This arduous process required a thorough reading of thousands of quantitative studies, since sometimes a religious commitment variable was included in the study in the tables of data but not alluded to in the discussion or results. Dave expected that the findings would follow a bell curve: a small number of findings with negative links, a large number that were neutral (the large part of the bell), and a few findings that were beneficial. He was amazed to discover that beneficial links amounted to 80 percent[7]—the opposite of what was taught in psychiatry residencies at the time. Convinced by these findings that a potential, primarily beneficial life dimension was often overlooked in health care, Dave decided to focus more of his career on investigating this "forgotten factor."[8]

Building on his experience at the NIH, Dave's drive led him to found the National Institute for Healthcare Research (NIHR). This nonprofit organization examined understudied variables, including religion and spirituality's potential links to physical and mental health. Leading this new organization meant leaving the government's employ with a salary cut, and heading an effort he repeatedly did not know would still remain afloat a few months down the road. But Dave's creative proposals, a productive track record, and generous funding by the John Templeton Foundation, King Pharmaceuticals, and others made possible efforts that helped alter the climate of medical research, education, and clinical care. Medicine began to more fully recognize the potential significance of religion/spirituality in prevention, coping, and even recovery from illness.

Dave's dauntless drive involved passionate, tireless commitment to his work. To almost any event we attended he would bring a research draft in his sport coat tucked into his belt at the back, ready to pull out before the event started—or during intermission or sometimes even during the presentation. I would occasionally tap him on the knee to signal he was creating distracting noise from turning pages during a concert.

Dave wanted to remain physically fit and alert throughout the day to tackle his work. He avoided devouring large lunches that would make him sluggish. This led to developing his own personal "Dr. Larson's Diet." He ate only fruit all day until dinner time. Consequently, on his many trips he hauled Granny Smith apples. This once led to problems in international travel when he was apprehended at customs for trying to bring fruit across the border.

Dave's chosen method of exercise became the exercise bike since he suffered with muscle pain in his joints from ankylosing spondylitis and had undergone seven ankle surgeries. This exercise choice was also partly due to the fact that he could work while biking 100 miles a week. He would often edit papers or make phone calls regarding various projects while he pedaled. His verve for his work was unstoppable.

Perhaps it is no surprise that Dave literally died with his running shoes on.[9]

PERVASIVE INTEGRITY

Along with his dauntless drive, Dave had integrity that permeated to the depth of his soul. As his wife, I saw him make difficult choices that only a man of such integrity would make. I admired his up-front honesty. He also desired to improve projects and build consensus through teamwork, gratefully making sure others received thanks, appreciation, and credit.

Dave desired to be unflinchingly honest, taking great pains to be above board despite the cost. One example at Duke stands out for me in particular.

After completing his residency, Dave was selected to serve as the first chief resident at a newly formed inpatient psychiatry unit that would be administrated by Duke at the county hospital. The new director had just joined the Duke medical faculty from the West Coast to head this unit.

Although Dave knew it might cost him his job, he decided he needed to give the new director some information about his relationship with one of the psychiatrists slated to become an attending physician for the new unit. This attending physician had served as one of Dave's supervisors for his group therapy training and had given Dave a "much less than enthusiastic" evaluation. Dave decided for the good of the new unit that he needed to inform the new director of these circumstances, offering to step down as chief resident if the director so desired.

The new director then asked Dave about the supervision, discovering that the attending physician had neither sat in on a session nor listened to a tape of any of the group sessions Dave had conducted. As a result, the director told Dave that he did not feel the evaluation had basis. He then told Dave about some of his own interactions with this individual, and that he felt this attending physician had some serious problems. Dave had chosen to reveal to the director the potential conflict with his up-front honesty even if it meant losing his position. As it turned out, this disclosure actually brought him closer to the new director.

An aspect of Dave's integrity involved thankfulness and teamwork. He would make sure he took time to express how much he appreciated people, so they knew they were not taken for granted. He also made sure that anyone he worked with received the credit they deserved. He collaborated with others in order to improve efforts and build consensus.

Dave's commitment to calling to say thanks once surprisingly helped him weather a career crisis. While at NIH, Dave served in the Uniformed Commissioned Corps of the U.S. Public Health Service, which is similar to serving in the armed forces. One receives orders to fill a particular position in a branch of the Public Health Service. At one point, Dave had been "detailed" from NIH to the U.S. Department of Health and Human Services into the office of the Assistant Secretary for Planning and Evaluation (ASPE). His immediate superior was a political appointee. After a presidential election and change of administration, Dave's boss left his appointment, as is customary. Dave's position was a job created by the U.S. Congress, so it was not subject to the change of political winds. Or so he thought.

Soon Dave received several repeated calls from a person at St. Elizabeth's psychiatric hospital talking to Dave about a position. Dave had been a researcher and out of clinical practice for nearly a decade, so he was not interested. But rather than ignoring the calls after the first one, he called back to thank them several times for their continuing kind offers.

"Don't you know what's going on?" the person at St. Elizabeth's finally told him. "Someone in ASPE told the U.S. Public Health Service that your position has been eliminated and is having you transferred." Dave was incredulous. He then discovered indeed this person at ASPE was removing Dave behind his back and having him reassigned either to provide mental health care to inmates in a prison in Pennsylvania, or to Eskimos in Alaska, or to patients at St. Elizabeth's. Dave's former boss came to his aid, confronting this person at ASPE and insisting that he not follow through on his shenanigans to end Dave's research career. The ASPE person at first denied his actions, but then admitted his duplicity. He told Dave he would give him no more than three days to find a new job in research. Miraculously, Dave did. With the stress of it all, Dave soon landed in the hospital with an infection requiring intravenous antibiotics. Had Dave not taken time to call back St. Elizabeth's one more time to thank them, he never would have known about the backroom dealings that might have derailed his research career.

Dave's team-building skills excelled from his college years onward. Furthermore, he made sure whomever he worked with was credited and encouraged. He strove to build consensus as a collaborator rather than garner glory as a prima donna. An effort's advancement mattered to him more than his ego.

Attending universities in Philadelphia, Dave had the chance to develop his networking skills. With so many schools in close proximity, Dave organized collaborative efforts between colleges and medical schools to bring in speakers and develop "open university" courses in which a group of schools could participate.

These intercollegiate endeavors, along with experience in planning field-building conferences at NIMH, helped Dave hone his skills for the crucial Scientific Progress in Spirituality Conferences that he organized. Held over the course of eighteen months with working committees in between, these three national consensus conferences brought researchers together in diverse fields of physical health, mental health, addictions, and neuroscience to examine findings on the potential benefits or harms of religious/spiritual practices and beliefs. The researchers summarized findings, assessed research strengths and weaknesses, then mapped out next steps to further develop the field of religion, spirituality, and health. The resulting consensus report, *Scientific Research on Spirituality and Health,*[10] helped spark interest in further research and in development of curricula for medical schools and residency programs by acknowledging the potential relevance of a patient's spiritual dimension in coping.

This report led to several other collaborative efforts. These included another ground-breaking conference held at the NIH in 2003 and co-sponsored by the National Cancer Institute and University of Pennsylvania. Presenters in fifty areas of physical, mental, and social health discussed findings on research regarding the relevance of religion and spirituality. Collaboration with the Association of American Medical Colleges resulted in the development of new curriculum objectives for medical students involving recognition of the importance of patients' spiritual beliefs.[11] Collaboration with members of the American Psychiatric Association produced a model curriculum for psychiatry residency training.[12] Each of these collaborative steps helped to develop the field of religion, spirituality, and health through consensus building.

WILEY INSIGHT

The television character Lieutenant Columbo of the Los Angeles Police Department ranked as one of Dave's heroes. Columbo ingeniously figured out cases by asking disarming questions that led to the discovery of information that pointed to decisive conclusions.

Dave often followed the "Columbo" approach. He thus excelled at ferreting out hidden emotions as well as hidden agendas. This "keeping one's cool" in letting a scenario play out became part of his professional toolbox early in his training. While in his residency, Dave would occasionally serve as a psychiatrist at a state prison. Convicted criminals can often be a trifle manipulative. Dave would listen to their stories patiently, ask questions, and act as if he was naively swallowing their every word. In a sense, he was reeling out the line to better catch the fish. Often their stories became so preposterous in their hopes for Dave to write prescriptions for drugs that they did not really need, that the manipulation would become obvious. Dave could then confront them.

Later in his numerous research presentations to medical audiences, Dave would often receive hostile "questions" that were really attacks on the research findings or on him for pursuing this "questionable" area of research. He would attempt to diffuse these calmly. He chose to let the peer-reviewed, published data speak for itself, and discerningly allow the questioner's own agenda to surface.

INDELIBLE DEVOTION

Not only was Dave daring and dauntless, with pervasive integrity and wiley insight, he was indelibly devoted to loving our family in ways that helped us grow.

When we were dating, Dave had told me that he did not want to have children. Knowing the pain of losing his dad, he was afraid he would die young and leave them struggling without a father. But then the prospect of becoming a dad outweighed the fear of the pain and he was overjoyed at the arrival of our son Chad and daughter Kristen. I discovered that one of the bonuses of marrying a psychiatrist is that he suggested ideas such as, "Let's pray they have complementary personalities." He was emotionally discerning and his encouragement abounded. He did not let either child get away with destructive patterns, keeping them accountable. He also affirmed their strengths.

Dave sought to respond to each child based on his or her unique personality, really thinking through what would help each one best. When reading to both of them and finding Kristen fidgeting, he changed course and took time to read to each based on individual interests. To Chad he read historical sagas. To Kristen, with her colorful imagination, he centered more on fantasy tales. He read their interests well. Chad majored in history at Princeton, continuing on to law school. Kristen majored in radio, TV, film, and entrepreneurship at Syracuse, becoming a media spokesman with the Oscar Mayer Wienermobile.

Dave was committed to expanding our minds and helping us to appreciate the world around us. He brought books with him to read passages to us when we went out for dinner. He'd ask us trivia questions to keep us on our toes. On vacations, he brought videotapes to teach us constellations and astronomy.

Dave truly was a jester in our lives, furthering openness and honesty and fun. At times when I was away and called home, he and Chad would get on the phone together and sound like a comedy team.

We were blessed by the fact that, unlike his own father, Dave was able to parent his children into their early twenties. He was a tremendously insightful, playfully life-giving, rock-solid source of emotional support for Chad, Kristen, and me. He was more than the proverbial "island in the storm." In addition to providing a sense of safety and protection, he would discuss ways to fortify us. This might include thinking through strategies on how to better handle a difficult person or situation. He also modeled how to wrestle with problems from a spiritual perspective, delving into scripture for guidance and asking for help in prayer. He pointed us to a source of strength beyond his own.

He never took his relationships with our children for granted. He showed unswerving devotion by making time available anytime they needed to talk. He thoroughly relished his relationships with them, perhaps all the more because he knew what it was like to grow up without a dad.

He also amused us with his amazing tallies of numerical accounts.

PLAYFUL LOVE OF NUMBERS

When Dave counted the days and hours until our wedding, I surmised this as romance. Little did I realize then that, besides his love for me, he had a love affair with numbers. Personally and professionally Dave was a devoted number-cruncher. He adored quantitative research. He was enthralled with statistical analysis. He thrived on data.

Personally, Dave took the admonition of "count your blessings" to new statistical significance. Anything that one can count, one can examine through observation over time and chart direction or progress. Anything positive that one can enumerate, one can revel in and feel grateful for in some way.

Dave grappled with how much life counted by counting. He could tell you how many hundreds of days he had worked at a particular place. When he went on a three-day trip to present research, he would count the exact number of hours from when we left home to when we returned, marveling that we had packed so much into so few hours. He counted his phone calls and tasks per day, per week, and per month, and compared them from year to year. He counted how many miles he jogged, celebrating when he reached 1,000. He counted the thousands of push-ups he did each year. He journaled how many miles he traveled on exercise bikes each week.

Dave would often ask numbers questions. When the family went skiing, he would inevitably inquire, "How many times did you ski down the mountain?"

To systematically count blessings at Thanksgiving dinner, Dave launched us through the alphabet with each of us stating something that we were thankful for that began with "a," then with "b" through "z."

At times I was baffled by the extensiveness of Dave's counting and keeping numerical track. Looking back, I think counting helped Dave persevere. Counting also helped him to set goals and to revel when he reached them as dreams came true. His life pulsated with hope, and each item he counted was evidence of that hope coming to fruition. Each number was a potential blessing worthy of gratitude.

Reflecting on Dave's drive to enumerate, I think Dave felt that when we take the trouble to count something we hold it closer to our hearts. We appreciate it—like when we count yearly anniversaries or birthdays. Counting helps us rejoice. Keeping count also helps us to realize how much has been accomplished, usually much more than one might have realized if one had not kept track. Counting can also serve as survival pegs to hold onto in tough times, marking not just milestones but millimeters of progress.

When I felt emotionally shattered after Dave's extremely abrupt graduation to Heaven in March 2002, I found myself driving along counting the number of pear trees in bloom in order to reach my destination with at least some equanimity. Light dawned. So maybe that is why Dave was so committed to counting. To keep going when times were tough. To mark things to celebrate when times were bleak. To find what is joyful amid pain. To realize how far you have come no matter how far yet you have to go.

David—

As white dogwoods dapple the spring-green trees and cherry blossoms fall like pink snow, I miss you more than ever. I miss your tall stature, deep blue eyes, profound faith, and wacky sense of humor. I marvel at your drive, integrity, and insight. I miss the devotion with which you loved me, Chad, and Kristen. You said you believed in me more than I did in myself. That was so true. I miss your stabilizing, strengthening, joyful company.

Thank you for traveling through twenty-six years of time as my husband— my Daring, Dauntless, Devoted White Knight.

You've forever shaped my heart.

I love you,

Susan

Susan Larson
Dave's Wife of 26 years, 65 days
Spring 2003

Susan S. Larson, MAT, is co-author of *The Forgotten Factor in Physical and Mental Health: What Does the Research Show?* and *The Costly Consequences of Divorce: Assessing the Clinical, Economic, and Public Health Impact of Marital Disruption in the United States.* A freelance science writer, she is author or co-author of more than forty articles in scientific journals and medical textbooks. She and her late husband David B. Larson, MD, MSPH, collaborated on numerous research reviews and medical education projects. A former newspaper reporter, she has also written numerous magazine articles.

As editor of *Research Reports* for the National Institute for Health-care Research, she summarized medical journal research findings for newspaper and Web site audiences regarding the potential relevance of religious faith in prevention and coping with illness. A Phi Beta Kappa graduate with a double major in English and Comparative Literature from Indiana University, she obtained a master's degree in teaching English from Duke University.

NOTES

1. Freud S. (1959). Obsessive actions and religious practices [1907]. In *The Standard Edition of the Complete Psychological Works of Sigmund Freud, Vol. IX* (pp. 126-127). Edited and translated by J Strachey. London, England: Hogarth.

2. Deikman A. (1977). Comments on the GAP Report on Mysticism. *Journal of Nervous and Mental Disease* 165:214.

3. Sherrill KA, Larson DB. (1994). The anti-tenure factor in religious research in clinical epidemiology and aging. In Levin JS (Editor), *Religion in Aging and Health: Theoretical Foundations and Methodological Frontiers* (pp. 149-177). Thousand Oaks, CA: Sage Publications.

4. Larson DB, Koenig HG, Kaplan BH, Greenberg RS, Logue E, Tyroler HA. (1989). The impact of religion on men's blood pressure. *Journal of Religion and Health* 28:265-278.

5. Strunk W Jr, White EB. (1999). *The Elements of Style,* Fourth Edition. Boston, MA: Allyn and Bacon.

6. Koenig KG, McCullough ME, Larson DB. (2001). *Handbook of Religion and Health.* New York: Oxford University Press.

7. Larson DB, Sherrill KA, Lyons JS, Craigie FC, Thielman SB, Greenwold MA, Larson SS. (1992). Dimensions and valences of measures of religious commitment found in the *American Journal of Psychiatry* and the *Archives of General Psychiatry*: 1978 through 1989. *American Journal of Psychiatry* 149:557-559.

8. Larson DB, Larson SS. (1994). *The Forgotten Factor in Physical and Mental Health: What Does the Research Show?: An Independent Study Seminar.* Rockville, MD: National Institute for Healthcare Research.

9. Dave collapsed while working out at a gym. The autopsy identified the cause of death as cardiac tamponade secondary to aortic dissection associated with anky-losing spondylitis.

10. Larson DB, Swyers JP, McCullough ME. (Editors) (1998). *Scientific Research on Spirituality and Health: A Consensus Report.* Rockville, MD: National Institute for Healthcare Research.

11. Puchalski CM, Larson DB. (1998). Developing curricula in spirituality and medicine. *Academic Medicine* 73:970-974.

12. Larson DB, Lu FG, Swyers JP. (Editors) (1996). *Model Curriculum for Psychiatry Residency Training Programs: Religion and Spirituality in Clinical Practice.* Rockville, MD: National Institute for Healthcare Research.

Chapter 16

Curriculum Vitae

David Bruce Larson, MD, MSPH, FAPA

Personal Information

Date of Birth:	March 13, 1947
Place of Birth:	Glen Ridge, New Jersey
Married:	Susan S. Larson, MAT, December 20, 1975
Children:	David Chad Larson (born May 23, 1978)
	Kristen Joan Larson (born October 21, 1980)

Military Experience

U.S. Public Health Service (PHS): May 25, 1985-February 11, 1994

Reserve Active Duty Military in the Commissioned Corps, PHS

Navy Rank Equivalent Achieved: Captain

Army Rank Equivalent: Colonel

Education and Clinical Training

09/65-06/69 BS in Humanities and Technology
Drexel University
Philadelphia, PA

09/69-05/73 MD
Temple University Medical School
Philadelphia, PA

06/73-07/74 Rotating Internship
MacNeal Memorial Hospital
Berwin, IL

07/74-07/77 Residency in Psychiatry
Duke University Medical Center
Durham, NC

06/81-06/82 MSPH in Epidemiology
University of North Carolina School of Public Health
Chapel Hill, NC

Clinical and Research Fellowships

07/75-07/77 Psychosomatics Teaching Fellow
Supervisor: Jeffrey L. Houpt, MD
Professor of Psychiatry
Department of Psychiatry
Duke University Medical Center
Durham, NC

07/76-06/78 Postdoctoral Fellow in the Behavioral Sciences
    Research Training Program in Mental Health
Supervisor: George L. Maddox, PhD
Professor of Sociology and Professor of Medical Sociology
Department of Psychiatry
Duke University Medical Center
Durham, NC

07/77-06/79 Chief Resident in Psychiatry
Durham County General Hospital
Milieu/Family-Oriented Inpatient Psychiatry Unit
Supervisor: Frederick T. Melges, MD
Professor of Psychiatry
Department of Psychiatry
Duke University Medical Center
Durham, NC

07/79-06/81 Clinical Fellowship in Geropsychiatry
Supervisor: Alan D. Whanger, MD
Professor of Psychiatry
Department of Psychiatry
Duke University Medical Center
Durham, NC

07/82-07/83 National Institute of Mental Health Epidemiology
  Fellow
Supervisor: Berton H. Kaplan, PhD
Professor of Epidemiology
University of North Carolina School of Public Health
Chapel Hill, NC

07/83-06/85 National Institute of Mental Health Epidemiology
  Fellow
Clinical Services Research Branch
Chief: Barbara J. Burns, PhD
Division of Biometry and Epidemiology
Director: Darrel A. Regier, MD, MPH
Rockville, MD

Faculty Positions

07/79-05/80 Clinical Associate
Department of Psychiatry
Division of Community and Social Psychiatry
Duke University Medical Center
Durham, NC

05/80-01/81 Clinical Assistant Professor
Department of Psychiatry
Duke University Medical Center
Durham, NC

01/81-02/90 Assistant Professor
Department of Psychiatry
Duke University Medical Center
Durham, NC

02/90-06/91 Adjunct Assistant Professor
Department of Psychiatry
Division of Community and Social Psychiatry
Duke University Medical Center
Durham, NC

06/91-08/95 Adjunct Associate Professor
Department of Psychiatry
Division of Community and Social Psychiatry
Duke University Medical Center
Durham, NC

02/94-03/02 Adjunct Professor
Department of Preventive Medicine and Biometrics
Uniformed Services University of the Health Sciences
Bethesda, MD

11/94-03/02 Adjunct Professor
Department of Psychiatry and the Behavioral Sciences
Northwestern University Medical School
Chicago, IL

08/95-03/02 Adjunct Professor
Department of Psychiatry and the Behavioral Sciences
Duke University Medical Center
Durham, NC

Administrative Positions

07/79-08/82 Assistant Director
Department of Psychiatry
Durham County General Hospital
Milieu/Family-Oriented Inpatient Psychiatry Unit
Durham, NC

07/79-04/80 Acting Director
Department of Psychiatry
Durham County General Hospital
Milieu/Family-Oriented Inpatient Psychiatry Unit
Durham, NC

05/85-02/91 Research Psychiatrist
Mental Health Services Research Branch

Division of Applied and Services Research
National Institute of Mental Health
Rockville, MD

08/88-02/91 Section Chief
Primary Care Research Section
Mental Health Services Research Branch
Division of Applied and Services Research
National Institute of Mental Health
Rockville, MD

02/91-03/93 Senior Policy Analyst
Office of the Assistant Secretary for Planning and Evaluation
Office of Family, Community, and Long-Term Care
Division of Family and Community Policy
Office of the Secretary
Department of Health and Human Services
Washington, DC

10/91-02/94 Senior Research Consultant
National Institute for Healthcare Research
Arlington, VA

03/93-02/94 Senior Analyst
Office of the Director
National Institutes of Health
Bethesda, MD

02/94-08/01 President
National Institute for Healthcare Research
Rockville, MD

08/01-03/02 President
International Center for the Integration of Health
    and Spirituality
Rockville, MD

Private Practice Positions

01/76-12/78   Monthly Psychiatric Consultation, Caledonia State Prison, Halifax, NC

07/78-06/79   Weekly Psychiatric Consultation, Durham Medical Center, Internal Medicine Private Group Practice, Durham, NC

07/78-06/80   Bi-Monthly Psychiatric Consultation, Federal Correctional Institute at Butner, Butner, NC

07/79-05/80   Associate on the Inpatient Staff, Department of Psychiatry, Durham County General Hospital, Durham, NC

12/80-06/82   Private Diagnostic Clinic, Department of Psychiatry, Duke University Medical Center, Durham, NC

05/80-06/82   Attending on the Inpatient Staff, Department of Psychiatry, Durham County General Hospital, Durham, NC

7/83-12/93   Outpatient Private Practice, Rockville, MD

Awards and Recognition

Scholarships Awarded

1965-1969 Drexel University
Pennsylvania Higher Education Assistance Scholarship
Hatboro Rotary Scholarship
Kermit Fischer Scholarship

Recognition: Clinical, Administration, Teaching, and Research

1973-1974	Intern of the Year Award, MacNeal Memorial Hospital
1976-1977	Elected President, Duke Psychiatry Residents' Group
1980-1982	American Academy of Family Physicians, Teaching Recognition Awards
May 1980	Elected into Sigma Xi: Scientific Research Society, Duke University Chapter, Durham, North Carolina.
June 1982	Finalist, Teacher of the Year Award, Department of Psychiatry, Duke University Medical Center
July 1989	Fifteen Year Service Award, Duke University Medical Center
December 1992	Ten Year Service Award, United States Government
April 1996	Elected to Hall of Fame, Hatboro-Horsham Senior High School, Horsham, PA
May 1996	Elected Fellow, American Psychiatric Association (FAPA)
February 1997	Named Honorary Fellow, Miami Obstetrical and Gynecological Society
September 1997	Elected Fellow, Southern Psychiatric Association
November 1997	Templeton Exemplary Papers: Co-author on two awards: "Modeling the cross-sectional relationships between religion, physical health, social support, and depressive symptoms." *American Journal of Geriatric Psychiatry* 1997; 5(2):131-144; and "Marriage and family therapists and the clergy: A need for more clinical collaboration, training, and research." *Journal of Marital and Family Therapy* 1997; 23(1):13-25.

November 1998   Templeton Exemplary Papers: Co-author on two awards: "Attendance at religious services, interleukin-6, and other biological indicators of immune function in older adults." *International Journal of Psychiatry in Medicine* 1997; 27(3): 233-250; and "Religious influences on child and adolescent development." In Alessi NE, ed., *The Handbook of Child and Adolescent Psychiatry,* Volume 4. New York: Basic Books; 1997:206-219.

November 1999   Templeton Exemplary Papers: Co-author on three awards: "Prayer." In Miller WR, ed., *Integrating Spirituality into Treatment: Resources for Practitioners.* Washington, DC: American Psychological Association Press; 1999:85-110; "The relationship between religious activities and blood pressure in older adults." *International Journal of Psychiatry in Medicine* 1998; 28(2):189-213; and "Is religion taboo in psychology?: A systematic analysis of research on religion in seven major APA Journals: 1991-1994." *The Journal of Psychology and Christianity* 1998; 17(3):220-232.

December 2001   American Psychiatric Association (APA) Oskar Pfister Award: The Oskar Pfister Award is given annually honoring an individual's contributions in psychiatry and religion. Award Lecture given at Annual Meeting of the APA in May 2002.

December 2001   International Center for the Integration of Health and Spirituality Awarded Maryland Nonprofits' Standards for Excellence Seal. Baltimore, MD: ICIHS was awarded the Seal of Excellence by the Maryland Association of Nonprofit Organizations. This Seal designates successful compliance with the Standards for Excellence: An Ethics and Accountability Code for the Nonprofit Sector. A group of independent peer reviewers completed an ethics "check-up" during which time all of ICIHS' operations, work, and accomplishments were evaluated. ICIHS passed the review with flying colors. The Seal of Excellence symbolizes well-managed, responsibly governed organizations that are deserving of the public's trust. The Standards for Excellence set a high benchmark. They go beyond the minimum requirements of current laws. The Standards mandate that organizations have procedures in place to help nonprofits demonstrate honesty in management, financial integrity, and objective evaluation of the effectiveness of their programs and services.

Commissioned Corps Awards and Recognition

January 1989   Commissioned Corps Commendation Medal: For the innovative development and the effective use of the Research Development Workshop methodology: a collaborative public-private sector, cost-effective, approach for increasing successful federal grant funding within an underfunded field of mental health research.

January 1990

Commissioned Corps Recognition Co-Step Preceptor: For providing an excellent learning and educational environment and experience in supervising Commissioned Corps co-step students.

February 1990   Commissioned Corps Unit Commendation Award: ADAMHA Administrator's Award for Meritorious Achievement: For the extremely successful development of mental health services research field grant-development initiatives and for stimulating a very successful field response. Also, for developing and supporting much needed research growth in mental health services research.

November 1991   Commissioned Corps Commendation Medal: For sustained achievement in the initiation, development, and effective research application of the Systematic Review (SR) method during the 1985-1990 years. The SR is an innovative, quantitative review methodology that can comprehensively review the frequency and quality of assessment of either a research factor or a research issue within an individual field (or multiple fields) of study.

February 1993   Commissioned Corps Commendation Medal: For effective leadership in conceptualizing, developing, and finalizing needed family policy research efforts. For providing outstanding administrative and research expertise in successfully guiding the needed research projects through ASPE's demanding administrative review process along with its comprehensive peer-panel contract review process. Finally, in achieving the needed contract outcomes and in presenting these findings at federal and national professional organization meetings.

Directories of Biographical Reference

March 1988   *Who's Who in the EAST*

March 1990   *Who's Who in America 1990/91*

June 1990   *Who's Who of Emerging Leaders in America*

August 1990   *Who's Who Among Human Services Professionals*

March 1992   *Who's Who in America 1992/93*

March 1994	*Who's Who in America 1994*
August 1994	*Who's Who in America 1995*
March 1995	*Who's Who in Theology and Science,* Second Edition
April 1995	*Who's Who in the World 1996*
July 1995	*Who's Who in Science and Engineering,* Third Edition
November 1995	*Who's Who in Medicine and Healthcare,* First Edition
January 1996	*Who's Who in the World 1997*
July 1996	*Who's Who in America 1997*
January 1997	*Who's Who in America 1998*
July 1997	*Who's Who in Medicine and Healthcare 1997,* Second Edition
December 1997	*Who's Who in the World 1998*
April 1998	*Who's Who in America 1999*
May 1998	*Who's Who in Executives and Businesses, 1998-99*
October 1998	*International Who's Who of Professionals*
January 1999	*Who's Who in America 2000*
January 1999	*The Capital Directory of Who's Who*
September 1999	*International Who's Who of Professionals*
September 1999	*Lexington Who's Who,* Millennium Edition
November 2000	*Who's Who in Executives and Professionals*

Community and Foundations Service and Consultation

1977-1982	Lecturer, Contact Durham Telephone Ministry, Durham, NC
1980-1987	Reviewer, Medical Assistance Programs-Reader's Digest (MAP-RDIF) Medical Student Fellowships, Wheaton, IL

1984-1992	Research Consultant, Prison Fellowship International, Reston, VA
1990-1992	Founding Board Member, the Paul Tournier Institute, the Christian Medical and Dental Society, Dallas, TX
1991-1994	Senior Research Consultant, National Institute for Healthcare Research (NIHR), Rockville, MD
1991-1994	Liaison Committee on Charitable Medical Care, Washington, DC
1992-1997	Advisory Board, the John Templeton Foundation, Radnor, PA
1994-1999	Planning Committee, the John Templeton Foundation, Radnor, PA
1995-1996	Editorial Advisory Board, *Better Ways to Health,* New York, NY
1999-2000	Fellow, George H. Gallup International Institute, Princeton, NJ
1998-2000	Editorial Advisory Board, *Science and Spirit,* Concord, NH
1999-2001	Advisory Board, the John Templeton Foundation, Radnor, PA
2001-Present	Advisory Board, the Danielsen Institute, Boston University, Boston, MA

Continuing Medical Education (CME) Recognition

American Medical Association (AMA) Physician Recognition Award in CME and the American Psychiatric Association (APA) CME Award:

First Award:	June 1, 1979, through June 30, 1982
Second Award:	April 1, 1982, through March 31, 1985

Third Award: April 1, 1985, through March 31, 1988
Fourth Award: February 1, 1988, through February 28, 1991
Fifth Award: March 1, 1991, through February 28, 1994
Sixth Award: March 1, 1994, through February 28, 1997
Seventh Award: March 1, 1997, through February 29, 2000
Eighth Award: March 1, 2000, through February 28, 2003

Teaching Responsibilities

1973-1976   Rotating Intern and Psychiatry Resident: Actively involved in the teaching of medical students from the University of Illinois and Duke University Medical Centers, respectively.

1977-1979   Chief Resident: Responsible for the teaching and the supervision of teaching of medical students and psychiatry and family practice residents from Duke University Medical Center.

1979-1982   Assistant (and Acting) Director of the Psychiatry Unit: Responsible for the teaching and the supervision of teaching of medical students and psychiatry and family practice residents, Duke University Medical Center.

1987-1988   Supervision of Commissioned Corps Co-Steps in the Division of Applied and Services Research, National Institute of Mental Health.

1986-1989   Supervision of ADAMHA/NIMH Guest Workers in the Division of Applied and Services Research, National Institute of Mental Health.

1991-2002   Supervision, consultation and assistance to national/ international leading researchers interested in studying and publishing concerning spirituality and religious commitment, National Institute for Healthcare Research, and then the International Center for the Integration of Health and Spirituality, Rockville, MD.

Licenses and Certifications

National Board of Medical Examiners	#133784 —	Issued 07/74
Medical License: North Carolina	#20306 —	Issued 08/75
Board Certified in Psychiatry	#20388 —	Issued 02/80
North Carolina Marital/Family Therapy License	#036 —	Issued 10/80
Board Certified in Administrative Psychiatry	#829 —	Issued 05/83
Medical License: Maryland	#D2935 —	Issued 06/84

Commissioned Corps Review Boards

February 1989	Commissioned Corps Medical Co-Steps Review Board
April 1989	Commissioned Corps Medical Co-Steps Review Board
September 1989	Commissioned Corps Medical Review Board
February 1990	Commissioned Corps Medical Co-Steps Review Board

Professional Affiliations

Southern Medical Association
American Medical Association
Southern Psychiatric Association
American Psychiatric Association
American Public Health Association
Sigma Xi: Scientific Research Society
Christian Medical and Dental Association
Society for the Scientific Study of Religion
American Association for Social Psychiatry
Christian Association for Psychological Studies
American Association for the Advancement of Science
American Society of Psychosocial and Behavioral Oncology/
    AIDS

Conferences, Task Forces, and Workshops
Where Participation Was Invited

I. Issues Concerning Spirituality, Health, and the Family

1. Invitee, National Research Forum on Family Issues: The White House Conference on Families, Washington, DC, April 1980.
2. Invitee, Duke University Medical Center Conference on the Therapeutic Usefulness of Faith, Durham, NC, March 1981.
3. Invitee, National Research Committee of the Association for Clinical Pastoral Education (ACPE), Chicago, IL, October 1984.
4. Co-Chair, Section on Research, International Congress on Christian Counseling, Atlanta, GA, November 1988.
5. Invitee, Spring Research Forum, the Independent Sector, Chicago, IL, March 1989.
6. Member, American Psychological Association Task Force on Religion and Family Issues, Washington, DC, August 1990-December 1992.
7. Planning Committee, Workshop on the Impact of the Media on Children and the Family, Pittsburgh, PA, November 9-11, 1990.
8. Co-Chair, Division of Family and Community Policy, Office of the Assistant Secretary for Planning and Evaluation, Advisory Group Meeting, Washington, DC, August 8-9, 1991.
9. Co-Coordinator, Department of Health and Human Services Working Group on Family Data, Washington, DC, October 1991-March 1993.
10. Invitee, National Institutes of Health Advisory Committee to Plan and Set Objectives Concerning the Use of Unconventional Medical Practices (UMPs), Bethesda, MD, May 1992-2002.
11. Member, Ad Hoc Advisory Panel on the Future of Research in the Veterans Administration (VA) Chaplaincy, Hampton, VA, July 1992-December, 1993.

12. Consultant, Department of Veteran Affairs Team-Building and Policy Development Conference for the National Veterans Administration (VA) Chaplain Center, Hampton, VA, September 1992.

13. Co-Chair, "Spiritual Dimensions in Clinical Research," sponsored by the National Institute for Healthcare Research (NIHR) and the John Templeton Foundation, Leesburg, VA, April 20-23, 1995.

14. Co-Chair, Model Curriculum Committee for Psychiatry Residency Training Programs on Religion and Spirituality in Clinical Practice, supported by the John Templeton Foundation and the National Institute for Healthcare Research (NIHR), Rockville, MD, January 1995-March 1996.

15. Chair and Moderator, "Religious, Social, and Environmental Factors That Influence Disease States," Presenters: J.S. Levin, H.G. Koenig, K.I. Pargament, D.A. Matthews, and H. Benson, American Association for the Advancement of Science (AAAS) Annual Meeting, Baltimore, MD, February 11, 1996.

16. Chair, "Spiritual Intervention in Clinical Practice," sponsored by the National Institute for Healthcare Research and the John Templeton Foundation, Leesburg, VA, April 18-21, 1996.

17. Chair, Conference series on "Scientific Progress in Spiritual Research," sponsored by the John Templeton Foundation and the National Institute for Healthcare Research (NIHR), Washington, DC, July 1996-July 1997.

18. Co-Chair, Mental Health Section, Conference series on "Scientific Progress in Spiritual Research," sponsored by the John Templeton Foundation and the National Institute for Healthcare Research (NIHR), Washington, DC, July 1996-July 1997.

19. Co-Chair, "Spirituality and Medicine: Curricular Development" Conference, cosponsored by the John Templeton Foundation, the National Institute for Healthcare Research (NIHR), and the Association of American Medical Colleges (AAMC), Washington, DC, April 25-26, 1997.

20. Co-Chair, "Spirituality, Cross-Cultural Issues, and End of Life Care: Curricular Development" Conference, cosponsored by the John Templeton Foundation, the National Institute for

Healthcare Research (NIHR), and the Association of American Medical Colleges (AAMC), Washington, DC, March 20-21, 1998.

21. Invitee, Clergy and Physician Partnership Conference, sponsored by the George Washington University and the Robert Wood Johnson Foundation, Washington, DC, June 17, 1999.

22. Committee Member, "Spirituality, Cross-Cultural Issues, and End of Life Care: Curricular Development" Conference, cosponsored by the John Templeton Foundation, the National Institute for Healthcare Research (NIHR), and the Association of American Medical Colleges (AAMC), Denver, CO, September 24-25, 1999.

23. Chair and Moderator, "Mortality and Religious Involvement: A Review and Critique of the Results, the Methods, and the Measures," cosponsored by the John Templeton Foundation and the National Institute for Healthcare Research (NIHR), Harvard Faculty Club, Cambridge, MA, October 4, 1999.

24. Participant, Spirituality, Religion, and Health Workshop, National Institutes of Health (NIH), Bethesda, MD, October 26-27, 1999.

25. Chair and Moderator, "A Forgotten Factor in Public Health: The Relevance of Faith and Faith-based Services" Symposium, American Public Health Association (APHA), Chicago, IL, November 8, 1999.

26. Member, Model Curriculum Committee for Primary Care Residency Training Programs on Spirituality in Clinical Practice, cosponsored by the John Templeton Foundation and the National Institute for Healthcare Research (NIHR), Rockville, MD, November 1997-December 1999.

27. Chair, NIHR-JTF Consensus Conference II Advisory Group, "Spiritual Intervention in Clinical Practice," cosponsored by the National Institute for Healthcare Research (NIHR) and the John Templeton Foundation, Herndon, VA, March 16-18, 2001.

28. Consultant, "So Help Me God: Substance Abuse, Religion, and Spirituality," A CASA White Paper. The National Center on Addiction and Substance Abuse (CASA), Columbia University, New York, NY, May-October 2001. Released November 14, 2001.

II. Primary Care and Consultation-Liaison Mental Health Issues

1. Consultant, American Psychiatric Association Task Force on Cost-Effectiveness in Consultation-Liaison Psychiatry, Rockville, MD, May 1984-June 1987.
2. Coordinator, First NIMH Research Development Workshop in C-L Psychiatry, Rockville, MD, September 1984.
3. Coordinator, Second NIMH Research Development Workshop in C-L Psychiatry, Tampa, FL, March 1985.
4. Invitee, Meeting of the National Committee on Traumatic Brain Injury, Washington, DC, October 1986.
5. Invitee, Consortium on Consultation-Liaison Psychiatry, Brooks Lodge, Kalamazoo, MI, June 1989.
6. Co-Coordinator, "Mental Health Services for Children and Adolescents in Primary Care Settings: A Research Conference," Yale University, New Haven, CT, June 1989.
7. Co-Coordinator, National Institute of Mental Health Workshop on DSM-IV Psychiatric Classifications in General Medicine, Rockville, MD, July 1989.
8. Member, Task Force on Consultation-Liaison Funding Opportunities, Academy of Psychosomatic Medicine, Chicago, IL, October 1989-December 1990.
9. Member, Office of Substance Abuse Treatment Improvement: Intergovernmental Primary Care Linkage Initiative Committee, Washington, DC, March 1990-December 1990.
10. Chair, Fourth Annual NIMH International Research Conference on the Classification and Treatment of Mental Disorders in General Medical Settings, Bethesda, MD, June 11-12, 1990.
11. Co-Coordinator, NIMH Research Workshop: Field Testing Mental Disorder Classifications for Children and Adolescents in Primary Care Settings, Bethesda, MD, December 4, 1990.
12. Co-Coordinator, NIMH Consultation-Liaison Research Development and Research Training Workshop, Bethesda, MD, July 15, 1991.
13. Member, Annual Meeting of Resident Award Committee, Southern Psychiatric Association, Birmingham, AL, January 1992-March 2002.

14. Co-Chair, Panel Task Force Report, Office of Alternative Medicine, Bethesda, MD, July 1993-July 1994.
15. Co-Chair, Technologies Assessment Meeting, Office of Alternative Medicine, NIH, Rockville, MD, September 7-8, 1993.
16. Co-Chair, Conference on Examining Research Assumptions in Alternative Medical Systems, Office of Alternative Medicine, NIH, Bethesda, MD, July 11-13, 1994.
17. Co-Chair, Editorial Review Board, Report to the National Institute of Health on the Status of Alternative Medicine, Bethesda, MD, July 1993-December 1994.
18. Section Co-Chair, Research Reviews Section, Office of Alternative Medicine, Research Methodology Conference, Bethesda, MD, April 27-28, 1995.
19. Invitee, "Future of Medicine" Summit, Christian Medical and Dental Society, St. Simon's Island, GA, October 20-24, 1999.
20. Invitee, "Complementary and Alternative Therapies in the Academic Medical Center: Issues in Ethics and Policy," sponsored by the University of Pennsylvania School of Medicine and the National Institutes of Health (NIH), Philadelphia, PA, November 10-12, 1999.
21. Committee Member, Alternative Medicine Project, "Complementary and Alternative Medicine: The Scientific and Pluralistic Challenge," sponsored by the Hastings Center and the Nathan Cummings Foundation, Boston, MA, December 9-10, 1999.

III. Specialty Mental Health Services Sector Issues

1. Chairperson, Department of Psychiatry, Duke University Medical Center Medical Peer Review, Durham, NC, July 1977-December 1978.
2. Section Secretary, Psychiatry, Southern Medical Association, Birmingham, AL, July 1984-June 1987.
3. Co-Coordinator, First NIMH Minority Mental Health Services Research Development Workshop, Rockville, MD, January 1987.
4. Invitee, NIMH Conference on the Future of Mental Health Services Research, Tampa, FL, February 1987.

5. Co-Coordinator, Second NIMH Minority Mental Health Services Research Development Workshop, Rockville, MD, June 1987.
6. Section Co-Chair, Psychiatry Section, Southern Medical Association, Birmingham, AL, July 1987-June 1988.
7. Invitee, the American Psychiatric Association Future of Psychiatry Conference, Washington, DC, December 1987.
8. Section Chair, Psychiatry Section, Southern Medical Association, Birmingham, AL, July 1988-June 1989.
9. Member, National Institute of Mental Health Psychotherapy and Rehabilitation Research Consortium, Rockville, MD, June 1989-February 1991.
10. Chair, Psychotherapy, Rehabilitation, and Mental Health Services Research Workgroup, National Institute of Mental Health Psychotherapy and Rehabilitation Research Consortium, Rockville, MD, January 1990-February 1991.
11. Chair, ADAMHA Research Technical Assistance Workshop on Services for Persons with Mental Disorders that Co-Occur with Alcohol and Drug Abuse Disorders, Alexandria, VA, April 27, 1990.

IV. Mental Health Services and Issues for Persons in Nursing Homes

1. Consultant, American Psychiatric Association Task Force on Nursing Homes, Washington, DC, May 1985-June 1986.
2. Consultant, American Psychiatric Association Task Force on Geriatric Psychiatry and Public Sector Mental Health Systems, Washington, DC, October 1988-June 1990.

V. Mental Health Needs of Those with AIDS/HIV Infection

1. Member, Public Health Service Subgroup on AIDS Patient Care/Health Service Delivery, Washington, DC, March 1986-January 1989.
2. Invitee, "Coolfont: Public Health Service Conference Plan for the Prevention and Control of AIDS and the AIDS Virus," Com-

mittee on Patient Care and Health Services Delivery, Berkeley Springs, WV, June 1986.
3. Member, Committee on Health Resources and Services Administration (HRSA) AIDS Services Demonstrations, Rockville, MD, October 1986.
4. Member, National Institute of Mental Health (NIMH) AIDS Work Group, Rockville, MD, January 1987-February 1991.
5. Member, Intra-Governmental Task Force on AIDS Health Care Delivery, Rockville, MD, January 1987-September 1987.

Presentations at Professional Meetings

I. Issues Concerning Spirituality, Health, and the Family

1. "The maltreated child grown up," Southern Psychiatric Association Annual Meeting, Pinehurst, NC, September 1977.
2. "Alternative strategies of family interventions: Issues and answers," Center for the Study of Aging, Workshop on the Family, Duke University Medical Center, Durham, NC, April 1979.
3. "The religious life of alcoholics," Southern Medical Association Annual Meeting, Las Vegas, NV, November 1979.
4. "Problems of family life" and "How marriages go wrong," Duke University Medical Center Conference on Evaluating and Managing Marriage and Family Problems, Durham, NC, November 1980.
5. "Marital therapy in the prison setting," American Association of Marital and Family Therapy Annual Meeting, San Diego, CA, October 1981.
6. "Religious life of drug addicts," Southern Medical Association Annual Meeting, New Orleans, LA, November 1981.
7. "Religion and some early American psychiatrists: Perennial issues in theory and practice" and "Mental health and Christian disciplines," Presented by: SB Thielman and MR Lyles, Christian Association for Psychological Studies Annual Meeting, Atlanta, GA, April 1982.
8. "Marital status and religious commitment—How is each associated with personal well-being, psychiatric morbidity, and mortality?" The National Leadership Forum on Family Well-Being, Washington, DC, June 1984.

9. "Patients and parishioners: Who goes to whom for help?" American Psychological Association Annual Meeting, Toronto, Ontario, Canada, August 1984.
10. "Quantifying religious research in four major psychiatric journals: 1978-1982," Southern Psychiatric Association Annual Meeting, Hot Springs, VA, October 1984.
11. "The physician's marriage," Christian Medical Foundation Annual Meeting, Tampa, FL, October 1984.
12. "Quantifying and assessing religious variables in the behavioral sciences," Christian Association of Psychological Studies, First Eastern Regional Meeting, Mt. Bethel, PA, October 1984.
13. "The religious life of substance abuse disorders," Duke University Medical Center Conference on Religious Interventions in the Treatment of Drug Addiction and Alcoholism, Chapel Hill, NC, March 1985.
14. "The measurement of religion in psychiatric research," American Psychiatric Association Annual Meeting, Dallas, TX, May 1985.
15. "The religious life of individuals with affective disorders," Southern Medical Association Annual Meeting, Orlando, FL, November 1985.
16. "The influence of religious practice on adolescent delinquency and suicide," Interagency Panel on Research and Development on Children and Adolescents, Washington, DC, December 1985.
17. "A systematic review of nursing home research in three U.S. psychiatry journals: 1966-1985," American Psychiatric Association Annual Meeting, Washington, DC, May 1986.
18. "The couch and the cloth: Weaving and upholstering," Anton T. Boisen Lecture, American Psychiatric Association of Mental Health Clergy Annual Meeting, Washington, DC, May 1986.
19. "The role of spiritual commitment in the lives of adult burn patients," Presenter: KA Sherrill, Southern Medical Association Annual Meeting, Atlanta, GA, November 1986.
20. "The impact of religious commitment on health and mental health: The individual and the family" and "Research as ministry," Kettering Medical Center Conference on Dynamic Is-

sues in Christianity and Psychiatry, Kettering, OH, October 1987.

21. "Research on the psychosocial impact of abortion: A systematic review," Presenter: JS Lyons, Family Research Council Conference on Values and Public Policy, Washington, DC, October 1987.

22. "Coping style, religiosity, and distress in older adult males with cancer of the head/neck," Co-presenter: AD Ackerman, Southern Medical Association Annual Meeting, San Antonio, TX, November 1987.

23. Keynote Speaker, "The impact of religious commitment on health and mental health: The individual and the family" and "Research as ministry," Christian Association of Psychological Studies, Midwest Regional Meeting, Toledo, OH, August 1988.

24. "The couch and the cloth: Estimating frequencies of clergy and mental health professional use in five catchment area surveys," Southern Psychiatric Association Annual Meeting, Colorado Springs, CO, October 1988.

25. "Psychiatric factors predicting the use of the clergy," Presenter: AA Hohmann, American Public Health Association Annual Meeting, Boston, MA, November 1988.

26. "Psychiatric, psychosocial, and health services utilization characteristics of frequent church attenders in Puerto Rico," Presenter: J Gartner, American Public Health Association Annual Meeting, Boston, MA, November 1988.

27. "Obtaining funding from the National Institute of Mental Health," "Results from systematic analyses on the use of religious variables in clinical journals," and, "Research as ministry," Co-presenters: WP Wilson, S White, and G Rekers, International Congress on Christian Counseling, Atlanta, GA, November 1988.

28. "The policy implications for religious activities and volunteerism," Spring Research Forum, Independent Sector Annual Meeting, Chicago, IL, March 1989.

29. "Religion and psychological distress in a community sample," Presenter: DR Williams, American Psychological Association Annual Meeting, New Orleans, LA, August 1989.

30. "The religious community's response to mental illness: Pathways to partnership," Third Annual Conference of Pathways to Promise: Interfaith Ministries for Prolonged Mental Illnesses and the National Alliance for the Mentally Ill (NAMI), St. Louis, MO, September 1989.
31. Presenter, "Religion and mental health—A research agenda," and Moderator, "Religion and Mental Health," American Public Health Association Annual Meeting, Chicago, IL, October 1989.
32. Panel participant, "Religious values in psychotherapy and mental health: Empirical findings and issues," Society for Psychotherapy Research Annual Meeting, Charlottesville, VA, June 1990.
33. Panel participant, "Rehabilitation, recidivism, and religion: Empirical studies," American Psychological Association Annual Meeting, Boston, MA, August 1990.
34. Panel participant, "Religion's quest into the clinical and behavioral research domains: Unanalyzed and misinterpreted," Association of Sociology of Religion Annual Meeting, Washington, DC, August 1990.
35. Panel participant, "Prevention and offender rehabilitation: Religious programs and their effects," American Society of Criminology Annual Meeting, Baltimore, MD, November 1990.
36. Plenary speaker, "Researching religious commitment's impact on clinical status: A high road 'much less' traveled," Paul Tournier Lecture, Annual Meeting of the Christian Medical and Dental Society House of Delegates, Chicago, IL, May 1991.
37. "Dimensions and valences of religious commitment measures in the *American Journal of Psychiatry* and the *Archives of General Psychiatry:* 1978-1989," Southern Psychiatric Association Annual Meeting, Boca Raton, FL, October 1991.
38. Keynote speaker, "The state and traits of studying religion in health and mental health research," Christian Association of Psychological Studies, Eastern Regional Meeting, North East, MD, September 1991.
39. "The quantity and quality of religious content in DSM-III-R's Appendix C: The glossary of technical terms," Southern Psy-

chiatric Association Annual Meeting, Boca Raton, FL, October 1991.

40. "The Christian doctor in academia," Christian Medical and Dental Society Inaugural Conference of the Paul Tournier Institute, Washington, DC, November 1991.

41. Keynote speaker, "Research as ministry" and "The impact of religious commitment on health, mental health, and social status," American Association of Pastoral Counselors Centers and Training Conference, Fort Lauderdale, FL, January 1992.

42. American Psychiatric Association course: "Religion: Research and clinical overview," Additional course faculty: SL Deppe, ES Bowman, and SM Graves, Washington, DC, May 4, 1992.

43. Discussant, "Family data from the National Center for Health Statistics," National Center for Health Statistics Data Users Conference, Bethesda, MD, August 1992.

44. Invited Speaker, "Research priorities for the AAMFT," American Association for Marital/Family Therapy (AAMFT) Annual Meeting, Miami, FL, October 1992.

45. "Grant writing for family therapists," Co-presenters: FP Piercy and S Moon, American Association for Marital/Family Therapy (AAMFT) Annual Meeting, Miami, FL, October 1992.

46. "A method for reviewing policy research: The systematic review," Co-presenter: JS Lyons, and "Federal family policy, research directions: Assessing the quantity and quality of marriage and family factors in peer-reviewed research," American Statistical Association Annual Meeting, Fort Lauderdale, FL, January 1993.

47. "The nearly neglected factor in clinical research: The social support clinical benefits of family and religion," the Steinhart Annual Lecture, University of Nebraska, Lincoln, NE, April 22, 1993.

48. "Religion: Research and clinical overview," Additional course faculty: SL Deppe, ES Bowman, and SM Graves, American Psychiatric Association Course, May 1993.

49. "Needs of underserved pediatric populations: Methodologic issues," Co-presenter: JS Lyons, American Academy of Pedi-

atrics Annual Meeting, Special Session of the Ethics Committee, Washington, DC, November 1993.

50. "Systematic review findings on spirituality," Spiritual Dimensions in Clinical Research Conference, Sponsored by the National Institute for Healthcare Research (NIHR) and the John Templeton Foundation, Leesburg, VA, April 20-23, 1995.

51. "Religion and health: Does clinical research count? A summary of findings from published systematic reviews," Association for the Sociology of Religion, Washington, DC, August 1995.

52. "The role of faith in correctional management," Co-presenter: BR Johnson, Nineteenth National Conference on Correctional Health Care, Washington, DC, November 1995.

53. "Family factors and criminality: A systematic review of the literature," Presenter: BR Johnson, American Society of Criminology Annual Meeting, Boston, MA, November 1995.

54. "The forgotten factor in physical and mental health: What does the research show?" Spirituality and Healing in Medicine Conference, Harvard Medical School, Mind/Body Medical Institute, and Deaconess Hospital, Boston, MA, December 3-5, 1995.

55. "Making the case for spiritual interventions in mental health," Spiritual Intervention in Clinical Practice Conference, Sponsored by the National Institute for Healthcare Research (NIHR) and the John Templeton Foundation, Leesburg, VA, April 1996.

56. Keynote speaker, "Religion: The forgotten factor in physical and mental health," Perspectives in Public Health Conference, Texas Department of Public Health, Austin, TX, September 20, 1996.

57. Keynote speaker, "Making the case for religion in clinical care: A look back," Spiritual Care Research: What Are We Learning Conference, Mayo Medical Center, Rochester, MN, November 8, 1996.

58. Discussant, "Public health and faith community alliances: Concepts and philosophies," American Public Health Association Annual Meeting, New York, NY, November 17-21, 1996.

59. "Spirituality and medical outcomes," Spirituality and Healing in Medicine Conference, Harvard Medical School, Mind/Body Medical Institute, and Deaconess Hospital, Boston, MA, December 15-17, 1996.
60. "Health: What's God got to do with it?" and "Making the case for spiritual interventions in mental health," Fuller Theological Seminary, Fuller Annual Award Lecture Series, Pasadena, CA, January 22-24, 1997.
61. "Perspectives and experiences with teaching spirituality in residency training," Spirituality in Health Care conference, University of New Mexico, Albuquerque, NM, February 27-March 1, 1997.
62. "Why is this important?" Spirituality and Medicine: Curricular Development Conference, Cosponsored by the John Templeton Foundation, the National Institute for Healthcare Research (NIHR), and the Association of American Medical Colleges (AAMC), Washington, DC, April 25-26, 1997.
63. "The development of a model curriculum: A case study," Co-presenter: FG Lu, Spirituality and Medicine: Curricular Development Conference, Cosponsored by the John Templeton Foundation, the National Institute for Healthcare Research (NIHR), and the Association of American Medical Colleges (AAMC), Washington, DC, April 25-26, 1997.
64. "Spirituality and mental health," Grand Rounds, Department of Psychiatry, Texas A&M University, Temple, TX, May 30, 1997.
65. "The forgotten factor in mental health: What does the research show?" Grand Rounds, Department of Psychiatry, University of Utah, Salt Lake City, UT, September 22, 1997.
66. "The forgotten factor in physical and mental health: What does the research show?" Brigham Young University Forum, Provo, UT, September 23, 1997.
67. "The forgotten factor in mental health: What does the research show?" Mayo Medical Center, Psychiatry Grand Rounds, Rochester, MN, November 11, 1997.
68. "The forgotten factor: What does the research show?" Mayo Medical Center, Grand Rounds, Department of Medicine, Rochester, MN, November 12, 1997.

69. "Religion and crime," Presenter: BR Johnson, American Society of Criminology Annual Meeting, San Diego, CA, November 19-22, 1997.
70. "Spirituality and medical outcomes," HG Koenig, DB Larson, and DA Matthews, Spirituality and Healing in Medicine Conference, Harvard Medical School, Mind/Body Medical Institute and Beth Israel Deaconess Medical Center, Boston, MA, December 14, 1997.
71. "Spirituality and medical outcomes," HG Koenig, DB Larson, and DA Matthews, Spirituality and Healing in Medicine Conference, Harvard Medical School, Mind/Body Medical Institute and Beth Israel Deaconess Medical Center, Houston, TX, March 22-24, 1998.
72. "Is God good for your health?" Association of Teachers of Preventive Medicine, American College of Preventive Medicine, San Francisco, CA, April 2, 1998.
73. "Health—What does God have to do with it?" Third Annual *Alternative Therapies in Health and Medicine* Symposium, San Diego, CA, April 3, 1998.
74. "Is God good for your health: What does the research say?" Center for Theology and the Natural Sciences Annual Lecture, Yale University, New Haven, CT, April 8-9, 1998.
75. "The role of spirituality in assessing and treating depression," Masonic Geriatric Healthcare Center, Wallingford, CT, April 28, 1998.
76. "The forgotten factor in physical and mental health: What does the research show?" Center for Mind, Body and Spirit, Baptist Medical Center, Oklahoma City, OK, May 11-12, 1998.
77. "Spiritual resources in healthcare," Colloquium on Spirituality and Health, the Park Ridge Center, Chicago, IL, May 28, 1998.
78. "Spirituality/religion in the medical school curriculum," American Psychiatric Association, Toronto, Ontario, Canada, May 30-June 4, 1998.
79. "Current perspectives on psychiatry and religion," American Psychiatric Association Toronto, Ontario, Canada, May 30-June 4, 1998.

80. "Spiritual/religious assessment: Why and how?" American Psychiatric Association, Toronto, Ontario, Canada, May 30-June 4, 1998.
81. "Religion, spirituality and addictions," American Psychiatric Association, Toronto, Ontario, Canada, May 30-June 4, 1998.
82. "The forgotten factor in physical and mental health," the Center for Mind/Body Studies, Allegheny University of the Health Sciences (Hahnemann Campus), Philadelphia, PA, October 2, 1998.
83. "End-of-life issues and spirituality," Organization of Student Representatives Plenary Presentation, Association of American Medical Colleges Annual Meeting, New Orleans, LA, October 31–November 3, 1998.
84. "Religious factors and criminality," BR Johnson and DB Larson, American Society of Criminology Annual Meeting, Washington, DC, November 1998.
85. "Summary of the research on the efficacy of faith-based factors," DB Larson and BR Johnson, Can Churches Save the Inner City Conference, the Manhattan Institute, New York, NY, November 13, 1998.
86. Spirituality and medical outcomes," HG Koenig, DB Larson, and DA Matthews, Spirituality and Healing in Medicine Conference with Special Emphasis on Death and Dying, Harvard Medical School, Mind/Body Medical Institute and Beth Israel Deaconess Medical Center, Boston, MA, December 12-14, 1998.
87. "The faith factor: Is God good for your health?: What does the research show?" The Faith Factor in Social Policy Conference, the Brookings Institution, Washington, DC, January 13, 1999.
88. "Is God good for your health?: What does the research say?" Tenth Annual Art and Science of Health Promotion Conference, American Journal of Health Promotion, Amelia Island, FL, March 3-4, 1999.
89. "The forgotten factor: What does the research show?" Healing Prescriptions for Body, Mind, and Spirit Educational Conference, the Institute of Religion and Health, Charleston, South Carolina, March 5, 1999.

90. "Spirituality and medical outcomes," HG Koenig, DB Larson, and DA Matthews, Spirituality and Healing in Medicine Conference, Harvard Medical School, Mind/Body Medical Institute, and Beth Israel Deaconess Medical Center, Chicago, IL, March 19-22, 1999.

91. "Spirituality in healthcare," The Circle of Life: Spirituality and Aging, Fairhill Center for Aging, Fairhill Hospital, Cleveland, OH, March 31, 1999.

92. "Researching the forgotten factor: A brief overview" and "Researching the forgotten factor: Highlights and future directions," Healing, Health and Spirituality, Eighth Annual Wheaton Theology Conference, Wheaton College, Wheaton, IL, April 8-10, 1999.

93. "Spirituality and health: Research, education and future direction," Society of General Internal Medicine Annual Meeting, San Francisco, CA, April 29, 1999.

94. "Spiritual/religious assessment in clinical work," American Psychiatric Association Annual Meeting, Washington, DC, May 18-20, 1999.

95. Presenter, Clergy and Physician Partnership Conference, Sponsored by the George Washington University and the Robert Wood Johnson Foundation, Washington, DC, June 17, 1999.

96. "Is God good for your health?: What does the research show?" Plenary presentation, Fifth National Meeting, Society for Spirituality and Social Work, St. Louis University, St. Louis, MO, June 27, 1999.

97. "The forgotten factor: Is God good for your health?" Third Annual Integrative Wholistic Healing Retreat, Moline, IL, July 15, 1999.

98. "Is God good for your health and mental health?" American Association of Christian Counselors, 1999 World Conference, Nashville, TN, September 8-11, 1999.

99. Grand Rounds, Departments of Surgery and Family Medicine, University of Texas Medical Branch (UTMB), Galveston, TX, September, 15, 1999.

100. Grand Rounds, Department of Family Medicine, and Grand Rounds, Department of Psychiatry, Cleveland Clinic Foundation, Cleveland, OH, September 23, 1999.

101. "Spirituality in dementia care," Keynote presentation, Understanding Dementia Conference Sponsored by Heather Hill Hospital, Health and Care Center, Cleveland, OH, October 11-12, 1999.
102. "Is God good for your health?: What does the research show?" Keynote presentation, Faith, Health, and Community Life Symposium Sponsored by Carilion Health System and Roanoke College, Salem, VA, October 12-13, 1999.
103. "A forgotten factor in public health: The relevance of faith and faith-based services," Workshop, American Public Health Association (APHA), Chicago, IL, November 8, 1999.
104. "Health: What's God got to do with it?" Presentation to Student American Medical Association, University of Maryland School of Medicine, Baltimore, MD, November 19, 1999.
105. "Spirituality in clinical care," Complementary and Alternative Medicine: The Scientific and Pluralistic Challenge, Sponsored by the Hastings Center and the Nathan Cummings Foundation, Boston, MA, December 9-10, 1999.
106. "Spirituality and medical outcomes," Spirituality and Healing in Medicine 1999, Sponsored by Harvard Medical School and Beth Israel Deaconess Medical Center, Boston, MA, December 11, 1999.
107. "Is God good for your health?" 2000 Convocation Series: Science—Perspectives and Possibilities, Gordon College, Wenham, MA, February 25, 2000.
108. "Spirituality and medical outcomes," Sponsored by Harvard Medical School and Beth Israel Deaconess Medical Center, Denver, CO, March 19-21, 2000.
109. "Is religion good for your health?" Capitol Hill Lecture Series, Washington, DC, March 28-29, 2000.
110. "Spirituality and medical outcomes—Part I and II," Spirituality and Healing Conference, Counseling and Mediation Center, Wichita, KS, April 6-7, 2000.
111. "Spirituality and health," Visiting Professor Grand Rounds, the University of Kansas School of Medicine, Wichita, KS, April 7, 2000.
112. "The forgotten factor in mental health and physical health," Hope: Empowering Recovery, First Annual Conference of

Medicine, Mental Health and Ministry, East Tennessee State University, Johnson City, TN, April 29, 2000.

113. "Spirituality and medicine: From research to clinical care," Society of General Internal Medicine 23rd Annual Meeting, Boston, MA, May 4-6, 2000.

114. "Is God good for your health?" North Atlantic Regional Medical Command, Fourth Annual Substance Abuse Symposium, Walter Reed Army Medical Center, Washington, DC, May 11, 2000.

115. Symposium: "Religion as a Wedge Between Doctor and Patient," with Presentation: "The forgotten factor in mental health," American Psychiatric Association 2000 Annual Meeting, Chicago, IL, May 15, 2000.

116. Symposium: "Model Residency Programs on Religion and Spirituality," and Workshop: "Spiritual/religious assessment in clinical work," American Psychiatric Association 2000 Annual Meeting, Chicago, IL, May 17-18, 2000.

117. "Wrestling with alligators: Reviewing a research career in spirituality and mental health," Invited Address, 2000 KJ Lee Fellowship Lecture, Columbia-Presbyterian Medical Center, College of Physicians and Surgeons, New York, NY, June 2, 2000.

118. "Spirituality and health," Invited presentation to National Fellows on Religion and the Media, Knight Center for Specialized Journalism, University of Maryland, College Park, MD, June 6, 2000.

119. Grand Rounds, Department of Psychiatry, St. Vincent's Hospital and Medical Center, New York, NY, July 5-7, 2000.

120. Discussant, "The future of human health and happiness," World Forum 2000, New York Hilton and Towers, New York, NY, September 6-9, 2000.

121. "Is religion good for your health?" Science and Religion Lecture Series, St. Bonaventure University, Olean, NY, September 20, 2000.

122. "The forgotten factor in mental and physical health" and "Is God good for your health?: What does the research show?" ACT International Conference 2000, Glorieta, NM, September 28-29, 2000.

123. "Spirituality in medicine," Connecticut Academy of Family Physicians 2000 Scientific Symposium, Hartford, CT, October 25, 2000.

124. The Philip Hochberg Annual Memorial Lecture and "Wrestling with the alligators: Reviewing a research career in spirituality and health," Day Kimball Hospital, Woodstock, CT, October 25, 2000, and Pastoral Care Day, Danbury Hospital, Danbury, CT, October 26, 2000.

125. "Wrestling with alligators: Reviewing the relationships between spirituality and health," University of North Florida College of Health, Jacksonville, FL, October 30, 2000.

126. "Is God good for your health?" Invited Address, Mayo Clinic, Walker Auditorium, Jacksonville, FL, October 31, 2000.

127. "Is God good for your health?: What does the research show?" and "The forgotten factor in mental health," Fall Psychiatric Regional Symposium, Knoxville, TN, November 3, 2000.

128. "Is God good for your health?: What does the research show?" 107th Annual Meeting of the Association of Military Surgeons of the United States (AMSUS), Inter-Allied Confederation of Reserve Medical Officers (CIOMR) Section Meeting, Las Vegas Hilton, Las Vegas, NV, November 8, 2000.

129. "Wrestling with alligators: Reviewing a research career of changes in spirituality and mental health," Grand Rounds, Department of Psychiatry, University of Minnesota Medical Center, Minneapolis, MN, November 14-15, 2000.

130. "The roles of spirituality in health: A brief review of the research," Wake Forest University Medical Center, December 8, 2000.

131. Plenary: "Role of spirituality in health: The data," and Workshop: "Research in spirituality and health: State-of-the-art and future directions," Spirituality and Healing in Medicine Conference, the Fairmont-Copley Plaza, Boston, MA, December 15-18, 2000.

132. "Wrestling with alligators: Looking back on a career in spirituality, mental health, and health," Lecture Series at Osprey Point Leadership Center, Royal Oak, MD, January 27-28, 2001.

133. SALUS Lecture: "The forgotten factor in health and mental health" and "A brief introduction to some of the findings on

the forgotten factor," Yale University, New Haven, CT, February 17, 2001.

134. "What is the relationship between spirituality and wellness," White House Commission on Complementary and Alternative Medicine Policy, Meetings on Complementary and Alternative Medicine in Self-Care and Wellness and Information Development and Dissemination, Washington, DC, March 27, 2001.

135. "Roles and relationships of spirituality and health," Harvard Medical School Mind-Body Medical Clinic and Institute, Harvard Spirituality and Healing in Medicine Conference, Clearwater, FL, March 30-31, 2001.

136. "Is God good for your health?: What does the research show?" Focus on Respiratory Critical Care Nursing Conference, Cleveland, OH, April 7, 2001.

137. "Spirituality and religion in physical health, mental health, and suicide," American Association of Suicidology Thirty-Fourth Annual Conference: Mind, Body, & Soul: Three Dimensions of Suicide, Atlanta, GA, April 19-20, 2001.

138. "Reviewing the research in spirituality and health," "Reviewing and reminiscing on a career in health and spirituality," and, "The forgotten factor in health and mental health: Spirituality—what does the research say?" State University of New York, Upstate Medical University, Syracuse, NY, April 25-26, 2001.

139. "Research in spirituality and health," Science and Mind-Body Medicine Conference, Harvard Medical School Mind-Body Medical Clinic and Institute, Boston, MA, May 3-5, 2001.

140. "Spiritual/religious assessment in clinical care" and "Model residency programs in religion and spirituality," American Psychiatric Association 154th Annual Meeting, New Orleans, LA, May 7-10, 2001.

141. "Reviewing the research on possible links between spirituality and health?" and "Is God good for your health: What does the research show?" College of Health, University of North Florida, Jacksonville, FL, May 12-15, 2001.

142. "Spirituality and health: What does the research say?" Spirituality and Health Conference, University of Calgary, Health Sciences Centre, Calgary, Alberta, Canada, May 23-25, 2001.

143. Fusion Health Roundtable, "Merging diverging paths in health-care," Symposium Sponsored by Fusion Health, Inc., Detroit, MI, May 30, 2001.
144. "Spirituality: The forgotten factor in health" and "Spirituality and health: The Data," Thirtieth Annual Southwest Heart Symposium, Santa Ana Pueblo, NM, August 31-September 1, 2001.
145. "Public health and spirituality: Collaborative opportunities," Emory University, Rollins School of Public Health, Atlanta, GA, October 10, 2001.
146. "Spirituality: Where are the opportunities in research and treatment?" the Danielsen Institute, Boston University, Boston, MA, October 17, 2001.
147. "Spirituality and health: What about business?" The Business Journal's Excellence in Healthcare and Wellness Awards Luncheon, University of North Florida, College of Health, Jacksonville, FL, November 2, 2001.
148. Invited Plenary: "Spiritual meaning, faith, and illness," Academy of Psychosomatic Medicine Forty-Eighth Annual Meeting, San Antonio, TX, November 15, 2001.
149. Grand Rounds: "Wrestling with alligators: Looking back on a career in spirituality, mental health, and health," Langley Porter Auditorium, Department of Psychiatry, University of California San Francisco, San Francisco, CA, November 28, 2001.
150. Symposium: "Spirituality: The forgotten factor: What does the research show?" Carr Auditorium, San Francisco General Hospital, the Spiritual Emergence Network, and the Department of Psychiatry, University of California San Francisco, San Francisco, CA, November 29, 2001.
151. Faculty Seminar: "The forgotten factor in healthcare: An introduction to the research in spirituality and medicine," University of Toronto, Ontario, Canada, December 5, 2001.
152. "Recognizing the relevance and roles of spirituality in substance abuse treatment and prevention," CSAT Targeted Capacity Expansion (TCE) Grantee Meeting, Washington, DC, January 23, 2002.

II. Primary Care and Consultation-Liaison Mental Health Issues

1. "Consultation liaison education revisited," Presenter: T Orleans, Academy of Psychosomatic Medicine Annual Meeting, Washington, DC, April 1978.
2. "Measuring cost and cost effectiveness in psychiatry: What was learned from an NIMH workshop on measuring clinical outcomes and cost-effectiveness in consultation-liaison psychiatry," Hospital and Community Psychiatry Annual Meeting, Denver, CO, October 1984.
3. "Research grant development in consultation-liaison psychiatry: The National Institute of Mental Health using liaison, consultation and intervention," American Society for Psychosomatic Obstetrics and Gynecology Annual Meeting, Philadelphia, PA, April 1986.
4. "The research development workshop: The case of consultation-liaison psychiatry and the National Institute of Mental Health," Southern Psychiatric Association Annual Meeting, Charleston, SC, October 1986.
5. "Cost-effectiveness findings in consultation-liaison psychiatry: National Institute of Mental Health initiatives" and "Combined psychiatry-medicine programs: Research in progress," American Psychiatric Association Annual Meeting, Chicago, IL, May 1987.
6. "Depression and timing of psychiatric consultation on depressed medical patients' lengths of stay," Presenter: AD Ackerman, Southern Medical Association Annual Meeting, San Antonio, TX, November 1987.
7. "Symptom management in the patient with cancer," American Psychiatric Association Annual Meeting, Montreal, Quebec, Canada, May 1988.
8. "Process and outcome measures in consultation-liaison research," Presenter: JS Lyons, VXII European Conference on Psychosomatic Research, Marburg, West Germany, September 1988.
9. "Psychotropic medication in the U.S.—1985: How much is given, who prescribes, and who receives?" Presenter: AA Hohmann, American Public Health Association Annual Meeting, Boston, MA, November 1988.

10. "Federal funding for primary care research: An insider's view," Co-presenters: JA Mayfield, W Mayer, Society of General Internal Medicine Annual Meeting, Arlington, VA, April 1989.
11. "Methodology in co-morbidity research: A classification of epidemiologic methods biases," Presenter: JL Levenson, Academy of Psychosomatic Medicine Annual Meeting, Las Vegas, NV, October 1989.
12. "Outcomes of a research development workshop—a second look," American Psychiatric Association Annual Meeting, New York, NY, May 1990.
13. "Spiritual assessment in clinical research," Conference on Examining Research Assumptions in Alternative Medical Systems, Bethesda, MD, July 1994.
14. "Spirituality, religion, and ritual," Complementary and Alternative Therapies in the Academic Medical Center: Issues in Ethics and Policy, sponsored by the University of Pennsylvania School of Medicine and the National Institutes of Health (NIH), Philadelphia, PA, November 11, 1999.

III. Specialty Mental Health Services Sector Issues

1. Moderator, Session on "Psychotherapy as a mental health service," Society for Psychotherapy Research Annual Meeting, Toronto, Ontario, Canada, June 1989.
2. Participant, Workshop on "Mental health services research," Society for Psychotherapy Research Annual Meeting, Charlottesville, VA, June 1990.
3. Co-Chair, Symposium on "Treating substance abuse among chronic mentally ill patients, the dually diagnosed," American Psychological Association Annual Meeting, Boston, MA, August 1990.

IV. Mental Health Services and Issues for Persons in Nursing Homes

1. "The 1984 national nursing home survey pre-test: An opportunity to survey mental disorder prevalence and service needs,"

Presenter: ID Goldstrom, American Public Health Association Annual Meeting, Anaheim, CA, November 1984.
2. "Mental disorder among nursing home patients: Findings from the national nursing home survey pretest," Presenter: BJ Burns, World Psychiatric Association, Section of Epidemiology and Community Psychiatry, Edinburgh, Scotland, September 1985.
3. "Impact of OBRA-87 on nursing home populations," Presenter: JS Lyons, American Public Health Association Annual Meeting, New York, NY, October 1990.

V. Mental Health Needs of Those with AIDS/HIV Infection

1. "Prevalence and treatment of mental disorders among persons with AIDS and HIV infections," Presenter: J Hidalgo, American Public Health Association Annual Meeting, Boston, MA, November 1988.
2. "Psychiatric and social services for persons with AIDS in the general hospital," Southern Psychiatric Annual Meeting, Asheville, NC, October 1989.

Journal Publications

I. Issues Concerning Spirituality, Health, and the Family

1. Larson DB, Wilson WP. (1980). Religious life of alcoholics. *Southern Medical Journal* 73(6):723-727.
2. Wilson WP, Larson DB. (1981). The physician and spouse I: Physician, know thyself—and thy mate. *North Carolina Medical Journal* 42(2):106-109.
3. Wilson WP, Larson DB. (1981). The physician and spouse II: Happiness, marriage, and family life. *North Carolina Medical Journal* 42(3):176-180.
4. Wilson WP, Larson DB. (1981). The physician and spouse III: Problems and some comments on solutions. *North Carolina Medical Journal* 42(4):274-277.
5. Cancellaro LA, Larson DB, Wilson WP. (1982). Religious life of narcotic addicts. *Southern Medical Journal* 75(10):1166-1168.

6. Lyles MR, Wilson WP, Larson DB. (1983). Mental health and discipleship. *Journal of Psychology and Christianity* 2(1): 62-69.
7. Wilson WP, Larson DB, Meier PD. (1983). Religious life of schizophrenics. *Southern Medical Journal* 76(9):1096-1100.
8. Thielman SB, Larson DB. (1984). Christianity and early American care for the insane: The work of Dr. Benjamin Rush. *Journal of Psychology and Christianity* 3(3):27-34.
9. Larson DB, Pattison EM, Blazer DG, Omran AR, Kaplan BH. (1986). Systematic analysis of research on religious variables in four major psychiatric journals, 1978-1982. *American Journal of Psychiatry* 143(3):329-334.
10. Wilson WP, Larson DB, Larson SS. (1986). The maltreated child grown up. *Wellness Perspectives* 3(2):21-27.
11. Bishop LC, Larson DB, Wilson WP. (1987). Religious life of individuals with affective disorders. *Southern Medical Journal* 80(9):1083-1086.
12. Sherrill KA, Larson DB. (1988). Adult burn patients: The role of religion in recovery. *Southern Medical Journal* 81(7):821-825.
13. Larson DB, Hohmann AA, Kessler LG, Meador KG, Boyd JH, McSherry E. (1988). The couch and the cloth: The need for linkage. *Hospital and Community Psychiatry* 39(10): 1064-1069.
14. Craigie FC, Liu IY, Larson DB, Lyons JS. (1988). A systematic analysis of religious variables in the *Journal of Family Practice*, 1976-1986. *Journal of Family Practice* 27(5):509-513.
15. Larson DB, Donahue MJ, Lyons JS, Benson PL, Pattison EM, Worthington EL, Blazer DG. (1989). Religious affiliation in mental health research samples as compared with national samples. *Journal of Nervous and Mental Disease* 177(2):109-111.
16. Larson DB, Koenig HG, Kaplan BH, Greenberg RS, Logue E, Tyroler HA. (1989). The impact of religion on men's blood pressure. *Journal of Religion and Health* 28(4):265-278.
17. Strayhorn JM, Weidman CS, Larson DB. (1990). A measure of religiousness, and its relation to parent and child mental health variables. *Journal of Community Psychology* 18(1):34-43.

18. Craigie FC, Larson DB, Liu IY. (1990). References to religion in the *Journal of Family Practice*: Dimensions and valence of spirituality. *Journal of Family Practice* 30(4):477-480.

19. Gartner JG, Harmatz M, Hohmann AA, Larson DB, Gartner AF. (1990). The effect of patient and clinician ideology on clinical judgement: A study of ideological countertransference. *Psychotherapy* 27(1):98-106.

20. Pressman P, Lyons JS, Larson DB, Strain JJ. (1990). Religious belief, depression, and ambulation status in elderly women with broken hips. *American Journal of Psychiatry* 147(6):758-760.

21. Larson DB, Gartner J, Vachar-Mayberry CD. (1990). A systematic review of the quantity and quality of empirical research published in four pastoral counseling journals: 1975-1984. *Journal of Pastoral Care* 44(2):115-123.

22. Gartner JG, Lyons JS, Larson DB, Serkland J, Peyrot M. (1990). Supplier induced demand for pastoral care services in the general hospital: A natural experiment. *Journal of Pastoral Care* 44(3):266-270.

23. Gartner J, Harmatz M, Hohmann AA, Larson DB, Gartner AF. (1990). The effect of client and counselor values on clinical judgement. *Counseling and Values* 35:58-62.

24. Galanter M, Larson DB, Rubenstone E. (1991). Christian psychiatry: The impact of evangelical belief on clinical practice. *American Journal of Psychiatry* 148(1):90-95.

25. Worthington EL, Larson DB, Lyons JS, Brubaker MW, Colecchi CA, Berry JT, Morrow D. (1991). Mandatory parental involvement prior to adolescent abortion. *Journal of Adolescent Health* 12(2):138-142.

26. Gartner J, Larson DB, Allen GD. (1991). Religious commitment and mental health: A review of the empirical literature. *Journal of Psychology and Theology* 19(1):6-25.

27. Williams DR, Larson DB, Buckler RE, Heckman RC, Pyle CM. (1991). Religion and psychological distress in a community sample. *Social Science and Medicine* 32(11):1257-1262.

28. Larson DB, Sherrill KA, Lyons JS, Craigie FC, Thielman SB, Greenwold MA, Larson SS. (1992). Associations between dimensions of religious commitment and mental health reported in the *American Journal of Psychiatry* and the *Archives of*

General Psychiatry: 1978-1989. *American Journal of Psychiatry* 149(4):557-559.

29. Sherrill KA, Larson DB, Greenwold MA. (1993). Is religion taboo in gerontology?: A systematic review of research on religion in three major gerontology journals, 1985-1991. *American Journal of Geriatric Psychiatry* 1(2):109-117.

30. Levin JS, Lyons JS, Larson DB. (1993). Prayer and health during pregnancy: Findings from the Galveston Low Birth Weight Survey (GLOWBS). *Southern Medical Journal* 86(9): 1022-1027.

31. Larson DB, Thielman SB, Greenwold MA, Lyons JS, Post SG, Sherrill KA, Wood GG, Larson SS. (1993). Religious content in the DSM-III-R Glossary of Technical Terms. *American Journal of Psychiatry* 150(12):1884-1885.

32. Skill T, Robinson JD, Lyons JS, Larson DB. (1994). The portrayal of religion and spirituality on fictional network television. *Review of Religious Research* 35(3):251-267.

33. Patterson-Keels L, Quint E, Brown D, Larson DB, Elkins TE. (1994). Family views on sterilization for their mentally retarded child. *Journal of Reproductive Medicine* 39(9):701-706.

34. Rutledge CM, Levin JS, Larson DB, Lyons JS. (1995). The importance of religion for parents coping with a chronically ill child. *Journal of Psychology and Christianity* 14(1):50-57.

35. Young MC, Gartner J, O'Connor T, Larson DB, Wright K. (1995). Long-term recidivism among federal inmates trained as volunteer prison ministers. *Journal of Offender Rehabilitation* 22(1,2):97-118.

36. Koenig HG, Larson DB, Matthews DA. (1996). Religion and psychotherapy with older adults. *American Journal of Geriatric Psychiatry* 29(3):155-184.

37. Johnson BR, Larson DB. (1995). Proposing a full range of intermediate sanctions: The potential benefit of the faith factor. *IARCA Journal* 6(6):28-31.

38. Larson DB, Milano MAG. (1995). Are religion and spirituality clinically relevant in health care? *Mind/Body Medicine* 1(3):147-157.

39. Larzelere RE, Schneider WN, Larson DB, Pike PL. (1996). The effects of discipline responses in delaying toddler mis-

behavior recurrences. *Child and Family Behavior Therapy* 18(3):35-57.

40. Weaver AJ, Koenig HG, Larson DB. (1997). Marriage and family therapists and the clergy: A need for clinical collaboration, training, and research. *Journal of Marital and Family Therapy* 23(1):13-25.

41. Larson DB, Milano MAG. (1997). Making the case for spiritual interventions in clinical practice. *Mind/Body Medicine* 2(1):20-30.

42. Matthews DA, Larson DB. (1997). Faith and medicine: Reconciling the twin traditions of healing. *Mind/Body Medicine* 2(1):3-6.

43. Bienenfeld D, Koenig HG, Larson DB, Sherrill KA. (1997). Psychosocial predictors of mental health in a population of elderly women: Test of an explanatory model. *American Journal of Geriatric Psychiatry* 5(1):43-53.

44. Koenig HG, Hays JC, George LK, Blazer DG, Larson DB, Landerman LR. (1997). Modeling the cross-sectional relationships between religion, physical health, social support, and depressive symptoms. *American Journal of Geriatric Psychiatry* 5(2):131-144.

45. Johnson BR, Larson DB, Pitts TC. (1997). Religious programs, institutional adjustment, and recidivism among former inmates in Prison Fellowship programs. *Justice Quarterly* 14(1):145-166.

46. Levin JS, Larson DB, Puchalski CM. (1997). Religion and spirituality in medicine: Research and education. *Journal of the American Medical Association* 278(9):792-793.

47. Weaver AJ, Samford JA, Kline AE, Lucas LA, Larson DB, Koenig HG. (1997). What do psychologists know about working with the clergy?: An analysis of eight APA journals: 1991-1994. *Professional Psychology: Research and Practice* 28(5): 471-474.

48. Koenig HG, Cohen HJ, George LK, Hays JC, Larson DB, Blazer DG. (1997). Attendance at religious services, interleukin-6, and other biological indicators of immune function in older adults. *International Journal of Psychiatry in Medicine* 27(3):233-250.

49. Matthews DA, McCullough ME, Larson DB, Koenig HG, Swyers JP, Milano MG. (1998). Religious commitment and health status: A review of the research and implications for family medicine. *Archives of Family Medicine* 7(2):118-124.
50. Larzelere RE, Sather PR, Schneider WN, Larson DB, Pike PL. (1998). Punishment enhances reasoning's effectiveness as a toddler discipline response. *Journal of Marriage and the Family* 60(5):388-403.
51. Weaver AJ, Flannelly LT, Flannelly KJ, Koenig HG, Larson DB. (1998). An analysis of research on religious and spiritual variables in three major mental health nursing journals: 1991-1995. *Issues in Mental Health Nursing* 19(3):263-276.
52. Weaver AJ, Kline AE, Samford JA, Lucas LA, Larson DB, Gorsuch R. (1998). Is religion taboo in psychology?: A systematic analysis of research on religious variables in seven major American Psychological Association journals: 1991-1994. *Journal of Psychology and Christianity* 17(3):220-233.
53. Koenig HG, George LK, Cohen HJ, Hays JC, Blazer DG, Larson DB. (1998). The relationship between religious activities and blood pressure in older adults. *International Journal of Psychiatry in Medicine* 28(2):189-213.
54. Weaver AJ, Samford JA, Larson DB, Lucas LA, Koenig HG, Patrick V. (1998). A systematic review of research on religion in four major psychiatric journals: 1991-1995. *Journal of Nervous and Mental Disease* 186(3):187-190.
55. Puchalski CM, Larson DB. (1998). Developing curricula in spirituality and medicine. *Academic Medicine* 73(9):970-974.
56. Koenig HG, George LK, Cohen HJ, Hays JC, Larson DB, Blazer DG. (1998). The relationship between religious activities and cigarette smoking in older adults. *Journal of Gerontology: Medical Sciences* 53A(6):M426-M434.
57. Koenig HG, Larson DB, Weaver AJ. (1998). Research on religion and serious mental illness. *New Directions for Mental Health Services* 80:81-95.
58. Koenig HG, Larson DB. (1998). Use of hospital services, religious attendance, and religious affiliation. *Southern Medical Journal* 91(10):925-932.
59. Koenig HG, Larson DB, Hays JC, McCullough ME, George LK, Branch PS, Meador KG, Kuchibhatla M. (1998). Reli-

gion and survival in 1,010 male veterans hospitalized with medical illness. *Journal of Religion and Health* 37:15-29.

60. Koenig HG, Branch PS, George LK, Kuchibhatla M, Larson DB, McCullough ME. (1999). Depressive symptoms and nine-year survival of 1,010 veterans hospitalized with medical illness. *American Journal of Geriatric Psychiatry* 7(2):124-131.

61. Larson SS, Larson DB, Swyers JP. (1999). Does divorce take a clinical toll?: A research review of potential physical and emotional health risks for adults and children. *Marriage and Family: A Christian Journal* 2(1):105-121.

62. McCullough ME, Larson DB, Koenig HG, Lerner R. (1999). The mismeasurement of religion in a systematic review of mortality research. *Mortality* 4(2):183-194.

63. McCullough ME, Larson DB. (1999). Religion and depression: A review of the literature. *Twin Research* 2:126-136.

64. Koenig HG, Hays JC, Larson DB, George LK, Cohen HJ, McCullough ME, Meador KG, Blazer DG. (1999). Does religious attendance prolong survival?: A six-year follow-up study of 3,968 older adults. *Journal of Gerontology: Medical Sciences* 54A(7):M370-M376.

65. Harris AHS, Thoresen CE, McCullough ME, Larson DB. (1999). Spiritually and religiously oriented health interventions. *Journal of Health Psychology* 4(3):413-433.

66. Koenig HG, Idler E, Kasl S, Hays JC, George LK, Musick M, Larson DB, Collins TR, Benson H. (1999). Religion, spirituality, and medicine: A rebuttal to skeptics. *International Journal of Psychiatry in Medicine* 29(2):123-131.

67. Weaver AJ, Samford JA, Morgan VJ, Lichton AI, Larson DB, Garbarino J. (2000). Research on religious variables in five major adolescent research journals: 1992-1996. *Journal of Nervous and Mental Disease* 188(1):36-44.

68. Johnson BR, Li SD, Larson DB, McCullough ME. (2000). A systematic review of the religiosity and delinquency literature: A research note. *Journal of Contemporary Criminal Justice* 16(1):32-52.

69. Larson DB, Koenig HG. (2000). Is God good for your health?: The role of spirituality in medical care. *Cleveland Clinic Journal of Medicine* 67(2):80-84.

70. Post SG, Puchalski CM, Larson DB. (2000). Physicians and patient spirituality: Professional boundaries, competency and ethics. *Annals of Internal Medicine* 132(7):578-583.

71. Johnson BR, Larson DB, Jang SJ, Li SD, Jang SJ. (2000). Escaping from the crime of inner cities: Church attendance and religious salience among disadvantaged youth. *Justice Quarterly* 17(2):377-391.

72. Hill PC, Pargament KI, Hood RW, McCullough ME, Swyers JP, Larson DB, Zinnbauer BJ. (2000). Conceptualizing religion and spirituality: Points of commonality, points of departure. *Journal for the Theory of Social Behaviour* 30(1):51-78.

73. McCullough ME, Hoyt WT, Larson DB, Koenig HG, Thoresen C. (2000). Religious involvement and mortality: A meta-analytic review. *Health Psychology* 19(3):211-222.

74. George LK, Larson DB Koenig HG, McCullough ME. (2000). Spirituality and health: What we know, what we need to know. *Journal of Social and Clinical Psychology* 19(1):102-116.

75. Johnson BR, Jang SJ, Li SD, Larson DB. (2000). The "invisible institution" and black youth crime: The church as an agency of local social control. *Journal of Youth and Adolescence* 29(4):479-498.

76. Larson DB, Larson SS, Puchalski CM, Koenig HK. (2000). Patient spirituality in clinical care: Clinical assessment and research findings: Part I. *Primary Care Reports* 6(20):165-172.

77. Larson DB, Larson SS, Puchalski CM, Koenig HK. (2000). Patient spirituality in clinical care: Clinical assessment and research findings: Part II. *Primary Care Reports* 6(21):173-180.

78. Musick M, Traphagan J, Koenig HG, Larson DB. (2000). Spirituality in physical health and aging. *Journal of Adult Development* 7(2):73-86.

79. Johnson BR, Jang SJ, Larson DB, Li SD. (2001). Does adolescent religious commitment matter?: A reexamination of the effects of religiosity on delinquency. *Journal of Research in Crime and Delinquency* 38(1):22-44.

80. Koenig HK, Larson DB, Larson SS. (2001). Religion and coping with serious medical illness. *Annals of Pharmacotherapy* 35(3):352-359.

81. McCullough ME, Kilpatrick SD, Emmons RA, Larson DB. (2001). Is gratitude a moral affect? *Psychological Bulletin* 127(2):249-266.

82. Koenig HG, Larson DB. (2001). Religion and mental health: Evidence for an association. *International Review of Psychiatry* 13:67-78.
83. Puchalski CM, Larson DB, Lu FG. (2001). Spirituality in psychiatry residency training programs. *International Review of Psychiatry* 13:131-138.
84. Ironson G, Solomon GF, Balbin EG, O'Cleirigh C, George A, Kumar M, Larson DB, Woods TE. (2002). The Ironson-Woods Spirituality/Religiousness Index is associated with long survival, health behaviors, less distress, and low cortisol in people with HIV/AIDS. *Annals of Behavioral Medicine* 24(1):34-48.
85. Baetz, M, Larson DB, Marcoux G, Bowen R, Griffin R. (2002). Canadian psychiatric inpatient religious commitment: An association with mental health. *Canadian Journal of Psychiatry* 47:159-166.
86. Larson DB, Larson SS, Koenig HK. (2002). Mortality and religion/spirituality: A brief review of the research. *Annals of Pharmacotherapy* 36:1090-1098.
87. Flannelly K, Weaver AJ, Larson DB, Koenig HG. (2002). A review of mortality research on clergy and other religious professionals. *Journal of Religion and Health* 41(1):57-68.
88. Weaver AJ, Flannelly KJ, Larson DB, Stapleton CL. (2002). Mental health issues among clergy and other religious professionals: A review of the research. *Journal of Pastoral Care and Counseling* 56(4):393-403.
89. Weaver AJ, Samford JA, Morgan V, Larson DB, Koenig HG, Flannelly KJ. (2002). A systematic review of research in six primary marriage and family journals: 1995-1999. *American Journal of Family Therapy* 30:293-309.
90. Baetz, M, Larson DB, Marcoux G, Jokie R, Bowen R. (2002). Religious psychiatry: The Canadian experience. *Journal of Nervous and Mental Disease* 190(8):557-559.
91. Van Ness PH, Larson DB. (2002). Religion, senescence, and mental health: The end of life is not the end of hope. *American Journal of Geriatric Psychiatry* 10:386-397.
92. George LK, Ellison CG, Larson DB. (2002). Explaining the relationships between religious involvement and health. *Psychological Inquiry* 13(3):190-200.

93. Kendler KS, Liu XQ, Gardner CO, McCullough ME, Larson DB, Prescott CA. (2003). Dimensions of religiosity and their relationship to lifetime psychiatric and substance use disorders. *American Journal of Psychiatry* 160(3):496-503.
94. Larson DB, Larson SS. (2003). Spirituality's potential relevance to physical and emotional health: A brief review of quantitative research. *Journal of Psychology and Theology* 31(1):37-51.
95. Puchalski CP, Kilpatrick SD, McCullough, ME, Larson, DB. (2003). A systematic review of spiritual and religious variables in *Palliative Medicine, American Journal of Hospice and Palliative Care, Hospice Journal, Journal of Palliative Care,* and *Journal of Pain and Symptom Management. Palliative and Supportive Care* 1(1):7-13.
96. Maton KI, Dodgen D, Domingo MRS, Larson DB. (In press). Religion as a meaning system: Policy implications for the new millennium. *Journal of Social Issues.*
97. Flannelly KJ, Liu C, Oppenheimer JE Weaver AJ, Larson DB. (In press). An evaluation of the quantity and quality of empirical research in three pastoral counseling journals, 1990-1999: Has anything changed? *Journal of Pastoral Care and Counseling.*

II. Primary Care and Consultation-Liaison Mental Health Issues

1. Orleans CS, Houpt JL, Larson DB, Hine FR. (1981). Traditional versus consultation-liaison psychiatry clerkships: A closer look. *Journal of Psychiatric Education* 5(4):306-315.
2. McCartney CF, Larson DB, Wada CY, Cahill P. (1986). Effect of psychiatric liaison on consultation rates and reasons for consult in gynecologic oncology. *Journal of Psychosomatic Obstetrics and Gynecology* 5:253-261.
3. Lyons JS, Hammer JS, Larson DB, Visotsky HM, Burns BJ. (1987). The impact of a prospective payment system on psychosocial service delivery in the general hospital. *Medical Care* 25(2):140-147.
4. Goldstrom ID, Burns BJ, Kessler LG, Feuerberg MA, Larson DB, Miller NE, Cromer WJ. (1987). Mental health services

use by elderly adults in a primary care setting. *Journal of Gerontology* 42(2):147-153.

5. Schatzkin A, Jones DY, Hoover RN, Taylor PR, Brinton LA, Ziegler RG, Harvey EB, Carter CL, Licitra LM, Dufour MC, Larson DB. (1987). Alcohol consumption and breast cancer in the Epidemiologic Follow-up Study of the first National Health and Nutrition Examination Survey. *New England Journal of Medicine* 316(19):1169-1173.

6. Schatzkin A, Hoover RN, Taylor PR, Ziegler RG, Carter CL, Larson DB, Licitra LM. (1987). Serum cholesterol and cancer in the NHANES I Epidemiologic Follow-up Study. *Lancet* 2(8554):298-301.

7. Larson DB, Kessler LC, Burns BJ, Pincus HA, Houpt JL, Fiester S, Chaitkin L. (1987). A research development workshop to stimulate outcome research in consultation-liaison psychiatry. *Hospital and Community Psychiatry* 38(10):1106-1109.

8. McCartney CF, Larson DB. (1987). Quality of life in patients with gynecologic cancer. *Cancer* 60(8):2129-2136.

9. Schatzkin A, Hoover RN, Taylor PR, Ziegler RG, Carter CL, Albanes D, Larson DB, Licitra LM. (1988). Site-specific analysis of total serum cholesterol and incident cancer in the National Health and Nutrition Examination Survey I Epidemiologic Follow-up Study. *Cancer Research* 48:452-458.

10. Ackerman AD, Lyons JS, Hammer JS, Larson DB. (1988). The impact of coexisting depression and timing of psychiatric consultation on medical patients' length of stay. *Hospital and Community Psychiatry* 39(2):173-176.

11. Lyons JS, Larson DB, Burns BJ, Cope N, Wright S, Hammer JS. (1988). Psychiatric co-morbidities and patients with head and spinal cord trauma: Effects on acute hospital care. *General Hospital Psychiatry* 10(5):292-297.

12. Lyons JS, Hammer JS, Larson DB, Petraitis J, Strain JJ. (1988). Treatment opportunities on a consultation/liaison service. *American Journal of Psychiatry* 145(11):1435-1437.

13. Beardsley RS, Gardocki GJ, Larson DB, Hidalgo J. (1988). Psychotropic medication prescribing by primary care practitioners and psychiatrists. *Archives of General Psychiatry* 45 (12):1117-1119.

14. McCartney CF, Cahill P, Larson DB, Lyons JS, Wada CY, Pincus HA. (1989). The effect of a psychiatric liaison on consultation rates and on detection of minor psychiatric disorders in cancer patients. *American Journal of Psychiatry* 146(7): 898-901.
15. Kelleher KJ, Hohmann AA, Larson DB. (1989). Prescription of psychotropics to children in office-based practice. *American Journal of Diseases of Children* 143(7):855-859.
16. Lyons JS, Larson DB. (1989). A proposed value matrix for the evaluation of psychiatric consultations in the general hospital. *General Hospital Psychiatry* 11(5):345-351.
17. Bareta JC, Larson DB, Lyons JS, Zorc JJ. (1990). A comparison of manual and MEDLARS reviews of the literature on consultation-liaison psychiatry. *American Journal of Psychiatry* 147(8):1040-1042.
18. Levenson JL, Colenda C, Larson DB, Bareta JC. (1990). Methodology in consultation-liaison research: A classification of biases. *Psychosomatics* 31(4):367-376.
19. Bryant SG, Larson DB, Fisher S, Olins NJ. (1990). Postmarketing surveillance: Effects of compensation on patient self-monitoring. *Drug Information Journal* 24:469-476.
20. Larson DB, Lyons JS, Hohmann AA, Beardsley RS, Hidalgo J. (1991). Psychotropics prescribed to the U.S. elderly in the early and mid 1980s: Prescribing patterns of primary care practitioners, psychiatrists, and other physicians. *International Journal of Geriatric Psychiatry* 6:63-70.
21. Hohmann AA, Larson DB, Thompson JW, Beardsley RS. (1991). Psychotropic medication prescription in U.S. ambulatory medical care. *DICP, The Annals of Pharmacotherapy* 25:85-89.
22. Zorc JJ, Larson DB, Lyons JS, Beardsley RS. (1991). Expenditures for psychotropic medications in the United States in 1985. *American Journal of Psychiatry* 148(5):644-647.
23. Burton RW, Lyons JS, Devens M, Larson DB. (1991). Psychiatric consultations for psychoactive substance disorders in the general hospital. *General Hospital Psychiatry* 13(2):83-87.
24. Broadhead WE, Larson DB, Yarnall KSH, Blazer DG, Tse CJ. (1991). Tricyclic antidepressant prescribing for nonpsy-

chiatric disorders: An analysis based on data from the 1985 . National Ambulatory Medical Care Survey. *Journal of Family Practice* 33(1):24-32.

25. Bryant SG, Fisher S, Prinsley DM, Olins NJ, Larson DB. (1991). Effects of age on reporting of adverse clinical events (ACE's): Results from two postmarketing surveillance methods. *Pharmacotherapy* 11(3):249-255.

26. Bryant SG, Fisher S, Larson DB, Olins NJ. (1992). Age effects on patient drug attribution judgements: Results from two postmarketing surveillance methods. *Journal of Aging and Health* 4(1):101-111.

27. Brody DS, Larson DB. (1992). The role of primary care physicians in managing depression. *Journal of General Internal Medicine* 7(2):243-247.

28. Eaton WW, Mengel M, Mengel L, Larson DB, Campbell DR, Montague RB. (1992). Psychosocial and psychopathologic influences on management and control of insulin-dependent diabetes. *International Journal of Psychiatry in Medicine* 22(2):105-117.

29. Lyons JS, Larson DB. (1992). Regulations controlling costs of drugs: A perspective from the U.S. *PharmacoEconomics* 2(2):91-94.

30. Lyons JS, Larson DB, Hromco J. (1992). Clinical and economic evaluation of benzodiazepines: A value analysis. *PharmacoEconomics* 2(5):397-407.

31. Brown D, Elkins TE, Larson DB. (1993). Prolonged grieving after abortion: A descriptive study. *Journal of Clinical Ethics* 4:118-123.

32. Elkins TE, Brown D, Larson DB, Wood GG. (1993). The cost of choice: A price too high in the triple screen for Down Syndrome. *Clinical Obstetrics and Gynecology* 36:532-540.

33. Brody DS, Thompson TL, Larson DB, Ford DE, Katon WJ, Magruder KM. (1994). Strategies for counseling depressed patients by primary care physicians. *Journal of General Internal Medicine* 9:569-575.

34. Brown D, Roberts J, Elkins T, Larson DB, Hopkins M. (1995). Hard choices: The gynecologic cancer patient's end-of-life preferences. *Gynecologic Oncology* 55:355-362.

35. Brody DS, Thompson TL, Larson DB, Ford DE, Katon WJ, Magruder KM. (1995). Recognizing and managing depression in primary care. *General Hospital Psychiatry* 17:93-107.
36. Roberts JA, Brown D, Elkins T, Larson DB. (1997). Factors influencing views of patients with gynecologic cancer about end-of-life decisions. *American Journal of Obstetrics and Gynecology* 176:166-172.

III. Specialty Mental Health Services Sector Issues

1. Orleans CS, Houpt JL, Larson DB. (1980). Interpersonal factors in the psychiatry clerkship: New findings. *American Journal of Psychiatry* 137(9):1101-1104.
2. Larson DB, Orleans CS, Houpt JL. (1980). Evaluating a clinical psychiatry course using process and outcome measures. *Journal of Medical Education* 55(12):1006-1012.
3. Trent PJ, Orleans CS, Houpt JL, Larson DB. (1984). What medical students retain from a psychiatry clerkship: A two year follow-up study. *Journal of Psychiatric Education* 8(2): 64-74.
4. Costa PT, McCrae RR, Zonderman AB, Barbano HE, Lebowitz B, Larson DB. (1986). Cross-sectional studies of personality in a national sample: II. Stability in neuroticism, extraversion, and openness. *Psychology and Aging* 1(2):144-149.
5. Farmer ME, Locke BZ, Moscicki EK, Dannenberg AL, Larson DB, Radloff LS. (1988). Physical activity and depressive symptoms: The NHANES I Epidemiologic Follow-up Study. *American Journal of Epidemiology* 128(6):1340-1351.
6. Wolff N, Henderson PR, MacAskill RL, Rosenstein MJ, Milazzo-Sayre LJ, Larson DB, Manderscheid RW. (1989). Treatment patterns for schizophrenia in psychiatric hospitals. *Social Science and Medicine* 28(4):323-331.
7. Okpaku SO, Larson DB, Manderscheid RW. (1990). Recent legislative and court activities relating to the SSI and SSDI programs for the mentally ill. *Hospital and Community Psychiatry* 41(5):560-562.
8. Lyons JS, O'Mahoney MT, Larson DB. (1991). The attending psychiatrist as a predictor of length of stay. *Hospital and Community Psychiatry* 42(10):1064-1066.

9. Lyons JS, Pressman P, Pavkov T, Salk P, Larson DB, Finkel S. (1992). Psychiatric hospitalization of older adults: Comparison of a specialty geropsychiatric unit to general psychiatric units. *Clinical Gerontologist* 12(2):3-17.

10. Colenda CC, Goldstein MZ, Pincus H, Dial T, Lyons J, Larson DB. (1995). Changing characteristics of psychiatrists who treat geriatric patients. *American Journal of Geriatric Psychiatry* 3(4):330-338.

IV. Mental Health Services and Issues Regarding Persons in Nursing Homes

1. Finestone DH, Larson DB, Whanger AD, Cavenar JO. (1982). Hyperactivity in senile dementia. *Journal of the American Geriatrics Society* 30(8):521-523.

2. Rabins PV, Rovner BW, Larson DB, Burns BJ, Prescott C, Beardsley RS. (1987). The use of mental health measures in nursing home research. *Journal of the American Geriatrics Society* 35(5):431-434.

3. Burns BJ, Larson DB, Goldstrom ID, Johnson WE, Taube CA, Miller NE, Mathis ES. (1988). Mental disorder among nursing home patients: Preliminary findings from the National Nursing Home Survey pretest. *International Journal of Geriatric Psychiatry* 3(1):27-35.

4. Beardsley RS, Larson DB, Lyons JS, Gottlieb GL, Rabins PV, Rovner B. (1989). Health services research in nursing homes: A systematic review of three clinical geriatric journals. *Journal of Gerontology: Medical Sciences* 44(1):M30-M35.

5. Beardsley RS, Larson DB, Burns BJ, Thompson JW, Kamerow DB. (1989). Prescribing of psychotropics in elderly nursing home patients. *Journal of the American Geriatrics Society* 37(4):327-330.

6. Larson DB, Lyons JS, Bareta JC, Burns BJ, Blazer DG, Goldstrom ID. (1989). The construct validity of the ischemic score of Hachinski for the detection of dementias. *Journal of Neuropsychiatry* 1(2):181-187.

7. Larson DB, Lyons JS, Hohmann AA, Beardsley RS, Huckeba WM, Rabins PV, Lebowitz BD. (1989). A systematic review of nursing home research in three psychiatric journals: 1966-

1985, *International Journal of Geriatric Psychiatry* 4(3):129-134.
8. Eichmann MA, Griffin BP, Lyons JS, Larson DB, Finkel S. (1992). An estimation of the impact of OBRA-87 on nursing home care in the United States. *Hospital and Community Psychiatry* 43(8):781-789.

V. Mental Health Needs of Those with AIDS/HIV Infection

1. Lyons JS, Sheridan K, Larson DB. (1988). A model for AIDS education for health professionals. *Health Education* 19(6): 12-15.
2. Ell KO, Larson DB, Finch W, Sattler F, Nishimoto RH. (1989). Mental health services among ambulatory patients with human immunodeficiency syndrome infections. *Journal of Health and Social Policy* 1(1):3-17.
3. Lyons JS, Larson DB, Anderson RL, Bilheimer LT. (1989). Psychosocial services for AIDS patients in the general hospital. *International Journal of Psychiatry in Medicine* 19(4): 385-392.
4. Lyons JS, Larson DB, Bareta JC, Liu IY, Anderson RL, Sparks CH. (1990). A systematic analysis of the quantity of AIDS publications and the quality of research methods in three general medical journals. *Evaluation and Program Planning* 13(1):73-77.

Invited Reviews and Book Chapters

1. Drowns-Allen KS, Allen RM, Larson DB. (1980). *How to Perform a Structured Mental Status Interview: A Self-Instructional Program*. Chapel Hill, NC: Health Sciences Consortium.
2. Larson DB, Whanger AD, Busse EW. (1983). Geriatrics. In: Wolman BB (Editor), *The Therapist's Handbook: Treatment Methods of Mental Disorders*, Second Edition (pp. 343-388). New York, NY: Van Nostrand Reinhold Co.
3. Larson DB, Blazer D. (1984). Family therapy with the elderly. In: Blazer DG, Siegler I (Editors), *Working with the Family*

of Older Adults (pp. 95-111). Menlo Park, CA: Addison-Wesley Co.

4. Larson DB, Larson SS, Whanger AD. (1984). Personality, marital, family, psychosexual, and sleep disorders. In: Whanger AD, Meyers AC (Editors), *Mental Health Assessment and Therapeutic Intervention with Older Adults* (pp. 189-211). Rockville, MD: Aspen Systems Corporation.

5. Larson DB. (1985). Religious involvement: Its association with marital status, marital well-being, and mortality. In: Rekers GA (Editor), *Family Building* (pp. 121-147). Ventura, CA: Regal Books.

6. Larson DB. (1985). Marital status: Its association with personal well-being, economic status, and psychiatric status. In: Rekers GA (Editor), *Family Building* (pp. 237-258). Ventura, CA: Regal Books.

7. Larson DB, Pattison EM, Blazer DG, Omran AR, Kaplan BH. (1986). The measurement of religion in psychiatric research. In: Robinson LH (Editor), *Psychiatry and Religion: Overlapping Concerns* (pp. 156-178). Washington, DC: American Psychiatric Press.

8. Larson SS, Larson DB. (1988). The facts about AIDS. In: Lanning C (Editor), *Answers to Your Questions About Homosexuality* (pp. 7-31). Wilmore, KY: Bristol Books.

9. Lyons JS, Larson DB, Huckeba WM, Rogers JL, Mueller CP. (1988). Research on the psychosocial impact of abortion: A systematic review of the literature 1966 to 1985. In: Regier GP (Editor), *Values and Public Policy* (pp. 77-90). Shippensburg, PA: Destiny Image Publishers.

10. Worthington EL, Larson DB, Brubaker MW, Colecchi MW, Berry JT, Morrow, D. (1988). The benefits of legislation requiring parental involvement prior to adolescent abortion. In: Regier GP (Editor), *Values and Public Policy* (pp. 221-243). Shippensburg, PA: Destiny Image Publishers.

11. Hohmann AA, Larson DB. (1988). Grant funding in mental health services research: Methods and mechanisms. In: Harrison AO, Jackson JS, Munday C, Blieden NB (Editors), *A Search for Understanding: Michigan Research Conference on Mental Health Services for Black Americans* (pp. 79-87). Na-

tional Institute of Mental Health, the Michigan Department of Mental Health, and the Detroit Psychiatric Institute.

12. Larson DB, Lyons JS, Gartner J, Sherrill K, Larson SS. (1989). Demonstrating the neglect of religion in the social sciences and researching the effectiveness of religious volunteerism: Some steps in responding to a research identity crisis. In: *Working Papers: 1989 Spring Research Forum: Philanthropy and The Religious Tradition* (pp. 631-650). The Independent Sector and United Way Institute.

13. Larson DB, Lyons JS. (1989). Puzzling evidence: The use of systematic reviews in policy research. *Physician* 1(4):14-15.

14. Larson DB, Zorc JJ. (1989). Prescribing psychotropics in the nursing home. *Geriatric Medicine Today* 8(8):42-51.

15. Larson SS, Larson DB. (1990). Divorce: A hazard to health? *Physician* 2(3):13-17.

16. Larson SS, Larson DB, Anderson RA, Lyons JS. (1990). School-based clinics: A systematic review of the research. *Physician* 2(5):13-17.

17. Larson DB, Larson SS, Gartner J. (1990). Families, relationships, and health. In: Wedding D (Editor), *Behavior and Medicine* (pp. 135-147). St. Louis, MO: Mosby Year Book.

18. Pincus HA, Lyons JS, Larson DB. (1991). The benefits of consultation-liaison psychiatry. In: Judd FK, Burrows GD (Editors), *Handbook of Studies on General Hospital Psychiatry* (pp. 43-52). Amsterdam, Netherlands: Elsevier Science Publishers.

19. Cohen-Cole SA, Howell E, Barrett JE, Lyons JS, Larson DB. (1991). Consultation-liaison research: Four selected topics. In: Judd FK, Burrows GD (Editors), *Handbook of Studies of General Hospital Psychiatry* (pp. 79-98). Amsterdam, Netherlands: Elsevier Publishers.

20. Larson DB, Larson SS. (1991). Religious commitment and health: Valuing the relationship. *Second Opinion: A Journal of Health, Faith and Ethics* 17(1):26-40.

21. Pressman P, Lyons JS, Larson DB, Gartner J. (1992). Religion, anxiety, and fear of death. In: Schumaker JF (Editor), *Religion and Mental Health* (pp. 98-109). New York, NY: Oxford University Press.

22. Larson DB, Pastro LE, Lyons JS, Anthony PE. (1992). *The Systematic Review: An Innovative Approach to Reviewing Research.* Washington, DC: Department of Health and Human Services.

23. Larson SS, Larson DB. (1992). Reviewing and demonstrating the impact of religious commitment in clinical research. *Physician* 4(3):14-16.

24. Larson DB, Larson SS. (1992). Part I: Facts for faith: Clinical religious research—Who cares and what does it show? *Christian Medical and Dental Society Journal* 23(2):18-22.

25. Crouse GC, Larson DB. (1992). Cost of teenage childbearing: Current trends. *ASPE Research Note.* Washington, DC: Department of Health and Human Services.

26. Larson SS, Larson DB. (1992). Part II: Facts for faith: Clinical religious research—Religious commitment: A new disease risk factor. *Christian Medical and Dental Society Journal* 23(3):15-19.

27. Hohmann AA, Larson DB. (1992). Psychiatric factors predicting use of clergy. In: Worthington EL (Editor), *Psychotherapy and Religious Values* (pp. 71-84). Grand Rapids, MI: Baker Book House.

28. Muffler J, Langrod JG, Larson DB. (1992). There is a balm in Gilead: Religion and substance abuse treatment. In: Lowinson JH, Ruiz P, Millman RB, Langrod JG (Editors), *Substance Abuse: A Comprehensive Textbook,* Second Edition (pp. 584-595). Baltimore, MD: Williams and Wilkins.

29. Larson DB, Lyons JS. (1993). The psychiatrist in the nursing home. In: Copeland JRM, Abou-Saleh MT, Blazer DG (Editors), *Principles and Practice of Geriatric Psychiatry* (pp. 953-959). London, England: John Wiley and Sons.

30. Larson SS, Larson DB. (1993). Research shows that religion is good for your mental health. *Religious Counseling Today* 1(4):26-31.

31. Larson DB, Wood GG, Larson SS. (1993). A paradigm shift in medicine toward spirituality? *Advances* 9(4):39-49.

32. Larson DB. (1993). Religion doesn't harm; it often helps. *Physician* 5(6):20-22.

33. Lyons JS, Anderson RL, Larson DB. (1993). A systematic review of the effects of aggressive and nonaggressive pornography. In: Zillman D, Bryant J, Huston A (Editors), *Media,*

Children, and the Family: Social Scientific, Psychodynamic, and Clinical Perspectives (pp. 271-310). Hillsdale, NJ: Lawrence Ehrlbaum Associates.

34. Lyons JS, Anderson RL, Larson DB, Brule P, Ellison S, Walker S. (1993). Using the systematic review method to assess peer-reviewed scientific literatures concerning family, marital, and community variables across 20 fields of inquiry. In: Hendershot GE, LeClere FB (Editors), *Family Health: From Data to Policy* (pp. 43-60). Minneapolis, MN: National Council for Family Relations.

35. Larson DB, Sherrill KA, Lyons JS. (1994). The neglect and misuse of the *R* word: Systematic reviews of religious measures in health, mental health, and aging. In: Levin JS (Editor), *Religion in Aging and Health: Theoretical Foundations and Methodological Frontiers* (pp. 178-195). Thousand Oaks, CA: Sage Publications.

36. Sherrill KA, Larson DB. (1994). The anti-tenure factor in religious research in clinical epidemiology and aging. In: Levin JS (Editor), *Religion in Aging and Health: Theoretical Foundations and Methodological Frontiers* (pp. 149-177). Thousand Oaks, CA: Sage Publications.

37. VandenBerghe E with Larson DB. (1994). Religion and (its relationship with) life. *The Ensign* 24(10):32-45.

38. Pincus HA, Lyons JS, Larson DB. (1994). Research on clinical and economic outcomes in consultation-liaison psychiatry. In: Michels R (Editor), *Psychiatry* (pp. 1-9). Philadelphia, PA: J.B. Lippincott Company.

39. Johnson BR, Larson DB. (1994). Everything works, nothing works, something works: Some reflections on the past and future directions of research on correctional rehabilitation. *Correctional Psychologist* 26(3):9-12.

40. Larson DB, Greenwold MA. (1995). Ethical problems in the clinical study of religion and health. In: Kilner J, Cameron N, Schiedermayer D (Editors), *Bioethics and the Future of Medicine: A Christian Appraisal* (pp. 50-67). Grand Rapids, MI: William Eerdmans.

41. Larson DB, Larson SS. (1995). Families, relationships, and health. In: Wedding D (Editor), *Behavior and Medicine,* Second Edition (pp. 137-149). St. Louis, MO: Mosby-Year Book.

42. Larson DB, Greenwold MA, Brown D, Wood G. (1995). Mental health and religion. In: Reich WT, Post SG (Editors), *The Encyclopedia of Bioethics* (pp. 1704-1711). New York, NY: The Macmillan Publishing Company.
43. Larson DB. (1995). Have faith: Religion can heal mental ills. *Insight* (March 6):18-20.
44. Larson DB. (1995). Faith: The forgotten factor in healthcare. *American Journal of Natural Medicine* 2(4):10-15.
45. Greenwold MA, Larson DB, Lyons JS, Sherrill KA. (1995). Selected and interpretation bias in post-abortion research. In: Doherty P (Editor), *The Post Abortion Syndrome: Its Wide Ramifications* (pp. 39-46). Dublin, Ireland: Four Courts Press.
46. Anderson RL, Hanley DC, Larson DB, Sider RC. (1995). Methodological considerations in empirical research on abortion. In: Doherty P (Editor), *The Post Abortion Syndrome: Its Wide Ramifications* (pp. 103-115). Dublin, Ireland: Four Courts Press.
47. Larson DB, Greenwold MA, Wood G. (1995). Religion and health: What ought to be done, all things considered? In: Hollman J (Editor), *New Issues in Medical Ethics* (pp. 149-164). Bristol, TN: Christian Medical and Dental Society.
48. Milano MAG, Larson DB. (1995). What the research shows: Religion can be healthy. *Healthwise* (Fall):5-7.
49. Jones TL with Larson DB. (1995). Religion's role in health: What's God got to do with it? *Texas Medicine* 91(12):26-29.
50. Larson DB, Milano MAG, Barry C. (1996). Religion: The forgotten factor in health care. *World and I* (February):293-317.
51. Cox M, Larson DB. (1996). Health: What's God got to do with it? *Physician* 8(2):17.
52. Larson DB, Milano MAG. (1996). Religion and mental health: Should they work together? *Alternative and Complementary Therapies* (March/April):91-98.
53. Weaver AJ, Larson DB. (1996). It is time psychologists join hands with the clergy. *American Psychological Association Monitor* (August 27) (8):52.
54. Benson PL, Masters KS, Larson DB. (1997). Religious influences on child and adolescent development. In: Alessi NE (Editor), *The Handbook of Child and Adolescent Psychiatry,* Volume 4 (pp. 206-219). New York, NY: Basic Books.

55. Cox M, Burford M, with Larson DB and Larson SS. (1997). Divorce: The forgotten trauma. *Physician* (September/October):14-16.

56. Johnson BR, Larson DB. (1997). Linking religion to the mental and physical health of inmates: A literature review and research note. *American Jails* (September/October):28-36.

57. Greenwold MA, Larson DB, Lu FG. (1998). Religion and mental health: The need for cultural sensitivity and synthesis. In: Okpaku S (Editor), *Clinical Methods in Transcultural Psychiatry* (pp. 191-210). Washington, DC: American Psychiatric Association Press.

58. Koenig HG, Larson DB. (1998). Religion and mental health. In: Friedman HS (Editor), *Encyclopedia of Mental Health* (pp. 381-392). San Diego, CA: Academic Press.

59. McCullough ME, Larson DB. (1998). Frontiers of research in religion and mental health. In: Koenig HG (Editor), *Handbook of Religion and Mental Health* (pp. 95-107). San Diego, CA: Academic Press.

60. Musick MA, Koenig HG, Larson DB, Matthews DA. (1998). Religion, spiritual beliefs, and cancer. In: Holland J (Editor), *Psycho-oncology* (pp. 780-789). New York, NY: Oxford University Press.

61. Johnson BJ, Larson DB. (1998). The faith factor: Religion's relationship to the health of inmates. *Corrections Today* (June): 106-110.

62. Larson DB, Koenig HG. (1998). Religion and health: Is there a connection? *St. Louis Metropolitan Medicine* 20(12):18-19.

63. McCullough ME, Larson DB. Prayer. (1999). In: Miller WR (Editor), *Integrating Spirituality into Treatment: Resources for Practitioners* (pp. 85-110). Washington, DC: American Psychological Association Press.

64. McCullough ME, Weaver AJ, Larson DB, Aay KR. (2000). Psychotherapy with mainline protestants: Lutheran, Presbyterian, Episcopal/Anglican, and Methodist. In: Richards PS, Bergin AE (Editors), *Handbook of Psychotherapy and Religious Diversity* (pp. 105-129). Washington, DC: American Psychological Association Press.

65. Larson DB, Larson SS, Puchalski CM. (2000). The once forgotten factor in psychiatry: Part I: Residency training ad-

dresses religious and spiritual issues. *Psychiatric Times* 17(1): 18-23.

66. Larson DB, Milano MAG, Weaver AJ. (2000). The role of clergy in mental health care. In: Boehnlein JK (Editor), *Psychiatry and Religion: The Convergence of Mind and Spirit* (pp. 125-142). Washington, DC: American Psychiatric Association Press.

67. Larson DB, Larson SS, Koenig HG. (2000). Religious commitment and serious illness: Part II. *Psychiatric Times* 17(6): 38-40.

68. Josephson AM, Larson DB, Juthani N. (2000). What's happening in psychiatry regarding spirituality. *Psychiatric Annals* 30(8):533-541.

69. Puchalski CM, Larson DB, Lu F. (2000). Spirituality courses in psychiatry residency programs. *Psychiatric Annals* 30(8): 543-548.

70. Larson DB, Larson SS, Koenig HG. (2000). Longevity and mortality, Part III. *Psychiatric Times* 17(8):32-33.

71. Larson DB, Larson SS, Koenig HG. (2000). The once-forgotten factor in psychiatry, research findings on religious commitment and mental health, Part IV. *Psychiatric Times* 17(10): 78-79.

72. Larson DB, Larson SS. (2000). Health's forgotten factor: Medical research uncovers religion's clinical relevance. In: Herrmann RL (Editor), *God, Science, and Humility: Ten Scientists Consider Humility Theology* (pp. 228-278). Radnor, PA: Templeton Foundation Press.

73. Larson DB, Larson SS, Johnson BR. (2001). Families, relationships and health. In: Wedding D (Editor), *Behavior and Medicine* (pp. 13-30). Seattle, WA: Hogrefe and Huber Publishers.

74. Larson DB, Larson SS. (2001). The search for "Shalom." *Contact: A Publication of the World Council of Churches* (July 1):3-7.

75. Larson DB, Larson SS. (2001). Patient spirituality and mental health: A new focus in clinical care and research: I. *The Royal College of Psychiatrists Spirituality and Psychiatry Special Interest Group Newsletter* (September)(5):19-27.

76. Weaver AJ, Smith, WJ, Larson, DB. (2001). Psychological trauma: The need for a pastoral response. *New Theology Review: An American Catholic Journal of Ministry* 14(4):22-31.

77. Larson DB, Larson SS, Koenig HK. (2001). The patient's spiritual/religious dimension: A forgotten factor in mental health. *Directions in Psychiatry* 21(4):307-333.

78. Larson DB, Larson SS. (2001). Patient spirituality and mental health: A new focus in clinical care and research: II. *The Royal College of Psychiatrists Spirituality and Psychiatry Special Interest Group Newsletter* (December)(6):21-29.

79. Larson DB. (2002). From "Have Faith: Religion Can Heal Mental Ills," *Insight* (March 6, 1995). In: Slife B (Editor), *Taking Sides: Clashing Views on Controversial Psychological Issues*, Twelfth Edition (pp. 354-366). Guilford, CT: McGraw-Hill/ Dushkin.

80. Larson DB, Larson SS. (2002). Spirituality in clinical care: A brief review of patient desire, physician response, and research opportunities. In: Callahan D (Editor), *The Role of Complementary and Alternative Medicine: Accommodating Pluralism* (pp. 84-106). Washington, DC: Georgetown University Press.

81. Larson DB, Larson SS. (2002). Patient spirituality: Clinical relevance, assessment and research. *American Academy of Family Physicians (AAFP) Home Study Self-Assessment* (January): 1-7.

82. Larson DB, Swyers JP. (2002). Do religion and spirituality contribute to marital and individual health? In: Wall J, Browning DS, Doherty WJ, Post SG (Editors), *Marriage, Health, and the Professions: If Marriage Is Good for You, What Does This Mean for Law, Medicine, Ministry, Therapy, and Business?* (pp. 283-304). Grand Rapids, MI: William B. Eerdmans Publishing Company.

83. Shih KC, Larson DB. (In press). Spirituality and cancer. In: Micozzi M (Editor), *Complementary and Alternative Therapies in Cancer*. UK: Harcourt Health Sciences.

Letters to the Editor

1. Grant DH. (1986). In response to Larson, Pattison, Blazer, et al.: Systematic analysis of research on religious variables in four major psychiatric journals, 1978-1982; The relationship between psychiatrists and the clergy. *American Journal of Psychiatry* 143(10):1317-1318.
2. Lyons JS, Larson DB, Anderson RL. (1988). Services for AIDS patients. *Hospital and Community Psychiatry* 39(11): 1214.
3. James PA. (1989). In response to Craigie, Liu, Larson, Lyons: A systematic analysis of religious variables in the *Journal of Family Practice,* 1976-1986; Religion and family medicine. *Journal of Family Practice* 28(5):625.
4. Worthington EL, Larson DB, Brubaker MW, Colecchi C, Berry JT, Marrow D. (1989). The benefits of legislation requiring parental involvement prior to adolescent abortion. *American Psychologist* 44(12):1542-1545.
5. Gruber E, Anderson MM. (1990). In response to Worthington, Larson, Brubaker, et al.: The benefits of legislation requiring parental involvement prior to adolescent abortion: Legislating parental involvement in adolescent abortion; Re-examining the arguments of Worthington and colleagues. *American Psychologist* 45(10):1174-1176.
6. Hohmann AH, Larson DB. (1990). Peer review: The unblind grading the blind. *Journal of NIH Research* 2(10):12-13.
7. Lyons JS, Larson DB, Bareta JC, Zorc JJ. (1991). In response to Gagnon K: Manual and computer assisted literature searches. *American Journal of Psychiatry* 148(4):549.
8. Lyons JS, Larson DB, Bareta JC. (1991). In response to Warling B, Gilman LB: Manual versus MEDLINE searches. *American Journal of Psychiatry* 148(5):686-687.
9. Lyons JS, Larson DB, Bareta JC. (1991). In response to Baxter WE, Hefner SR: Computerized literature searches. *American Journal of Psychiatry* 148(8):1107-1108.
10. Johnson WC. (1991). In response to Galanter, Larson, Rubenstone: A survey of U.S. evangelical psychiatrists: Aspects of their clinical practice, personal values and religious beliefs;

Evangelical Christian psychiatrists. *American Journal of Psychiatry* 148(8):1108.

11. Galanter M, Larson DB. (1991). In response to Dalgarrondo P: Religious issues in psychiatry. *American Journal of Psychiatry* 148(10):1414-1415.

12. Pressman P, Larson DB, Lyons JS, Humes D. (1992). Impact of religious belief on psychological distress. *Psychosomatics* 33(4):470.

13. Larimore WL, Larson DB, Sherrill KA. (1992). In response to Rosenfeld JA: Emotional sequelae to therapeutic abortion. *American Family Physician* 46(3):665-666.

14. Vessey JT, Larson DB, Lyons JS, Rogers JL, Howard KI. (1994). In response to Carey RF, Herman WA, Retta SM, Rinaldi JE, Herman BA, Athey TW: Effectiveness of latex condoms as a barrier to Human Immunodeficiency Virus-sized particles under conditions of simulated use; Condom safety and HIV. *Sexually Transmitted Diseases* 21(1):59-60.

15. Trumbull DA, Ravenel D, Larson DB. (1995). In response to Wissow SL, Roter D: Toward effective discussion of discipline and corporal punishment during primary care visits: Findings from studies of doctor-patient interaction. *Pediatrics* 96(4):792-794.

16. Matthews DA, McCullough ME, Larson DB, Koenig HG, Swyers JP, Milano MG. (1999). In response to "Do people of different religious denominations have different average life expectancies?" *Archives of Family Medicine* 8(6):476.

17. Larson DB, Larson SS, Puchalski CM. (2000). In response to Ostow M: Residency training addresses religious and spiritual issues. *Psychiatric Times* 17(6):12-13.

18. Puchalski CM, Larson DB, Post SG. (2000). In response to Graner J: Physicians and patient spirituality. *Annals of Internal Medicine* 133(9):748-749.

19. Weaver AJ, Larson DB, Stapleton CL. (2001). In response to Stotland N: Tug-of-War: Domestic abuse and religion. *American Journal of Psychiatry* 158(5):822-823.

20. McCullough ME, Hoyt WT, Larson DB. (2001). In response to Sloan RP, Bagiella E: Small, robust, and important: Reply to Sloan and Bagiella (2001). *Health Psychology* 20(3):228-229.

Books, Monographs, Bibliographies, and National Reports

1. Intragovernmental Task Force on AIDS Health Care Delivery (including Larson DB). (1988). *AIDS Health Care Delivery: Report of the Intragovernmental Task Force.* Rockville, MD: U.S. Department of Health and Human Services, Public Health Service, Health Resources and Services Administration.

2. Larson DB, Larson SS. (1992, revised 1994). *The Forgotten Factor in Physical and Mental Health: What Does the Research Show?* Rockville, MD: National Institute for Healthcare Research.

3. Harris CK, Larson SS, Larson DB. (1993). *The Forgotten Factor in Physical and Mental Health: What Does the Research Show?: Study Guide.* Rockville, MD: National Institute for Healthcare Research.

4. Matthews DA, Larson DB, Barry CP. (1993). *The Faith Factor: An Annotated Bibliography of Clinical Research on Spiritual Subjects.* Rockville, MD: National Institute for Healthcare Research, 1993.

5. Larson DB. *The Faith Factor: An Annotated Bibliography of Systematic Reviews and Clinical Research on Spiritual Subjects,* Volume II. Rockville, MD: National Institute for Healthcare Research.

6. Lyons JS, Anderson RL, Larson DB, Penner J. (1993). *Of Parents and Pocket-Books: A Systematic Review of the Peer-Reviewed Scientific Literature of Family, Marital, and Community Variables Used in the Field of Juvenile Criminal Justice.* Washington, DC: Department of Justice.

7. Fogel BS, Colenda C, deFiguerido JM, Larson DB, Luchins D, Moak G, Olympia J, Pfeiffer E, Waxman H. (1993). *State Mental Hospitals and the Elderly.* Washington, DC: American Psychiatric Association Press.

8. Miranda J, Hohmann AA, Attkisson C, Larson DB. (1994). *Mental Disorders in Primary Care.* San Francisco, CA: Jossey-Bass, Inc.

9. Berman B, Larson DB. (Editors), (1994). *Alternative Medicine: Expanding Medical Horizons—A Report to the National Institutes of Health (NIH) on Alternative Medical Systems*

and Practices in the United States. Washington, DC: U.S. Government Printing Office.

10. Matthews DA, Larson DB. (1995). *The Faith Factor: An Annotated Bibliography of Clinical Research on Spiritual Subjects,* Volume III: *Enhancing Life Satisfaction.* Rockville, MD: National Institute for Healthcare Research.

11. Larson DB, Swyers JP, Larson SS. (1995). *The Costly Consequences of Divorce: Assessing the Clinical, Economic, and Public Health Impact of Marital Disruption in the United States.* Rockville, MD: National Institute for Healthcare Research.

12. Hanley DC, Anderson RL, Larson DB, Piersma HL, King SD, Sider RC. (1995). *Post-Traumatic Abortion-Related Stress in Psychiatric Outpatients: Comparisons Among Abortion-Distressed, Abortion-Non-Distressed, and No-Abortion Groups.* New York, NY: Pine Rest Foundation.

13. Larson DB, Lu FG, Swyers JP. (1996, revised 1997). *Model Curriculum for Psychiatry Residency Training Programs: Religion and Spirituality in Clinical Practice.* Rockville, MD: National Institute for Healthcare Research.

14. Larson DB, Swyers JP, McCullough ME. (Editors) (1998). *Scientific Research on Spirituality and Health: A Consensus Report.* Rockville, MD: National Institute for Healthcare Research.

15. Puchalski CM, Epstein LC, Fox E, Johnson MAC, Kallenberg GA, Kitchens LW Jr, Larson DB, Lu FG, McLaughlin MA, O'Donnell JF, Sarraf K, Swyers JP, Woolliscroft J, Anderson MB. (1999). *Report III: Contemporary Issues in Medicine: Communication in Medicine.* Medical School Objectives Project. Washington, DC: Association of American Medical Colleges.

16. Koenig HG, McCullough ME, Larson DB. (2001). *Handbook of Religion and Health.* New York, NY: Oxford University Press.

Unpublished Thesis

1. Larson DB. (1983). The frequency of church attendance, importance of religion, and blood pressure status. Master's Thesis, University of North Carolina School of Public Health.

Unpublished Manuscripts

1. Lyons JS, Pomp HC, Larson DB, Pavkov TW, Eichman M. A theoretical and empirical evaluation of the feasibility of risk-adjusted capitation funding of the seriously mentally ill in urban settings.
2. Larson DB, Lyons JS, Huckeba WM, Beardsley RS. A systematic review of the quantity and quality of nursing home research in three geriatric journals.
3. Lyons JS, Anderson RL, Von Roenn J, Sheridan EP, Larson DB. Comparing hospital and hospice charges for persons with AIDS: A preliminary investigation.
4. Ford DE, Larson DB, Anthony JC, Farmer ME. Seasonal variation of depression in a community sample.
5. Lyons JS, Talano JV, Larson DB, Martin G, Singer D. Mitral valve prolapse, anxiety sensitivity, and panic disorder.
6. Thompson JT, Larson DB, Douglas W, Harras A, Frazier S. Suicide in American Indian adolescents: Data validity and community response.
7. Williams DR, Chung AM, Jackson JS, Larson DB. Religion and psychological distress: Findings from the National Survey of Black Americans.
8. Gartner J, Hohmann AA, Larson DB, Canino GJ. Psychiatric, psychosocial and mental health services use: Characteristics of frequent church attenders in Puerto Rico in 1980.
9. Doukas DJ, Brown DR, Gornflo DW, Bartscht K, Elkins TE, Larson DB. The impact of physician values on the delivery of care for the elderly.
10. Pavkov TW, Lyons JS, Larson DB. Psychiatric consultations to minority patients with traumatic head injury.
11. Lyons JS, Anderson RL, Larson DB. Systematic review and meta-analysis of empirical research on the effects of acupuncture in the treatment of chronic pain.
12. Montague RB, Eaton WW, Larson DB, Mengel MC, Mengel LS, Campbell R. Depressive symptomatology in an IDDM treatment population.
13. Gartner A, Gartner J, Halgin R, Larson DB. Therapists' experiences with adolescent vs. adult patients in individual therapy.

14. McCullough ME, Kilpatrick SD, Puchalski CM, Larson DB. A systematic review of spiritual and religious variables in *JAMA, NEJM,* and *Lancet,* 1994-1998.
15. Kilpatrick SD, McCullough ME, Puchalski CM, Larson DB, Hays JC, Farran CJ. A systematic review of spiritual and religious measures in nursing research journals 1995-1999.
16. Kilpatrick SD, McCullough ME, Puchalski CM, Larson DB. A systematic review of spiritual and religious measures in social work research and healthcare journals 1995-1999.

Index

Page numbers followed by the letter "t" indicate tables.